Pocket Guide to
Laboratory and Diagnostic Tests

Pocket Guide to Laboratory and Diagnostic Tests

Kathleen Deska Pagana, R.N., M.S.N.

Department of Nursing, Lycoming College,
Williamsport, Pennsylvania; Doctoral Candidate,
University of Pennsylvania,
Philadelphia, Pennsylvania

Timothy James Pagana, M.D.

Surgical Oncologist,
Williamsport, Pennsylvania

Illustrated

The C. V. Mosby Company

St. Louis • Baltimore • Toronto   1986

MOSBY

A TRADITION OF PUBLISHING EXCELLENCE

Developmental Editor: Theresa Van Schaik
Assistant Editor: Maureen Slaten
Manuscript Editor: Connie Leinicke (Top Graphics)
Designer: Diane M. Beasley
Production: Susan Trail (Top Graphics)

Cover photograph © G. Robert Bishop 1985

Printed in the United States of America

Library of Congress Cataloging in Publication Data
Pagana, Kathleen Deska, 1952-
    Pocket guide to laboratory and diagnostic tests.

    Includes index.
    1. Diagnosis, Laboratory—Handbooks, manuals, etc.
2. Diagnosis—Handbooks, manuals, etc. 3. Nursing—
Handbooks, manuals, etc. I. Pagana, Timothy James,
1949- . II. Title. [DNLM: 1. Diagnosis, Laboratory—
handbooks. 2. Diagnosis, Laboratory—nurses' instruction.
QY 39 P128p]
RT48.5.P34   1986   616.07′5   85-31721
ISBN 0-8016-3760-0

The C.V. Mosby Company
11830 Westline Industrial Drive, St. Louis, Missouri 63146

C/D/D 9 8 7 6 5   02/A/228

Consultant Board

Preface

The *Pocket Guide to Laboratory and Diagnostic Tests* is one in a group of clinical handbooks designed for both the student and the practitioner. The fact that many clients are anxious regarding diagnostic/laboratory testing procedures can hardly be disputed. As a result, it is vitally important that the nurse be knowledgeable about diagnostic testing to ensure patient teaching, accurate test results, and appropriate patient care before, during, and after the tests.

A key feature of this pocket guide is that the diagnostic/laboratory studies are arranged according to a body systems approach. All types of tests related to a certain system (such as chest x-ray, sputum study, pulmonary angiography, and lung scan) are discussed in the same chapter. Each chapter is divided into the following categories: clinical laboratory tests (e.g., blood tests, stool tests), radiologic laboratory tests (e.g., x-ray films and nuclear scanning), and special studies (e.g., catheterization procedures). The format of each study includes the following components: normal values, deviations from normal, indications, contraindications, procedure, and nursing implications.

The *normal values* section includes pediatric and newborn results when applicable. Included in *deviations from normal* are conditions causing abnormal test results. The *indications* section succinctly lists the most common uses for the study. *Contraindications* are then listed for each study.

The *procedure* section includes information necessary for patient teaching and a concise description of the actual procedure. This section is invaluable because it includes patient sensation; the need for anesthesia or sedation; where the study is performed; who performs the study; and the duration of the procedure. (Note: The procedure for each study may vary in different institutions and in different areas of the country.) The *nursing implications* address specific nursing responsibilities before, during, and after each procedure. A special section, entitled *nurse alert,* focuses nursing attention on potential complications of certain studies.

Numerous illustrations are included to enhance the reader's understanding of the diagnostic procedures. Areas of pathology on x-ray film and nuclear scans are clearly marked. Appendix 1 provides a complete listing of commonly used abbreviations and symbols. Appendixes 2 and 3 list the normal values for blood, plasma, serum, and urine. Please note that normal values may vary because of different units of measurements or different laboratory methods. Since many laboratories are now using the system of international units (SI units), many common laboratory values are expressed in both conventional and in SI units.

It is our belief that the *Pocket Guide to Laboratory and Diagnostic Tests* should be invaluable as a quick reference book for nurses and nursing students. All types of laboratory/diagnostic studies (such as blood, urine, x-ray, nuclear scan, ultrasonography, endoscopy, and amniocentesis) are described to facilitate client preparation and safe performance of the studies. The systems approach and the uniform format of this text ensure quick and easy retrieval of information.

Kathleen Deska Pagana
Timothy James Pagana

Contents

APPENDIXES

Pocket Nurse Guide to
Laboratory and Diagnostic Tests

Cardiovascular System

1

Clinical laboratory tests
  Blood tests
    Cardiac enzyme studies
      Creatine phosphokinase (CPK), creatine kinase (CK)
      Serum aspartate aminotransferase (AST), formerly serum glu-
        tomic oxaloacetic transaminase (SGOT)
      Lactic dehydrogenase (LDH)
    Serum lipid studies
      Blood lipids, lipid profile, cholesterol, triglycerides, phospho-
        lipids
Radiologic laboratory tests
  X-ray tests
    Femoral arteriography (peripheral vascular arteriography)
    Venography (phlebography, venogram)
  Nuclear scanning tests
    Cardiac nuclear scanning (myocardial scan, cardiac scan, myo-
      cardial scintiphotography, nuclear cardiac scanning)
    ^{125}I fibrinogen uptake test
Special studies
  Cardiac catheterization (coronary angiography, angiocardiography,
    ventriculography)
    Computerized tomography of the chest (heart); CAT scanning
      (computerized axial tomography, CT scan of the heart, com-
      puterized axial transverse tomography, EMI scanning, elec-
      tronic musical instrument scanning)
  Ultrasound tests
    Doppler ultrasound and plethysmographic arterial study (nonin-
      vasive arterial studies)
    Doppler ultrasound and plethysmographic venous study
  Echocardiography (cardiac echo)
  Electrocardiography (ECG)

Exercise stress testing (stress, exercise, or electrocardiographic stress testing)
Holter monitoring
Event records
Oculoplethysmography (OPG)
Pericardiocentesis (pericardial fluid analysis)

Clinical Laboratory Tests

Blood Tests

Cardiac Enzyme Studies

Creatine phosphokinase (CPK); creatine kinase (CK)
Serum aspartate aminotransferase (AST); formerly serum glutamic oxaloacetic transaminase (SGOT)
Lactic dehydrogenase (LDH)

CREATINE PHOSPHOKINASE (CPK); CREATINE KINASE (CK)

CPK is fractionated into isoenzymes to measure the cardiac component of the total enzyme and thus provide a more specific index of cardiac muscle damage. An increase in the isoenzyme MB indicates myocardial damage.

Normal Values

- 5 to 75 mU/ml.

Deviations from Normal

- CPK level rises within 6 hours after damage to myocardial cells, peaks in approximately 18 hours, and returns to normal in 2 to 3 days.
- CPK may also be elevated with:
  Myopathy associated with chronic alcoholism;
  Electrical cardioversion;
  Cardiac catheterization;
  Hypothyroidism;
  Stroke;
  Surgery; or
  Clofibrate therapy.

SERUM ASPARTATE AMINOTRANSFERASE (AST); FORMERLY SERUM GLUTAMIC OXALOACETIC TRANSAMINASE (SGOT)

Normal Values

- 12 to 36 U/ml or 5 to 40 IU/L.

Deviations from Normal

- The AST level rises within 6 to 10 hours after myocardial injury, peaks at 12 to 48 hours, and returns to normal in approximately 3 to 4 days.
- Other conditions that may cause AST elevation include:
  Liver disease;
  Use of salicylates, opiates, or coumarin-type anticoagulants;
  Primary muscle disease;
  Cardiac operations;
  Acute pancreatitis;
  Extensive central nervous system damage;
  Hemolytic crisis;
  Toxemia of pregnancy;
  Crash injuries or burns;
  Hypothyroidism; or
  Infarction of the kidneys, spleen, or intestine.

LACTIC DEHYDROGENASE (LDH)

LDH is fractionated into isoenzymes to obtain a more specific index of cardiac muscle damage. The heart muscle is rich in LDH.

Normal Values

- 90 to 200 ImU/ml.

Deviations from Normal

- After myocardial infarction, the serum LDH level rises within 24 to 72 hours, peaks in 3 to 4 days, and returns to normal in approximately 14 days.
- LDH may also be elevated with:
  Pulmonary disease; or
  Congestive heart failure.

Procedure
Client preparation

1. The procedure and purpose of the study are explained.

Procedure

1. Following standard venipuncture procedure, one red-top tube of blood is drawn.
2. Pressure or a pressure dressing is applied to the venipuncture site(s) after completing the procedure.
3. The procedure is repeated per physician's orders.

Nursing implications

1. With repeated testing, rotate the venipuncture sites.
2. Observe site for bleeding.
3. Avoid hemolysis of blood.
4. Avoid giving a client with cardiac disease IM injections.
5. If the client received an IM injection before admission to the unit, indicate the date and time of injection on the lab slip.
6. On each lab slip, include the date and time blood was drawn.

Serum Lipid Studies
BLOOD LIPIDS, LIPID PROFILE, CHOLESTEROL, TRIGLYCERIDES, PHOSPHOLIPIDS (Table 1-1)
Normal Values

- Total lipids: 400 to 1000 mg/dl.
- Cholesterol: 150 to 250 mg/dl.
- Triglycerides: 40 to 150 mg/dl.
- Phospholipids: 150 to 380 mg/dl.
- Cholesterol lipoproteins: HDL, 45 mg/dl (men); 55 mg/dl (women). VLDL, 25% to 50%. LDL, 60 to 180 mg/dl.

Deviations from Normal

- Elevated LDL has a strong association with coronary artery disease.

Table 1-1   Patterns of hyperlipoproteinemia

Lipoprotein Type	Major Lipoprotein Elevation	Major Lipid Elevation
I (rare)	Chylomicrons	Triglycerides
IIa (common)	LDL	Cholesterol
IIb	LDL and VLDL	Cholesterol and triglycerides
III (uncommon)	Remnants	Triglycerides and cholesterol
IV (common)	VLDL	Triglycerides
V (uncommon)	VLDL and chylomicrons	Triglycerides and cholesterol

- Elevated HDL suggests a decreased risk of myocardial infarction.
- Elevated cholesterol levels occur with cardiovascular disease, atherosclerosis, obstructive jaundice, and uncontrolled diabetes.
- Decreased cholesterol levels occur with fat malabsorption, liver disease, and hyperthyroidism.

Indications

- To aid in the diagnosis of atherosclerotic disease.
- To help determine the dietary treatment of a client with atherosclerotic disease.

Contraindications

- None.

Procedure

Client preparation

1. The purpose of the study and the dietary restrictions imposed by the test are explained.
2. The client receives nothing by mouth, except water, for at least 12 hours before the test.
3. The physician may order the discontinuance of thyroid medications, steroidal contraceptives, and lipid-lowering drugs for at least 3 weeks before the test.

Procedure

1. Following standard venipuncture procedure, two tubes of blood (one red-top and one lavender-top) are drawn.
2. Pressure or a pressure dressing is applied to the puncture site.

Nursing implications

1. Following the venipuncture, observe the site for bleeding.

Radiologic Laboratory Tests

X-Ray Tests
FEMORAL ARTERIOGRAPHY (PERIPHERAL VASCULAR ARTERIOGRAPHY)
Normal Values

- Normal femoral arterial vasculature.

Deviations from Normal

- Arteriosclerotic vascular occlusive disease.
- Arterial emboli or acute thromboses (Fig. 1-1).
- Arterial trauma (e.g., lacerations).
- Aneurysm.
- Unusual arterial disorders (e.g., Buerger's disease).

Indications

- To identify and locate femoral artery occlusions.
- To diagnose conditions listed under ''Deviations from Normal'' above.

Contraindications

- An uncooperative client.
- A client allergic to contrast medium.

Procedure
Client preparation

1. Preferably, the client is kept fasting for 8 hours prior to the test.

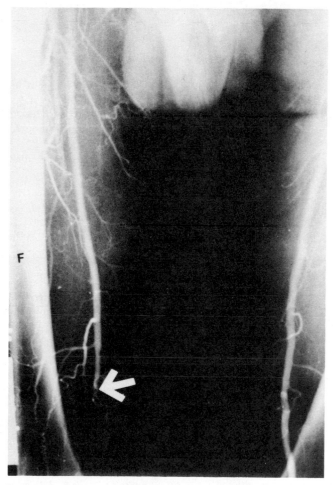

Figure 1-1
Femoral arteriogram. White arrow on left side indicates
area of right superficial femoral artery occlusion. Note
the normal left femoral artery (right side of photograph).
F, femur.

2. The client is told that the contrast medium may cause a discomforting and sometimes painful heat flash (usually less than 10 seconds).
3. If ordered, the client receives a sedative.

Procedure

1. The client is placed on a special, movable x-ray table in the supine position.
2. A radiopaque catheter is guided under x-ray visualization into the proximal iliac artery, through the aorta, and down the leg to be studied.
3. Radiopaque contrast medium is injected, and x-ray films of the thigh, calf, and ankle are taken immediately at a timed sequence.
4. After the x-ray films are taken, the catheter is removed, and a pressure dressing is applied to the puncture site.
5. A radiologist performs this test in approximately 40 minutes.

Nursing implications

1. Generally, keep the client on bed rest for approximately 8 hours after the procedure to allow complete sealing of the arterial puncture.
2. Observe the catheter insertion site for inflammation, hemorrhage, hematoma, or the absence of peripheral pulse.
3. Assess the involved extremity for numbness, tingling, pain, or loss of function.
4. Compare the color and temperature of the involved extremity with that of the uninvolved extremity.
5. Assess vital signs for evidence of bleeding (decreased blood pressure and increased pulse).
6. Site should be checked for hematoma formation.

Nurse alert

1. Complications of this study include:
   a. Hemorrhage at the site of the arterial puncture;
   b. Occlusion of the femoral vessel;
   c. Catheter dissection of the intimal lining of the artery; and
   d. Allergic reaction to the contrast medium.

VENOGRAPHY (PHLEBOGRAPHY, VENOGRAM)

Normal Values

- Negative (no venous thrombi).

Deviations from Normal

- Venous thrombosis.

Indications

- To identify and locate thrombi in the venous system of the lower extremities.

Contraindications

- An uncooperative client.
- A client allergic to iodinated contrast medium.

Procedure

Client preparation

1. The client is told that the contrast medium may cause a warm flush.

Procedure

1. The client is assessed for contrast medium allergies.
2. Catheterization of a superficial vein on the foot is performed.
3. The radiologist then injects an iodinated, radiopaque contrast medium into the vein and takes x-ray films to follow the course of the contrast medium up the leg.

Nursing implications

1. Medication may be indicated for the patient in pain to avoid movement during the procedure.
2. Handle the affected extremity gently because it will be sensitive to the touch.
3. After the study, assess the client for:
   a. Cellulitis (redness, swelling, pain, tenderness) from subcutaneous contrast medium infiltration; and
   b. Bacteremia (increased temperature, tachycardia, cutaneous flush, chills).

Nurse alert

1. Complications in venography include:
   a. Allergic reaction to iodinated contrast medium;
   b. Subcutaneous infiltration of contrast medium;
   c. Induction of venous thrombophlebitis;
   d. Bacteremia; and
   e. Embolism.

Nuclear Scanning Tests
CARDIAC NUCLEAR SCANNING (MYOCARDIAL SCAN, CARDIAC SCAN, MYOCARDIAL SCINTIPHOTOGRAPHY, NUCLEAR CARDIAC SCANNING)
Normal Values

- Normal myocardial cells.

Deviations from Normal

- "Hot" or "cold" spots dependent on the radiocompound used (Table 1-2).

Table 1-2   Myocardial scanning

Disease	Technetium 99m Pyrophosphate*	Thallium 201†
None (normal)	No uptake	Diffuse and even uptake
Acute myocardial infarction	"Hot" spot	"Cold" spot
Myocardial ischemia	"Warm" spot	Normal at rest "Cold" spot during exercise‡
Old myocardial infarction	No uptake	"Cold spot"§

*And related compounds, such as mercury 203, gallium 67, or any technetium 99m-labeled compound.
†And related compound, such as potassium 43, cesium 131, or rubidium 86.
‡Such as stress testing.
§Unable to differentiate "acute" from "old" myocardial infarction.

Indications

- To screen for "old" infarction.
- To evaluate chest pain and equivocal ECGs.
- To rule out acute myocardial infarction.
- To evaluate precoronary and postcoronary bypass surgery.
- To quantify and survey myocardial infarction.
- To evaluate ventricular function.

Contraindications

- An uncooperative client.
- A pregnant client because of the possibility of radiopaque contrast media causing fetal damage.

Procedure

Client preparation

1. The client is reassured that the procedure is safe and non-invasive and that the only uncomfortable part is the venous puncture.

Procedure

1. The client receives an intravenous injection of the appropriate radionuclide into a peripheral vein.
2. In less than 4 hours a gamma-ray detector is placed over the precordium.
3. The client is placed in the supine, lateral, and both oblique positions.

Nursing implications

1. Encourage verbalization of the client's fears.
2. Provide emotional support.

^{125}I FIBRINOGEN UPTAKE TEST

Normal Values

- Negative (no deep-vein thrombosis).

Deviations from Normal

- Areas of clot formation (e.g., venous thrombosis).

Indications

- To diagnose deep-vein thrombophlebitis.
- To detect subclinical, early thromboses.

Contraindications

- A client in whom the diagnosis of deep-vein thrombosis is needed in less than 24 hours.
- A client with ongoing inflammation of the leg (e.g., superficial phlebitis).
- A client with primary lymphedema.

Procedure

Client preparation

1. The procedure is explained to the client to reduce anxiety and enhance cooperation.

Procedure

1. The client receives an intravenous injection of ^{125}I-labeled fibrinogen.
2. A Geigerlike detector is placed over the client's ankles, calves, and lower thighs 24 hours later.
3. A radionuclear technician performs the test in the nuclear medicine department in approximately 1 hour.

Nursing implications

1. Before the study, assess the client's legs for evidence of inflammation, which will cause a false-positive result.

Nurse alert

1. Because the fibrinogen used for the test is obtained from donated blood, the possibility of hepatitis transmission exists. Following the test, observe for hepatitis symptoms (anorexia, nausea, vomiting, malaise, fever, jaundice, fatigue, hepatomegaly, abdominal and gastric discomfort, abnormal liver function, clay-colored stools and dark urine, arthralgia, myalgia, headache, photophobia, cough, pharyngitis). See incubation period (Table 3-1) for an estimate of the time interval in which the nurse should ex-

pect to start observing signs and symptoms of hepatitis. Note that these symptoms may precede the onset of jaundice by 1 to 2 weeks.

Special Studies

Cardiac Catheterization (Coronary Angiography, Angiocardiography, Ventriculography)

Normal Values

- Normal heart, blood vessels, pressures, and volumes.

Deviations from Normal

- Abnormal heart, blood vessels, pressures, and volumes suggest one or more of the conditions listed under "Indications" below.

Indications

- To identify atherosclerotic plaques within the coronary arteries.
- To identify acquired and congenital cardiac valve disorders and nonvalvular congenital disorders.
- To evaluate the success of previous heart surgery.
- To evaluate cardiac muscle function.
- To identify ventricular aneurysm.
- To identify congenital disorders of the great vessels.
- To evaluate an acute myocardial infarction and to facilitate infusion of streptokinase into the occluded artery.
- To allow for injection of contrast media into the coronary arteries so they can be seen (coronary cineangiography).

Contraindications

- An uncooperative client.
- A client who would refuse surgery if the lesion found were amenable to surgery.
- A client with iodine contrast media allergies who has not received the appropriate preventive treatment with prednisone and diphenhydramine (Benadryl).

Procedure
Client preparation

1. The procedure and dietary restrictions are explained.
2. The sensations the client is likely to experience are explained, including:
   a. The client lies still in a dark room on an x-ray table that may rotate in several positions.
   b. The client's arm may feel as though it is "going to sleep" if the brachial artery is used for access.
   c. The client may feel palpitations as the catheter touches the ventricles because of PVCs.
   d. The client may feel a warm flush when the radiopaque contrast medium is injected. The sensation is very uncomfortable and lasts 4 to 10 seconds.
   e. The client may cough as the catheter is passed into the pulmonary artery.
3. Food and fluid are withheld for 6 to 8 hours before the procedure to prevent vomiting and aspiration of vomitus during study.
4. The physician must obtain written and informed consent for this procedure.
5. The client is assessed for contrast media allergies.
6. The preprocedure medications are administered.

Procedure

1. The quality of peripheral pulses is noted and recorded as baseline data.
2. A local anesthetic is administered at the catheter insertion site.
3. ECG leads are placed on the four extremities.
4. A peripheral intravenous (IV) needle is inserted to allow venous access in the event that antiarrhythmic drugs are needed.
5. To study the right side of the heart, a sterile radiopaque catheter is inserted into the antecubital or femoral vein, into the superior or inferior vena cava, and through the right atrium and ventricle and into the pulmonary artery.
6. For left-sided heart catheterization, the catheter is usually passed retrograde from the femoral or brachial artery into

the aorta and then into the left ventricle. Left-sided catheterization can also be achieved transseptally by puncturing the atrial septum during right-sided catheterization with a needle and passing the catheter from the right atrium into the left atrium.

7. After the study of either side of the heart, the cardiac catheter is removed.
8. The catheter insertion site is immobilized for several hours.
9. Pressure is applied to the site.
10. A cardiologist performs the procedure under sterile conditions in the cardiac catheterization laboratory in 1 to 3 hours. The procedure may be performed at the bedside in the cardiac care unit or in the intensive care unit.

Nursing implications

1. Ask the client to explain the procedure and reinforce the client's understanding.
2. After the procedure, keep the extremity in which the catheter was placed straight and immobilized for several hours after catheterization.
3. Monitor the client's vital signs at frequent intervals for arrhythmias and hypotension.
4. Observe the arterial puncture site for hemorrhage, inflammation, hematoma, or absence of pulse.
5. Check the peripheral pulses and compare the quality of the pulses with the preprocedure baseline values.
6. Assess the extremity for signs of ischemia (numbness, tingling, pain, absence of peripheral pulses, and loss of function).
7. Regularly compare the color and temperature of the extremity with the color and temperature of the uninvolved extremities.
8. Following the procedure, enforce safety measures until the effect of the preprocedure medication has worn off.

Nurse alert

1. Possible complications include:
   a. Cardiac arrhythmias;
   b. Perforation of the heart by the catheter;

c. Stroke or myocardial infarction;
d. Peripheral arterial complications;
e. Allergic reaction to the contrast medium; and
f. Infection.

COMPUTERIZED TOMOGRAPHY OF THE CHEST (HEART); CAT SCANNING (COMPUTERIZED AXIAL TOMOGRAPHY, CT SCAN OF THE HEART, COMPUTERIZED AXIAL TRANSVERSE TOMOGRAPHY, EMI SCANNING, ELECTRONIC MUSICAL INSTRUMENT SCANNING)

Normal Values

- No evidence of pathologic conditions.

Deviations from Normal

- Vascular aneurysms.
- Occlusion(s) of coronary bypass grafts.

Indications

- To assist in the diagnosis of conditions listed under "Deviations from Normal."

Contraindications

- Pregnancy.
- A client allergic to iodinated intravenous contrast medium.
- An uncooperative client.

Procedure

1. See "CT of the Chest," p. 119.

Nursing implications

1. See "CT of the Chest," p. 119.

Nurse alert

1. See "CT of the Chest," p. 119.

Ultrasound Tests

DOPPLER ULTRASOUND AND PLETHYSMOGRAPHIC ARTERIAL STUDY (NONINVASIVE ARTERIAL STUDIES)

Normal Values

- Negative (no arterial occlusion).

Deviations from Normal

- Arterial occlusion.

Indications

- To locate peripheral arteriosclerotic occlusive disease.

Contraindications

- An uncooperative client.

Procedure
Client preparation

1. The test is explained to the client to reduce anxiety and increase cooperation.
2. The client is instructed to avoid smoking for at least 30 minutes before the study.

Procedure

1. To perform the Doppler ultrasound test, blood pressure cuffs are placed around the thigh, calf, and ankle while the client is in a semirecumbent position.
   a. The highest pressure at which the blood flow is heard is recorded as the systolic pressure of the artery located under the detector.
2. Next the cuffs are attached to a plethysmograph.
   a. The amplitudes of the wave at each cuff are measured and compared.
3. A technician performs this study in about 15 minutes.

Nursing implications

1. See ''Doppler Ultrasound and Plethysmographic Venous Study'' below.

DOPPLER ULTRASOUND AND PLETHYSMOGRAPHIC VENOUS STUDY

Normal Values

- Normal venous patency and venous volume.

Deviations from Normal

- No venous "swishing."
- Reduced plethysmographic recordings.

Indications

- To diagnose venous thrombosis.

Contraindications

- An uncooperative client.

Procedure

Client preparation

1. The procedure is explained to the client.

Procedure

1. Plethysmography is performed first on the client in the semirecumbent position.
   a. A large, inflatable "occlusion cuff" is placed high on the client's thigh.
   b. A second, smaller plethysmographic "monitor cuff" is placed on the calf.
   c. After taking a sustained deep breath, the client exhales, and respiratory waves are displayed on a pulse-volume recorder.
   d. The occlusion cuff is then inflated.
   e. After the highest volume is recorded, the occlusion cuff is rapidly deflated, and the leg should return to its preocclusion volume within 1 second.
2. Next, the Doppler ultrasound test is performed.
   a. The transducer "probe" is placed on the skin, and characteristic swishing sounds are sought, indicating movement of blood within an unoccluded and non-thrombosed vein.

3. A trained technician performs the study at the client's bedside or in the noninvasive vascular study laboratory in appropriately 15 minutes.

Nursing implications

1. After the study, gently remove the conduction lubricant from the client's extremities.

Nurse alert

1. Because of the danger of dislodging thrombi, the client's leg is not massaged after the procedure.

Echocardiography (Cardiac Echo)

Normal Values

- Normal position, size, and movements of cardiac valves and chambers.

Deviations from Normal

- Abnormal position, size, and movement of cardiac valves and chambers.

Indications

- To diagnose pericardial effusion, valve disease, subaortic stenosis, cardiomyopathy, cardiac tumor, congenital heart disease, aortic root disease, prolapse, and mural thrombosis.

Contraindications

- An uncooperative client.

Procedure

Client preparation

1. The client is told:
   a. The study is painless;
   b. A gel will be applied to the chest to enhance transmission of sound waves; and
   c. ECG leads will be applied.

Procedure

1. After undressing to the waist, the client is placed in the supine position on a bed in a darkened room.
2. The ultrasonographer applies mineral oil or glycerine to the skin over the fourth left intercostal space.
3. The pencil-like probe (transducer) is then placed on the skin, held there, and then tilted (rocked) into various positions to inscribe an arc that will demonstrate several areas of the heart sequentially.
4. An ECG is recorded simultaneously during echocardiography to time the events demonstrated by ultrasound with the cardiac cycle.
5. The ultrasonographer performs the study in approximately 15 to 45 minutes.

Nursing implications

1. To ensure comfort, expose only the client's arms and chest.
2. Make sure the request form for the study includes client history and the specific problem the referring physician suspects.
3. After the study, remove the gel from the client's chest.

Nurse alert

1. Because of danger of accidental shock or electrocution with any test involving electrical equipment, be sure equipment is in good working order and correctly grounded, with no wires frayed or tangled.

Electrocardiography (ECG)
Normal Values

- Normal rate (60 to 100 beats/min), rhythm, and wave deflections.

Deviations from Normal

- Altered or absent P waves.
- Prolonged PR interval.

- Shortened PR interval.
- Widened QRS complex.
- Elevated or depressed ST segment.

Indications

- To identify abnormal heart rhythms (arrhythmias).
- To diagnose acute myocardial infarction.
- To diagnose conduction defects.
- To diagnose ventricular hypertrophy.

Contraindications

- An uncooperative client.

Procedure
Client preparation

1. The purpose and procedure of the study is explained to the client.
2. The client is told that the ECG is painless and that electrical current flows *from*, not *to*, the client.

Procedure

1. The client is directed to lie still and not to talk during the ECG.
2. The client is placed in the supine position on the table or bed.
3. The skin areas designated for electrode placement are prepared with alcohol swabs or sandpaper. Fig. 1-2 illustrates areas for electrode placement.
4. A small amount of electrode gel is applied.
5. The limb leads are secured with straps or clamps.
6. The chest leads (suction cups) are applied.
7. Cardiac technicians and nurses perform this test in less than 5 minutes in the "heart station" or at the bedside.

Nursing implications

1. To maintain client comfort, expose only the client's arms and chest.
2. Only a small amount of electrode gel is applied to avoid producing wandering baseline.

3. Electrodes and wires are applied so tension on electrodes is avoided.
4. Straps are not tightly placed.
5. After the ECG is recorded, the electrodes are removed and the gel wiped off.

Nurse alert

1. Because of danger of accidental shock or electrocution with any test involving electrical equipment, be sure equipment is in good working order and correctly grounded, with no wires frayed or tangled.

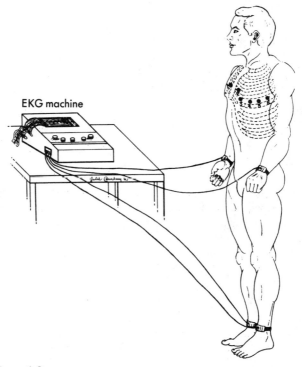

EKG machine

Figure 1-2
Placement of ECG electrodes.

Exercise Stress Testing (Stress, Exercise, or Electrocardiographic Stress Testing)

Normal Values

- Negative (no significant symptoms or ECG abnormalities).

Deviations from Normal

- Positive (recording paper shows a depression of the ST segment of 1 mm [0.1 mV] below the baseline).

Indications

- To evaluate chest pain.
- To determine limits of safe exercise.
- To detect labile or exercise-related hypertension.
- To detect exercise-related leg cramps.
- To evaluate the effectiveness of antiarrhythmic or antianginal treatment.

Contraindications

- A client with unstable angina.
- A client with valvular disease (such as aortic stenosis).
- A client with recent myocardial infarction (preceding few weeks).
- A client with advanced or untreated congestive heart failure.
- A client with severe arrhythmias.

Procedure

Client preparation

1. The test is explained to reduce anxiety and encourage cooperation.
2. Client instruction includes:
   a. Get adequate sleep the night before the study.
   b. Eat a light meal (no coffee, tea, or alcohol) 4 hours before the test, then nothing by mouth until test.
   c. No smoking for at least 4 hours before test.
   d. Wear loose-fitting clothes with a front-buttoning shirt to facilitate application of monitoring devices.
   e. Wear comfortable, well-fitting shoes with rubber soles (no slippers).

    f. Follow physician's orders regarding discontinuing certain drugs (e.g., beta blockers) that limit heart rate.

    g. Report any signs of chest pain, exhaustion, shortness of breath, or generalized fatigue during the test.

3. The physician obtains written informed consent for this study.

Procedure

1. The pre–stress test ECG is recorded.
2. During the test, ECG and heart rate are recorded continuously with monitoring devices.
3. Blood pressure is recorded intermittently.
4. The test is usually terminated when there are increasingly frequent PVCs, spurts of ventricular tachycardia, ST segment depression, drop in blood pressure, or worsening client complaints of chest pain, exhaustion, generalized fatigue, dyspnea, and dizziness.
5. After the test, ECG and vital sign recordings are made at intervals during a 5- to 10-minute recovery period.
6. A cardiologist performs the stress test in the cardiology clinic in 30 to 45 minutes.

Nursing implications

1. After the study, advise the client to rest for several hours and avoid stimulants or extreme temperature changes.
2. Further advise the client not to take a hot shower for at least 2 hours.
3. If test results are positive, encourage the client to discuss his or her feelings; provide emotional support.

Nurse alert

1. Although uncommon, complications including fatal cardiac arrhythmias and myocardial infarction can occur.
2. Appropriate emergency equipment, including a defibrillator, Ambu bag, and antiarrhythmia drugs, should be available in the testing room.
3. A staff member stands next to the client in case he or she becomes dizzy or falls.

Holter Monitoring

Normal Values

- See "Electrocardiography," p. 20.

Deviations from Normal

- See "Electrocardiography," p. 20.

Indications

- To correlate cardiac rhythm disturbances with symptoms of dizziness, syncopy, palpitations, or chest pain.
- To assess pacemaker function.
- To assess medication effectiveness.

Contraindications

- See "Electrocardiography," p. 21.

Procedure

Client preparation

1. The client is told that, as with ECG monitoring, this monitoring is painless.
2. The client is instructed to carry a monitor for 24 to 48 hours, as ordered.
3. The client is instructed to carry a diary and record daily activities in it.
4. The client is instructed to use an "event marker," if required, to record pain, syncopy, or palpitations as they occur.

Procedure

1. The monitor is attached to leads.
2. At the end of the prescribed monitoring time, the monitor and the ECG electrodes are disconnected.

Nursing implications

1. After disconnecting electrodes, wipe off gel.
2. See "Electrocardiography," p. 21.

Event Records

Normal Values

■ See "Electrocardiography," p. 20.

Deviations from Normal

■ See "Electrocardiography," p. 20.

Indications

■ To assist in diagnosis and management of clients with periodic "spells" or near syncope.

Procedure
Client preparation

1. The recording is explained to the client to ensure cooperation and reduce anxiety.
2. The client is instructed to hold an event recorder to the chest to record the ECG.
3. If transmission is to be "live," the client is instructed to call the physician's office during the event that is to be recorded.

Oculoplethysmography (OPG)

Normal Values

■ Normal and equal blood flow in both carotid arteries.

Deviations from Normal

■ Delayed blood flow to the eyes.

Indications

■ To evaluate symptoms of transient ischemic attacks, cardiac bruits, and neurologic deficits.
■ To follow up after carotid endarterectomy.

Contraindications

■ An uncooperative client.
■ A client who has recently had eye surgery.

- A client with cataracts.
- A client who has had retinal detachment.

Procedure

Client preparation

1. The client is told:
    a. A stinging sensation is felt when the ophthalmic drops are applied.
    b. A pulling sensation is felt when suction is applied on the eye.
    c. Vision may be temporarily lost during the suction application.
    d. ECG electrodes will be attached to the extremities.

Procedure

1. The client lies in the supine position. The blood pressure in both arms is taken before the test.
2. ECG electrodes are applied to the client's extremities.
3. Anesthetic eye drops are instilled in both eyes.
4. Small detectors are attached to the earlobes. Tracings for both ears are taken and compared.
5. Eye cups resembling contact lenses are applied directly to the eyeball.
6. Tracings of the pulsations within each eye are recorded.
7. A vacuum source is applied to the suction cup.
8. A technician usually performs the test in 20 to 30 minutes. When the suction source is stopped, the blood flow then returns to the eyes.

Nursing implications

1. After the study, inform the client:
    a. The eye anesthesia usually wears off in about 30 minutes;
    b. Do not rub eyes for at least 2 hours following the test and blot eyes dry if tears appear;
    c. Do not insert contact lenses for at least 2 hours after the test;
    d. Bloodshot eyes are a normal reaction and last for several hours.
2. Instill artificial tears to soothe eye irritation.

Nurse alert

1. Complications of OPG include conjunctival hemorrhage and corneal abrasions.
2. If corneal abrasions occur, the eye is patched and a lubricant such as Dacriose solution is applied.
3. Clients may also experience photophobia for a short time after the procedure.

Pericardiocentesis (Pericardial Fluid Analysis)

Normal Values

- Clear, straw-colored pericardial fluid without evidence of pathogens, blood, or malignant cells.

Deviations from Normal

- Large amounts of fluid.
- Fluid containing pus or blood.
- Abnormal pericardial fluid containing pathogens, blood, or malignant cells.

Indications

- To relieve cardiac tamponade.
- To remove a small sample of pericardial fluid for lab examination.
- To identify the cause of pericardial effusion.

Contraindications

- An uncooperative or uncontrollable client because the risk of laceration will be increased.
- A client with a bleeding disorder or on anticoagulant therapy.

Procedure

Client preparation

1. This procedure is frightening to most clients. It is explained to reduce anxiety and encourage cooperation.

Procedure

1. The client is placed in a supine position with the head of the bed elevated 60 degrees unless the physician requests another position.
2. A peripheral IV is started and maintained at keep-vein-open (KVO) rate of approximately 20 ml/h to administer preprocedure medications and to have venous access in the event of any complications.
3. An area in the fifth to sixth intercostal space at the left sternal margin (or subxyphoid) is antiseptically prepared and injected with a local anesthetic.
4. A pericardiocentesis needle attached to a three-way stopcock with a 50 cc syringe is introduced.
5. An ECG lead wire is then attached by an alligator clamp to the hub of the needle. As the needle is inserted through the chest wall into the pericardial sac, the ECG is observed for changes in the ST segment.
6. The pericardial fluid is then aspirated and specimen tubes are labeled and numbered.
7. When the needle is removed, pressure is immediately applied to the site with a sterile gauge pad for approximately 3 to 5 minutes. A bandage is then applied.
8. A physician performs this procedure in approximately 10 to 20 minutes.

Nursing implications

1. Assist the physician as necessary during the procedure.
2. During the procedure, observe the ECG for evidence of ST elevation. During the procedure, observe the aspirate for blood.
3. Carefully label and number the specimen tubes of pericardial fluid and send them to the lab immediately after the procedure. The specimen tubes usually contain an additive.
4. If bacterial culture and sensitivity tests are scheduled, record any antibiotic therapy the client is receiving on the lab slip.
5. After the procedure, observe the puncture site for bleeding and hematoma formation.
6. After the procedure, monitor the vital signs closely.

Nurse alert

1. Possible complications include:
   a. Laceration of a coronary artery or the myocardium;
   b. Ventricular fibrillation and other arrhythmias;
   c. Vasovagal arrest;
   d. Pleural infection;
   e. Pneumothorax; and
   f. Inadvertent puncture of the lung, liver, or stomach.
2. To minimize complications, an echocardiography is performed prior to pericardiocentesis to determine the appropriate fusion site.

Bibliography

Acierno, L.J., and Worrell, L.T.: Cardiac nuclear imaging, Radiol. Technol. **55**(2):616-621, Nov./Dec. 1983.

Acierno, L.J., and Worrell, L.T.: Radionuclide imaging in coronary artery disease, Radiol. Technol. **54**(4):79-87, March/April 1984.

Anderson, U.K.: Cardiovascular laboratory testing procedures. In Guzzetta, C.E., and Dossey, B.M.: Cardiovascular nursing: bodymind tapestry, St. Louis, 1984, The C.V. Mosby Co.

Anthony, C.P., and Thibodeau, G.A.: Textbook of anatomy and physiology, ed. 11, St. Louis, 1983, The C.V. Mosby Co.

Braunwald, E., and Alpert, J.S.: Acute myocardial infarction. In Petersdorf, R.G., and others, editors: Harrison's principles of internal medicine, ed. 10, New York, 1983, McGraw-Hill Book Co.

Braunwald, E., and Cohn, P.F.: Ischemic heart disease. In Petersdorf, R.G., and others, editors: Harrison's principles of internal medicine, ed. 10, New York, 1983, McGraw-Hill Book Co.

Brown, M.S., and Goldstein, J.L.: The hyperlipoproteinemias and other disorders of lipid metabolism. In Petersdorf, R.G., and others, editors: Harrison's principles of internal medicine, ed. 10, New York, 1983, McGraw-Hill Book Co.

Cohen, J.A., Pantaleo, N., and Shell, W.: A message from the heart: what isoenzymes can tell you about your cardiac patient, Nursing '82 **12**(4):46-49, 1982.

Criss, E.: Digital subtraction angiography, Am. J. Nurs. **82**:1706-1707, Nov. 1982.

Cudworth-Bergin, K.L.: Detecting arterial problems with a Doppler probe, RN **47**(1):38-41, Jan. 1984.

Dossey, B.M.: The person with pericarditis, pericardial effusion, and cardiac temporale. In Guzzetta, C.E., and Dorsey, B.M.: Cardiovascular nursing: bodymind tapestry, St. Louis, 1984, The C.V. Mosby Co.

Finesilver, C.: Reducing stress in patients having cardiac catheterization, Am J. Nurs. **80**(10):1805-1807, Oct. 1980.

Gruntzig, A.R., and others: Nonoperative dilatation of coronary-artery stenosis: percutaneous transluminal coronary angioplasty, N. Engl. J. Med. **301**:61, 1979.

Haughey, C.W.: Preparing your patient for echocardiography, Nursing '84 **14**:68-71.

Hirzel, H.O., and others: Short- and long-term changes in myocardial perfusion after percutaneous transluminal coronary angioplasty assessed by Thallium 201 exercise scintigraphy, Circulation **63**:1001, 1981.

Hoffman, S.J.: Serum enzyme studies. In Hudak, C.M., Lohr, T., and Gallo, B.M., editors: Critical care nursing, ed. 3, Philadelphia, 1982, J.B. Lippincott Co.

Kaye, W.: Invasive therapeutic techniques: emergency cardiac pacing, pericardiocentesis, intracardiac injections, and emergency treatment of tension pneumothorax, Heart Lung **12**(3):300-319, May 1983.

Kernicki, J.G., and Weiler, K.M.: Electrocardiography for nurses: physiological correlates, New York, 1981, John Wiley & Sons.

Marinelli-Miller, D.: What your patient wants to know about angiography—but may not ask, RN **46**(11):53-54, 1983.

Mautner, R.K., and Phillips, J.H.: Coronary arteriography prior to hospital discharge after first myocardial infarction, Heart Lung **12**(2):171-174, March 1983.

McCaffery, M.: Relieving pain with noninvasive techniques, Nursing '80 **10**:55, 1980.

Mulqueeney-Yamada, E.: Cardiovascular physiology, assessment, and incidence. In Beyers, M., and Dudas, S., editors: The clinical practice of medical-surgical nursing, ed. 2, Boston, 1984, Little, Brown & Co.

Myerburg, R.J.: Electrocardiography. In Petersdorf, R.G., and others, editors: Harrison's principles of internal medicine, ed. 10, New York, 1983, McGraw-Hill Book Co.

O'Neill, D.M.: Percutaneous transluminal angioplasty: development, technique, and application, Radiol. Technol. **55**(3):10-16, Jan./Feb. 1984.

Purcell, J.A., and Giffin, P.A.: Percutaneous transluminal coronary angioplasty, Am. J. Nurs. **81**(9):1620-1626, Sept. 1981.

Purcell, J.A., and Haynes, L.: For CE credit: using the ECG to detect MI, Am. J. Nurs. **84**(5):627-645, May 1984.

Ross, J., and Peterson, K.L.: Cardiac catheterization and angiography. In Petersdorf, R.G., and others, editors: Harrison's principles of internal medicine, ed. 10, New York, 1983, McGraw-Hill Book Co.

Sanderson, R.G.: Diagnostic techniques. In Sanderson, R.G., and Kurth, C.L., editors: The cardiac patient: a comprehensive approach, ed. 2, Philadelphia, 1983, W.B. Saunders Co.

Smith, C.E.: Nursing assessment: cardiovascular system. In Lewis, S.M., and Collier, I.C., editors: Medical-surgical nursing: assessment and management of clinical problems, New York, 1983, McGraw-Hill Book Co.

Tilkian, S.M., Conover, M.B., and Tilkian, A.G.: Clinical implications of laboratory tests, ed. 3, St. Louis, 1983, The C.V. Mosby Co.

Wheeler, H.: A modern approach to diagnosing deep vein thrombosis, J. Cardiovasc. Med. **5**:3, March 1980.

Wynne, J., O'Rourke, R.A., and Braunwald, E.: Noninvasive methods of cardiac examination. In Petersdorf, R.G., and others, editors: Harrison's principles of internal medicine, ed. 10, New York, 1983, McGraw-Hill Book Co.

Zeluff, G.W., and others: Evaluation of coronary arteries and myocardium by radionuclide imaging, Heart Lung **9**(2):344-347, March/April 1980.

Gastrointestinal System

2

Clinical Laboratory Tests

Blood Tests
CARCINOEMBRYONIC ANTIGEN TEST (CEA)
Normal Values

- <2 ng/ml.

Deviations from Normal

- Elevated CEA levels or rising CEA level.

Indications

- To monitor the client's response to therapy for colorectal cancer.
- To follow-up clients who have had potentially curative resections for tumor recurrence.

Contraindications

- None.

Procedure
Client preparation

1. The purpose of the study is explained to the client.

Procedure

1. Following standard venipuncture technique, a blood sample is collected.
2. After the venipuncture, apply pressure or a pressure dressing to the site.
3. The sample is sent to the lab immediately for analysis.

Nursing implications

1. Observe the site for bleeding.

SERUM GASTRIN DETERMINATION
Normal Values

- 40 to 150 pg/ml.

Deviations from Normal

- Mildly elevated in patients with pernicious anemia, anti-ulcer procedures, and gastric ulcers.
- Extremely high in patients with Zollinger-Ellison syndrome and in patients with G-cell hyperplasia.

Indications

- To aid in the diagnosis of gastric ulcers and Zollinger-Ellison syndrome.

Contraindications

- None.

Procedure
Client preparation

1. The procedure is explained to the client.

Procedure

1. Following the standard procedure for venipuncture, one red-top tube of blood is collected. The tube should contain no anticoagulant.
2. Pressure or a pressure dressing is applied to site after completing procedure.
3. The sample is sent to the lab immediately for analysis.

Nursing implications

1. Observe the site for bleeding.

D-XYLOSE TEST
Normal Values

- Blood: 20 to 52 mg/dl in 2 hours.
- Urine: 4 g in a 5-hour urine specimen.

Deviations from Normal

- A decrease in D-xylose absorption occurs with enterogenous steatorrhea associated with malabsorption disorders such as sprue and celiac diseases. A decrease in D-xylose absorption can also occur with myxedema, rheumatoid arthritis, alcoholism, and diabetic neuropathic diarrhea.

Indications

■ To assist in the diagnosis of malabsorption diseases.

Contraindications

■ None.

Procedure

Client preparation

1. The procedure and purpose of the study are explained.

Procedure

1. All fluids and food are withheld from the client after midnight the day of the test.
2. The client is asked to void and the urine is discarded just before the test begins.
3. The client is asked to drink a 25 g dose of D-xylose dissolved in 240 ml of water. The D-xylose dose is then followed by 250 ml of water.
4. The time of the D-xylose dose is recorded.
5. The client receives nothing by mouth until the test is completed.
6. The client is instructed to stay on bed rest until the test is completed.
7. Following standard venipuncture procedures, a 3 ml red-top tube of blood is drawn and sent to the laboratory 2 hours after the D-xylose dose is given.
8. Pressure is applied to the venipuncture site.
9. All urine voided after the dose of D-xylose is given is saved.
10. The last urine specimen is collected 5 hours after the test began.
11. The urine specimen is labeled and sent to the laboratory.

Nursing implications

1. Assess the venipuncture site for bleeding.
2. Post the hours of the urine collection on the client's door, above the bedpan hopper, and in the utility room to prevent accidental discarding of the specimen.

3. Remind the client to void before defecating to avoid contaminating the urine. Also remind the client not to put toilet paper in the urine.

Stool Tests
STOOL CULTURE (STOOL FOR CULTURE AND SENSITIVITY, C & S; STOOL FOR OVA AND PARASITES, O & P)
Normal Values

- Normal intestinal flora.

Deviations from Normal

- The presence of pathogenic intestinal flora.

Indications

- To diagnose *Staphylococcus aureus, Salmonella* organisms, *Shigella* organisms, *Ascaris* organisms, strongyloidiasis, and *Giardia lamblia*.

Contraindications

- None.

Procedure
Client preparation

1. The method of stool collection is explained to the client.
2. Collection method: stools for bacteria or parasites are collected in a clear, wide-mouth plastic or waxed container with a tight-fitting lid.
3. The client is instructed not to mix urine or toilet paper with the specimen.
4. The client is instructed to handle the specimen carefully because it may be infection causing.

Procedure

1. After the stool is collected, the lab slip is completed, indicating whether the client is taking any medications (e.g., antibiotics) that can alter the flora of the intestines.

2. The specimen is sent to the lab as soon as possible after collection.

Nursing implications

1. Generally, barium, oil, or laxatives containing heavy metals are not given 7 days prior to the stool collection.
2. If the client received a purgative medication, the complete stool specimen is usually collected.
3. If an enema must be administered to collect specimens, only normal saline or tap water should be used.
4. If the nurse assists with specimen collection, he or she should wear gloves.

EXAMINATION OF STOOL FOR OCCULT BLOOD
Normal Values

- Negative results; no occult blood detected.

Deviations from Normal

- Positive results; occult blood detected.

Indications

- To aid in the diagnosis of gastrointestinal benign or malignant tumors, ulceration, inflammation of the upper or lower gastrointestinal system, hematobilia, or the swallowing of nasopharyngeal blood.

Contraindications

- None.

Procedure
Client preparation

1. The client is told the number of stool specimens required and given the required number of containers.
2. If the nurse or physician is going to digitally retrieve the specimen, explain the examination to the patient (a gloved index finger is gently inserted into the rectum to remove a piece of stool).
3. The physician may prescribe a special diet before the test

(often high fiber with no red meat for 48 to 72 hours prior to the test).

4. The physician may also withhold medications such as iron preparations, iodines, colchicine, salicylates, steroids, and ascorbic acid.

5. The client is instructed not to mix urine or toilet paper with the stool.

Procedure

1. Test the stool for occult blood on the unit or send the specimen to the lab for analysis.

2. If testing the specimen on the unit, the nurse follows directions explicitly.

Nursing implications

1. Clients screened for occult blood who show a weak positive result are usually placed on a restricted diet and studied again later.

Radiologic Laboratory Tests

X-Ray Tests
BARIUM ENEMA STUDY (LOWER GI SERIES)
Normal Values

- Normal filling, contour, patency, positioning, and transit time of barium.

Deviations from Normal

- Abnormal filling, contour, patency, positioning, and transit time of barium.

Indications

- To detect the presence and location of polyps, tumors (Fig. 2-1), and diverticula (Fig. 2-2).
- To detect possible abnormalities (e.g., malrotation).
- To attempt to reduce nonstrangulated ileocolic intussusception in children.

Contraindications

- Clients suspected of having a perforated viscus because, if the barium leaks through, serious infection will result. In such cases, a water-soluble contrast medium (e.g., Gastrografin) is used.

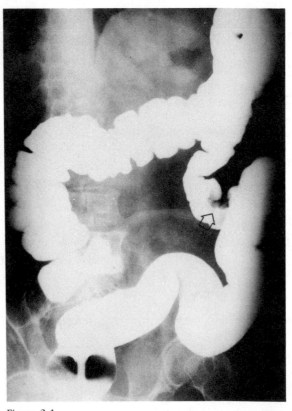

Figure 2-1
Barium enema demonstrating a cancer *(arrow)* in the descending colon.

Procedure
Client preparation

1. The client is told that the preparation and procedure may be exhausting.
2. Written instructions for the preparation are given to the client.

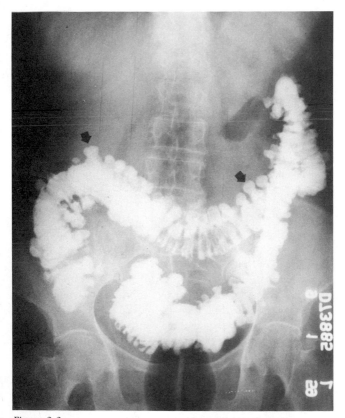

Figure 2-2
Barium enema demonstrating multiple diverticula *(arrows)* in the colon.

3. The client receives assistance as needed with the required preparation.

4. The radiologist performing the procedure may vary the above steps.

Procedure

1. The test begins with the rectal instillation of approximately 500 to 1500 ml of barium. Because the client often has difficulty retaining the barium, a rectal tube with an inflatable balloon is used.

2. The client is placed in supine, prone, and lateral positions.

3. The progress of the barium flow is followed on a fluoroscope.

4. Small polyps and early changes in ulcerative colitis are more easily detected with an *air-contrast barium enema* study. In this study, after the bowel mucosa is outlined with a thin coat of barium, air is insufflated to enhance the contrast and outline of small lesions.

5. After the x-ray films are taken, the client is allowed to expel the barium. This may take as long as 30 minutes.

6. After the barium is expelled, another film is taken for retention of the barium. The colon is examined again for pathologic conditions in the postevacuation film.

7. A different procedure is used for clients with a colostomy or ileostomy.

   a. The stoma is covered with a colostomy or bongart pouch to catch any backflow of barium.

   b. A cone from a colostomy irrigation kit is inserted into the stoma and then attached to irrigation tubing with a straight catheter.

   c. A clamp is opened and the contrast medium is instilled.

   d. A collection device (such as a bedpan) can be placed at the client's side to collect any overflow of contrast medium from the stoma. The end of the pouch can be brought down to rest in the collecting device.

   e. When the x-ray studies are completed, a clamp is placed at the bottom of the pouch.

8. A radiologist performs the study in the radiology department in approximately 45 minutes.

Nursing implications

1. Suggest that the client take reading material to the x-ray department.
2. The client may resume a regular diet after the procedure is completed.
3. Force oral fluids to avoid dehydration caused by cathartics.
4. After the study, assess the client for complete evacuation of the barium.
5. A cathartic or an oil-retention enema may be given.
6. A local anesthetic ointment may be ordered to relieve anal discomfort.
7. If the client is not too tired, a warm bath may be soothing.
8. Allow the client time to rest after the test.

BARIUM SWALLOW

Normal Values

- Normal size, contour, filling, patency, and positioning of the esophagus.

Deviations from Normal

- Defects in luminal filling, which may indicate tumor, strictures, or varices.
- Anatomical abnormalities (e.g., hiatal hernia).
- Left atria dilation, aortic aneurysm, and paraesophageal tumors (e.g., bronchial tumors).
- Esophageal reflux.

Indications

- To aid in the diagnosis of conditions such as esophageal tumors, strictures, and varices, and other conditions discussed under ''Deviations from Normal'' above.

Contraindications

- A client with suspected gastrointestinal perforation because a barium leak from a perforated organ results in intense inflammation and abscess. Instead of barium, a water-soluble contrast medium (e.g., Gastrografin) is used.

Procedure
Client preparation

1. The client is kept on nothing by mouth after midnight the day of the test.

Procedure

1. The fasting client swallows a flavored barium solution similar to that used in an upper GI series.
2. The radiologist follows the barium column through the entire esophagus.
3. Both frontal and lateral views are taken over a 15-minute period.

Nursing implications

1. Explain to the client the importance of rectally expelling all the barium.
2. Increased fluid intake, a mild laxative, or an enema may be necessary to prevent impaction.

UPPER GASTROINTESTINAL STUDY (UPPER GI, UGI)

Normal Values

- Normal size, contour, patency, filling, positioning, and transit time of barium.

Deviations from Normal

- Tumors, scarring, or varices.
- Malignant or benign ulceration and anatomical abnormalities.
- Benign or malignant obstruction.
- Hypermotility of the bowel.

Indications

- To detect ulcerations (benign and malignant) (Fig. 2-3), tumors, inflammation, or anatomical malposition of the organs visualized.

- To follow the healing process of ulcers through repeat UGI studies.
- To identify and define the anatomy of small bowel fistulas through a *small bowel follow-through* study.

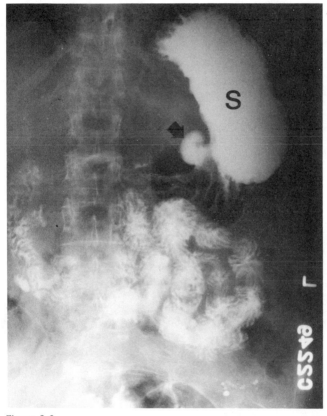

Figure 2-3
Upper gastrointestinal series demonstrating an ulcer *(black arrow)* on the lesser curvature of the stomach *(S)*.

Contraindications

- An uncooperative client.
- A client with complete bowel obstruction.
- A client with perforated viscera of stomach, duodenum, or small bowel.

Procedure

Client preparation

1. The client is kept on nothing by mouth after midnight the day of the test.

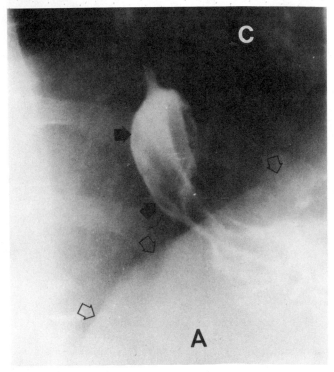

Figure 2-4
Upper gastrointestinal series demonstrating hiatal hernia. Note that proximal portion of the stomach *(solid black arrows)* is above the diaphragm *(arrow outlines)* and lying within the chest *(C)*. A, abdominal cavity.

2. The client is told that the test may take several hours and that, during this time, he or she cannot eat or drink.

Procedure

1. The fasting client swallows approximately 8 oz of barium, a white, chalky, radiopaque substance that is ingested in a milk-shake-like suspension.
2. After drinking the barium, the client is moved through several positional changes, such as prone, supine, and lateral, to promote barium flow by gravity through the upper GI tract.
3. As this contrast medium descends, the lower esophagus is examined for position, patency, and filling defects.
4. As the barium fills the stomach, the gastric wall is examined for ulceration, filling defects, and anatomical abnormalities such as hiatal hernia (Fig. 2-4).
5. As the barium leaves the stomach, the patency of the pyloric valve is evaluated.
6. If desired, a *small bowel follow-through* study may be performed by instructing the client to drink additional barium mixed with saline.
   a. Films are then taken at timed intervals to follow the progression of the barium through the small intestine.
7. If desired, a *small bowel enema* can be performed by placing a tube through the mouth, esophagus, stomach, and duodenum, and into the small intestines. Through this tube, barium is injected, allowing concentrated barium to flow through the small intestines. After the barium has been injected through the tube, the small bowel enema is carried out as described above.
8. A radiologist performs the test in approximately 30 minutes in the radiology department.

Nursing implications

1. Explain to the client the importance of rectally expelling all of the barium.
2. Increased fluid intake, a mild laxative, or an enema may be necessary to prevent impaction.

GASTROINTESTINAL (GI) SCINTIGRAPHY (ABDOMINAL SCINTIGRAPHY, GI BLEEDING SCAN)

Normal Values

■ No collection of radionuclide in the gastrointestinal tract.

Deviations from Normal

■ Pooling of the radionuclide indicates intestinal bleeding.

Indications

■ To localize the site of bleeding in clients with gastrointestinal hemorrhage.

Contraindications

■ None.

Procedure

Client preparation

1. The client should understand that only a small dose of nuclear material is administered.
2. The client is told to notify the technician if the client has a bowel movement during the test.

Procedure

1. Ten millicuries of freshly prepared technetium 99m sulfur colloid are administered intravenously to the client.
2. If technetium-labeled red blood cells are used, 3 ml of the client's blood is combined with technetium and reinjected into the client.
3. Immediately after the administration of the radionuclide, the client is placed under a scintillation camera. Multiple images of the abdomen are obtained at short intervals.
4. A radiologist performs this study in the nuclear medicine department in approximately 10 to 20 minutes.

Nursing implications

1. If the client is experiencing a major gastrointestinal bleed, closely monitor the vital signs during the test.

Special Studies

Endoscopic Procedures

COLONOSCOPY

Normal Values

- Normal intestines.

Deviations from Normal

- Benign and malignant neoplasms, mucosal inflammation or ulceration, and active hemorrhage.

Indications

- To detect lesions in the proximal colon.
- To aid in diagnosing neoplasms, inflammation, ulceration, and hemorrhage.
- To obtain biopsy specimens.
- To remove small tumors.
- To coagulate actively bleeding vessels.

Contraindications

- An uncooperative client.
- A client who is bleeding profusely from the rectum (see "Gastroscopy," p. 51).
- A client in whom bowel preparation has not completely removed all fecal material; the test is then delayed and rescheduled.

Procedure

Client preparation

1. The client is told that the examination is uncomfortable but that he or she will receive sedation by injection and intravenous infusion. Emotional support should be provided.
2. The client is told that he or she will be draped to avoid unnecessary embarrassment.
3. The client is told that because air is insufflated into the bowel during the procedure, he or she may have "gas pains."
4. The preparation regimen is explained to the client.

5. The client is assisted with the preparation.
6. The results from the cathartic and enemas are recorded.
7. Preprocedure medications are administered as ordered.

Procedure

1. An intravenous infusion is begun, and the client is premedicated.
2. With the client in the Sims' position, the scope is inserted into the rectum (or colostomy) and slowly advanced to the cecum.
3. As in all endoscopy, air is insufflated to distend the bowel for better visualization.
4. Endoscopic biopsy specimen or polyp removal is performed and the scope is removed.
5. The gastroenterologist performs the study in a specially equipped room. The study takes approximately 1 to 1½ hours to complete.

Nursing implications

1. Unless further studies are needed or bowel perforation is suspected, the client may resume a normal diet after the procedure.
2. Force fluids to avoid cathartic-induced dehydration.
3. If the client is not too tired, a warm bath may be soothing.
4. Allow the client to rest after the test. The cleansing regimen and fasting may make the client weak and tired.
5. Take safety precautions until the effect of the medications has worn off.

Nurse alert

1. Complications include:
   a. Bowel perforation;
   b. Persistent bleeding from biopsy site; and
   c. Oversedation resulting in respiratory depression.
2. Have Ambu bag ready in the event of respiratory depression.
3. After the test, observe for evidence of bowel perforation (abdominal pain, tenderness, and bleeding). Check stools for gross blood.

ESOPHAGOGASTRODUODENOSCOPY (UGI, ENDOSCOPY, GASTROSCOPY)

Normal Values

- Normal GI tract.

Deviations from Normal

- Tumor, varices, mucosal inflammation, hiatal hernias, polyps, ulcers, and obstructions.

Indications

- To examine esophagus, stomach, and duodenum for conditions listed under "Deviations from Normal" above.
- To extract specimens for biopsy for suspected pathologic conditions.
- To remove polyps and coagulate sources of active gastrointestinal bleeding.
- To evaluate the small intestine for arteriovenous malformation, tumors, enteropathies, and ulcerations by using *enteroscopy*.

Contraindications

- An uncooperative client.
- A client who has severe UGI bleeding because blood clots may cover the viewing lens and prevent good visualization. (The stomach should be lavaged and aspirated.)
- A client with esophageal diverticula because the scope can easily fall into the diverticulum and perforate its wall.

Procedure

Client preparation

1. The client is told that the test is not painful but may cause discomfort and vomiting when the gag reflex is initiated.
2. The client is told that he or she will be unable to speak when the scope is positioned in the GI tract.
3. Since the tube is passed through the mouth, oral hygiene procedures should be performed before and after the test.
4. The client is kept on nothing by mouth after midnight the day of the test.

5. The client's dentures and eyeglasses are removed before the test.
6. Diazepam (Valium) is administered as prescribed by the physician for sedation.
7. Atropine is administered as prescribed by the physician to decrease secretions.

Procedure

1. The client is placed in left lateral decubitus (Sims') position.
2. The client's posterior pharynx is anesthetized with lidocaine (Xylocaine) to inactivate the gag reflex and to lessen the discomfort caused by the passage of the scope.
3. The scope is then passed slowly into the mouth, esophagus, stomach, and duodenum.
4. Air is insufflated to maintain patency of the lumen.
5. Any tissue specimens are placed into an appropriately labeled container.
6. A gastroenterologist usually performs this procedure in the endoscopy room in approximately 30 minutes.

Nursing implications

1. Inform the client that after the anesthesia wears off, he or she may be hoarse and have a sore throat for several days.
2. After the client's throat has been anesthetized with lidocaine (Xylocaine), he or she is not permitted to eat or drink anything until the gag reflex returns (usually 2 to 4 hours).
3. Observe the client for bleeding, fever, abdominal pain, dysphagia, and dyspnea. Monitor the vital signs as ordered.
4. Observe safety precautions until the effects of the sedatives have worn off.

Nurse alert

1. A rare complication of endoscopy is perforation of the esophagus, stomach, and duodenum.
2. Other complications include bleeding from the site of the biopsy specimen extraction, aspiration of gastric contents

into the lungs, and respiratory arrest from diazepam overdose. Carefully monitor the vital signs.
3. Have an Ambu bag available in case of respiratory arrest.
4. Have medications available to counteract serious respiratory depression.

SIGMOIDOSCOPY (LOWER GI ENDOSCOPY)
Normal Values

■ Normal anus, rectum, and sigmoid colon.

Deviations from Normal

■ Abnormalities are described in "Indications."

Indications

■ To aid in diagnosing tumors, polyps, or ulcers.

Contraindications

■ An uncooperative client.
■ Clients with painful anorectal conditions (e.g., fissures, fistulae, or hemorrhoids).
■ Clients with severe rectal bleeding.

Procedure
Client preparation

1. The client is allowed a light breakfast on the morning of the test.
2. The client is assisted with, or given, enemas as ordered the evening before and the morning of the test.
3. The client is warned that the procedure is uncomfortable and that the passing of the sigmoidoscope creates the urge to defecate.
4. The client is told that the insufflation of air into the bowel during the procedure may cause "gas pains."

Procedure

1. The client is assisted in assuming the knee-chest position or, if this position is not possible, the lateral (Sims') po-

sition with buttocks 10 to 12 cm over the edge of the bed to allow complete rotation of the sigmoidoscope.
2. The client is draped to avoid unnecessary exposure and embarrassment.
3. The procedure begins with digital examination of the rectum, which slowly dilates the anal sphincter.
4. The well-lubricated instrument is gently passed about 25 cm (10 in) into the rectum and then into the sigmoid colon.
5. Air is insufflated to distend the bowel, allowing better visualization.
6. Small amounts of stool and mucus can be removed during the procedure with cotton swabs or by suctioning.
7. A physician usually performs the procedure in a specialized room.

Nursing implications

1. After the study, observe the client for fever, bleeding, abdominal distention, and unusual complaints of pain. Slight rectal bleeding may occur if biopsy specimens were taken.

Esophageal Function Studies (EFS)

Manometry studies (LES pressure, swallowing pattern)
Acid reflux
Acid clearing
Bernstein test (acid perfusion)

Manometry Studies
LES PRESSURE
Normal Values

- 10 to 20 torr.

Deviations from Normal

- Inadequate pressure suggests gastroesophageal reflux in adults, chalasia in infants.
- Increased pressure indicates achalasia.

SWALLOWING PATTERN
Normal Values

- Normal peristaltic waves.

Deviations from Normal

- Reduced or no swallowing waves suggests achalasia. Strong, asynchronous, nonpropulsive waves indicate diffuse esophageal spasm.

Acid Reflux
Normal Values

- Negative.

Deviations from Normal

- Clients with an incompetent LES will regurgitate gastric acid into the esophagus, causing a drop in the pH there.

Acid Clearing
Normal Values

- Less than 10 swallows.

Deviations from Normal

- Clients with decreased esophageal motility require a greater number of swallows to clear acid.

Bernstein Test (Acid Perfusion)
Normal Values

- Negative.

Deviations from Normal

- Pain with the instillation of hydrochloric acid into the esophagus indicates reflux esophagitis.

Indications

- To aid in diagnosing esophageal malfunctions.

Contraindications

■ An uncooperative client.

Procedure

Client preparation

1. Explain the initial gag response to the client.
2. The client is kept on nothing by mouth after midnight the day of the test.

Procedure

1. The fasting, unsedated client is asked to swallow three very thin tubes. The tubes are attached to transducers for pressure recordings. All tubes are passed into the stomach.
2. The three tubes are slowly pulled back into the esophagus and the LES pressure is recorded.
3. With all tubes in the esophagus, the client is asked to swallow. The swallowing pattern is then recorded.
4. The tubes are again passed into the stomach. A fourth tube (pH indicator) is passed into the esophagus. The stomach is filled with a solution of hydrochloric acid. A drop in esophageal pH indicates *acid reflux* from the stomach into the esophagus.
5. The tubes are returned to the esophagus. Hydrochloric acid is instilled through them. Counting the number of swallows required to completely clear the acid determines *acid clearing*.
6. Hydrochloric acid (0.1 N) and saline are alternately instilled into the esophagus for the *Bernstein test*. If the client volunteers symptoms of discomfort while the acid is running, the test is positive. If no discomfort is recognized, the test is negative.
7. Esophageal studies are usually performed in a room specially equipped with appropriate instruments and take approximately 30 minutes.

Nursing implications

1. Avoid sedating the client because sedation will cause a false decrease in LES pressure and because the client's

participation is essential for swallowing the tubes, for swallowing during the acid clearance test, and for describing any discomfort during the Bernstein test.

Examination for Gastric Cytology
Normal Values

- No malignancy.

Deviations from Normal

- A positive cytology report indicates malignancy.

Indications

- To aid in the diagnosis of gastric malignancy.

Contraindications

- If gastroscopy is used, refer to contraindications for that study, p. 51.

Procedure
Client preparation

1. The client is told that the nasogastric tube or gastroscope causes the discomfort associated with this test.
2. The client is kept on nothing by mouth after midnight the day of the test.

Procedure

1. Gastric aspiration for cytology can be obtained during gastroscopy (p. 51) or with the insertion of a nasogastric tube.
2. Approximately 100 ml of saline solution is instilled through the tube.
3. The client is asked to turn 360 degrees several times.
4. The fluid is aspirated and sent to the cytology laboratory in a covered container.
5. The nasogastric tube or gastroscope is removed.

Nursing implications

1. See "Gastroscopy," p. 52.

Gastric Analysis

Normal Values

■ See Table 2-1.

Deviations from Normal

■ Table 2-1 compares gastric acid output in normal patients and those with peptic ulcer or gastric cancer.
■ A BAO/MAO ratio greater than 0.6 indicates Zollinger-Ellison syndrome.

Indications

■ To determine whether the ulcer is benign or malignant (Table 2-1).
■ To determine the location of the ulcer.
■ To diagnose Zollinger-Ellison syndrome.
■ To determine the efficacy of therapy by measuring the reduction in acid output.

Table 2-1   Basal and Histalog-stimulated* gastric secretions in normal subjects and in patients with peptic ulcer or with gastric cancer

Condition	Basal Acid Output (BAO) (mEg/1 h)	Maximal Acid Output (MAO) (mEg/1 h)
Normal		
Male	2-5	10-20
Female	1-4	7-15
Duodenal ulcer		
Male	5-10	15-30
Female	3-8	10-20
Gastric ulcer		
Male	1-5	10-20
Female	1-3	5-15
Gastric cancer		
Male	0-3	0-10
Female	0-3	0-5

*Histalog given in dose of 1.5 mg/kg of body weight.

Contraindications

■ Clients with cardiac disease, carcinoid syndrome, and hypertension receive a decreased dose of betazole or histamine.
■ Clients allergic to histamine.

Procedure

Client preparation

1. The client is kept on nothing by mouth after midnight the day of the test.
2. The patient is not given anticholinergic medications for 24 hours before the test.
3. The client is told that smoking is prohibited before the test.

Procedure

1. A nasogastric tube is inserted and a 50 cc syringe is attached to the tube for aspiration.
2. The first specimen is aspirated and discarded.
3. At the appropriate time interval (usually every 15 minutes for four times), the entire gastric contents are aspirated.
4. The gastric contents are placed in a clean specimen container and numbered for sending to the chemistry lab for analysis.
5. The client is instructed to expectorate saliva during the entire procedure, since it may buffer the stomach's acid content.
6. As prescribed, a histamine phosphate (0.04 mg/kg) or betazole hydrochloride (Histalog) (1 to 2 mg/kg) is administered subcutaneously to stimulate maximal stomach acid production.
7. After the subcutaneous injection, the client's pulse and blood pressure are taken immediately. Usually, pulse increases and blood pressure decreases slightly.
8. Specimens are aspirated every 15 minutes for eight times. Aspirate is handled as in step 4 above.
9. When the test is completed, the nasogastric tube is clamped and withdrawn.

Nursing implications

1. After injecting the histamine, monitor the client for side effects, principally contraction of smooth muscle, promotion of gastric acid secretion, and dilation of capillaries (which is the most bothersome side effect and includes flushing, increase in skin temperature, itching, and a drop in blood pressure). The blood pressure drop is usually transient.
2. After completing the test, give nose and mouth care.
3. The client can usually assume a normal diet after the test.

Nurse alert

1. Following the subcutaneous injection of histamine, observe for symptoms of overdose:
   a. Drop in blood pressure;
   b. Intense headache;
   c. Dyspnea;
   d. Flushing;
   e. Vomiting;
   f. Diarrhea; and
   g. Shock.
2. Administration of epinephrine will prevent or quickly counteract these symptoms.

Hydrogen Breath Test
Normal Values

- No rise in exhaled hydrogen, above that obtained during fasting, following a high-lactose meal.

Deviations from Normal

- Lactose intolerance.
- Bacterial overgrowth syndrome.

Indications

- To assist in the diagnosis of lactose intolerance and bacterial overgrowth syndrome.

Contraindications

■ An uncooperative client.

Procedure
Client preparation

1. The procedure and purpose are explained, emphasizing that the test causes no discomfort.

Procedure

1. All antibiotics are discontinued for 7 to 10 days prior to the test or per physician's orders.
2. The client should not eat wheat bran 12 hours prior to the test.
3. The client is taken to the GI lab where a fasting hydrogen test is performed (see detail of procedure below).
4. For the evening meal prior to the test, the client receives a high-lactose meal, usually 6 oz cooked red meat, 3 cups cooked white rice, and as much water as desired.
5. Following the evening meal the client may only have water.
6. All foods and fluids are withheld after midnight.
7. The client is cautioned not to smoke for 2 hours before the test.
8. The client is instructed not to exercise in the morning prior to the test. Performing routine morning care is allowed.
9. The test is usually performed in the GI lab by a special trained nurse or technician.
10. Once in the lab the client is asked to have a normal inspiration. Before exhaling, a mouthpiece is inserted in the client's mouth.
11. Next the client is asked to exhale using normal force. The client is cautioned not to exhale forcefully.
12. The first portion of the exhalation is discarded. The latter is kept and the amount of hydrogen content is measured in parts per million by a gas chromatograph.
13. The client may be asked to repeat the procedure again.
14. The test usually takes 15 to 20 minutes.
15. The client is returned to his or her room.

Nursing implications

1. Notify the dietary department of the need for a special diet.
2. Place an NPO sign on the client's door and above the bed.
3. There should be no cleaning solvents, alcohol, or smoking in the room where the test is conducted.

Nutritional Assessment Studies

Triceps skin-fold thickness (TSF): estimates the amount of subcutaneous fat
Midarm circumference (MAC)
Midarm muscle circumference (MAMC): calculated using the MAC and TSF
Anthropometric measurements

Nutritional assessment studies are usually used in conjunction with the following tests:

Hemoglobin;
Hematocrit;
Total iron binding capacity;
Serum albumin;
Total protein;
Total lymphocyte count;
Blood urea nitrogen (BUN);
24-hour urine for creatinine; and
Serum triglycerides.

Normal Values

■ Vary with age and sex of client.

Deviations from Normal

■ Vary with age and sex of the client.

Indications

■ To aid in diagnosing nutritional disorders (e.g., anorexia nervosa, bulimia).

Contraindications

■ None.

Procedure

1. See individual studies.

Small Bowel Biopsy

Normal Values

- Normal mucosa and submucosa of the small bowel.

Deviations from Normal

- Abnormalities of small intestine can be found with Whipple's disease, giardiasis, amyloidosis, lymphoma, coccidiosis, mast cell disease, hypogammaglobulinemia, intestinal lymphangiectasia, constrictive pericarditis, sprue, and celiac disease.

Indications

- To assist in the diagnosis of the conditions listed under "Deviations from Normal."

Contraindications

- An uncooperative client.

Procedure

Client preparation

1. The procedure and purpose are explained.

Procedure

1. Twenty-four to forty-eight hours before the biopsy the client is put on a clear liquid diet.
2. All fluids and foods are withheld after the evening meal prior to the biopsy.
3. The client is taken to the x-ray department where the biopsy is performed.
4. The client is asked to swallow the small bowel biopsy capsule by drinking sips of water as the capsule and connecting tube are passed down the throat and progressed into the small intestine.
5. A flat plate x-ray film of the abdomen is performed to assure proper placement of the biopsy capsule.

6. After correct placement has been confirmed, the physician aspirates a biopsy of the small bowel's mucosa.
7. The biopsy aspirate is placed in a specimen container, labeled, and sent to pathology for histology.
8. The biopsy capsule is slowly withdrawn.
9. The client's vital signs are taken every 15 minutes for 1 hour, every 30 minutes for 1 hour, and every hour for 2 hours, or per physician's order.
10. The client is returned to his or her room.

Nursing implications

1. Observe the client for signs and symptoms of abdominal bleeding (e.g., increased pulse, decreased blood pressure, dizziness, fainting, emesis containing blood, coldness, sweating).
2. Order the client a diet per physician's orders.

Nurse alert

1. Notify the physician immediately of signs and symptoms of abdominal bleeding.

Bibliography

Arnell, I., and Nassberg, B.R.: A clean, quick way to administer a barium enema through a colostomy. Nursing '81 **11**(2), 81-83, 1981.

Braden, B.: Disturbances in ingestion. In Jones, D.A., Dunbar, C.F., and Jirovee, M.M., editors: Medical-surgical nursing: a conceptual approach, ed. 2, New York, 1982, McGraw-Hill Book Co.

Brunner, L.S., and Suddarth, D.S.: Textbook of medical-surgical nursing, ed. 5, Philadelphia, 1984, J.B. Lippincott Co.

Claggett, M.S.: Anorexia nervosa: a behavioral approach, Am. J. Nurs. **80:**1471, Aug. 1980.

Gilbertsen, V.A., and others: The earlier detection of colorectal cancer, Cancer **45:**2899, 1981.

Given, B.A., and Simmons, S.J.: Gastroenterology in clinical nursing, ed. 4, St. Louis, 1984, The C.V. Mosby Co.

Hartfield, M.J., and Casan, C.L.: Effects of information on emotional responses during barium enema. Nurs. Res. **30**(3):151, 1981.

Johnson, R., Quan, M., and Rodney, W.: Flexible sigmoidoscopy, J. Fam. Pract. **14**(4):757-770, 1982.

Lamphier, T., and Lamphier, R.: Upper GI hemorrhage: emergency evaluation and management, Am. J. Nurs. **81**(10):1814-1817, Oct. 1981.

Leicester, R.J., and others: Flexible fiberoptic sigmoidoscopy as an outpatient procedure, Lancet **8262**(1):34-35, Jan. 2, 1982.

Long, B.C., and Durham, N.: Assessment of upper gastrointestinal tract function. In Phipps, W.J., Long, B.C., and Woods, N.F.: Medical-surgical nursing: concepts and clinical practice, ed. 2, St. Louis, 1983. The C.V. Mosby Co.

Marks, R.G.: Anorexia and bulimia: eating habits that can kill, RN **47**(1):44-47, Jan. 1984.

Neville, J.: Assessment of nutritional status. In Phipps, W.J., Long, B.C., and Woods, N.F.: Medical-surgical nursing: concepts and clinical practice, ed. 2, St. Louis, 1983, The C.V. Mosby Co.

Neville, J.: Interventions for the person with impaired nutrition. In Phipps, W.J., Long, B.C., and Woods, N.F.: Medical-surgical nursing: concepts and clinical practice, ed. 2, St. Louis, 1983, The C.V. Mosby Co.

Richardson, T.P.: Anorexia nervosa: an overview, Am. J. Nur. **80**:1470, Aug. 1980.

Rohde, J., and others: Diagnosis and treatment of anorexia nervosa, J. Fam. Pract. **10**(6):1007, June 1980.

Schottelius, B.A., and Schottelius, D.D.: Textbook of physiology, ed. 19, St. Louis, 1983, The C.V. Mosby Co.

Silverstein, F.E., and Rubin, C.E.: Gastrointestinal endoscopy. In Petersdorf, R.G., and others, editors: Harrison's principles of internal medicine, ed. 10, New York, 1983, McGraw-Hill Book Co.

Suitor, C.W., and Hunter, M.F.: Nutrition-principles and application in health promotion, Philadelphia, 1980, J.B. Lippincott Co.

Tucker, S.M., and others: Patient care standards, ed. 3, St. Louis, 1984, The C.V. Mosby Co.

Winawar, S.J., and others: Current status of fecal occult blood testing in screening for colorectal carcinoma. CA **32**:100, 1982.

Hepatobiliary and Pancreatic System 3

Clinical laboratory tests
  Blood tests
    Blood ammonia test
    Hepatitis virus studies (hepatitis-associated antigen, HAA, Australian antigen)
  Liver enzyme studies
    Serum aspartate aminotransferase (AST), formerly serum glutamic oxaloacetic transaminase (SGOT)
    Serum alanine amino transferase (ALT), formerly serum glutanic pyruvic transaminase (SGPT)
    Lactate dehydrogenase (LDH)
    Alkaline phosphatase (ALP)
    5'-Nucleotidase
    Serum leucine aminopeptidase (LAP)
    Serum gamma-glutamyl transpeptidase (GGTP)
    Serum amylase test
    Serum bilirubin test
    Serum lipase test
    Serum proteins test
  Stool tests
    Fecal fat test
  Urine tests
    Urine amylase test
    Urine bilirubin test
    Urine urobilinogen test
Radiologic laboratory tests
  X-ray tests
    Oral cholecystography (gallbladder series, GB series, cholecystogram)

Cholangiography procedures
   Endoscopic retrograde cholangiopancreatography of the biliary duct (ERCP)
   Endoscopic retrograde cholangiopancreatography of the pancreatic duct
   Intravenous cholangiography (intravenous cholangiogram)
   Operative cholangiography
   Percutaneous transhepatic cholangiography (PTHC)
   T-tube cholangiography (postoperative cholangiography)
Nuclear scanning tests
   Cholescintigraphy (hepatobiliary scintigraphy, hepatobiliary imaging, biliary tract radionuclide scan, biliary scintigraphy, and DISIDA scanning)
   Liver scanning
Computerized tomography tests
   Computerized tomography of the abdomen (CT of the abdomen)
Special studies
   Liver biopsy
   Secretin-pancreozymin test
   Sweat electrolytes test (iontophoretic sweat test)
   Ultrasound tests
      Ultrasound examination of the liver and biliary system
      Ultrasound examination of the pancreas (pancreas echogram)

Clinical Laboratory Tests

Blood Tests
BLOOD AMMONIA TEST
Normal Values

- Adult: 15 to 110 µg/dl.
- Child: 40 to 80 µg/dl.
- Newborn: 90 to 150 µg/dl.

Deviations from Normal

- *Elevated levels* may occur with liver dysfunction, hepatic failure, erythroblastosis fetalis, cor pulmonale, pulmonary emphysema, congestive heart failure, and exercise.
- *Decreased levels* may occur with renal failure, essential or malignant hypertension, or the use of certain antibiotics (e.g., neomycin, tetracycline).

Indications

- Used primarily to assist in diagnosis of hepatic encephalopathy or coma.

Contraindications

- None.

Procedure

1. The client is kept on nothing by mouth for 8 hours before the blood sample is drawn.
2. Using standard technique for drawing a venous blood sample, 5 to 7 ml of venous blood are collected in a green-top tube.

Nursing Implications

1. Because many clients with liver disease have prolonged clotting times, assessing the venipuncture site for bleeding after drawing the sample is particularly important.
2. Because certain antibiotics can cause a decreased ammonia level and thus give inaccurate results, list any antibiotics the client is taking on the lab slip.

HEPATITIS VIRUS STUDIES (HEPATITIS-ASSOCIATED ANTIGEN, HAA, AUSTRALIAN ANTIGEN)

Normal Values

- Negative.

Deviations from Normal

- See Table 3-1.

Indications

- To aid in diagnosis of hepatitis A, B, and non-A, non-B.
- To track the client's recovery from hepatitis.
- To identify hepatitis "carriers."

Contraindications

- None.

Procedure

1. Using standard technique for peripheral venipuncture, one red-top tube of blood is drawn.
2. Pressure or a pressure dressing is applied to the venipuncture site after the blood is drawn.

Table 3-1 Hepatitis viruses and test indications

	Causal Virus		
	A (HAV)	B (HBV) (Dane Particle)	Non-A, Non-B (NANB) (Hepatitis C)
Original name	Infectious hepatitis	Serum hepatitis	
Incubation period	2-6 wks	5 wks to 6 mos	2-12 wks
Mode of transmission	Fecal-oral route	Blood transfusion, blood, saliva, semen	Blood transfusion, blood, saliva, semen
Prognosis	Usually complete recovery	May result in liver failure and death	Much less severe illness than Hepatitis B
Antigen/test available	None	HBsAg/yes (s = surface) HBcAg/no (c = core) HBeAg/yes	
Antibody/test available	IgM (HAV Ab/IgM)/ yes IgG (HAV/Ab IgG/yes	HBsAb/yes HBcAb/yes HBeAb/yes	

Nursing Implications

1. Handle the serum specimen as if it were capable of transmitting viral hepatitis.
2. Wash hands carefully after handling all equipment. Many labs suggest that the nurse or technician wear gloves during the venipuncture.

Liver Enzyme Studies
SERUM ASPARTATE AMINOTRANSFERASE (AST); FORMERLY SERUM GLUTAMIC OXALOACETIC TRANSAMINASE (SGOT)

Normal Values

- 5 to 40 IU/L.

Deviations from Normal

- High serum levels occur after myocardial infarction and liver damage.
- AST levels are also increased in clients with acute pancreatitis, acute hemolytic anemia, severe burns, acute renal disease, musculoskeletal disease, trauma, beriberi, and diabetic ketoacidosis, and in pregnant women.

Indications

- See "Deviations from Normal."

SERUM ALANINE AMINOTRANSFERASE (ALT); FORMERLY SERUM GLUTAMIC PYRUVIC TRANSAMINASE (SGPT)

Normal Values

- 5 to 35 IU/L.

Deviations from Normal

- Liver dysfunction is usually the cause of elevated ALT levels. AST and ALT levels are often compared. The AST/ALT ratio is usually >1 in alcoholic cirrhosis, liver congestion, and metabolic tumor to the liver. Ratios <1 may appear in patients with acute hepatitis, viral hepatitis, and infectious mononucleosis.

Indications

- To help confirm the liver origin of an AST increase.

LACTIC DEHYDROGENASE (LDH)

Normal Values

- 90 to 200 ImU/ml.

Deviations from Normal

- A wide variety of client situations increase LDH levels: acute myocardial infarction, congestive heart failure, cardiovascular surgery, hepatitis, untreated pernicious anemia, renal disease, muscle disease, pulmonary embolus, and malignant tumors.

Indications

- To aid in diagnosis of conditions listed under "Deviations from Normal."

ALKALINE PHOSPHATASE (ALP)

Normal Values

- Adults: 30 to 85 ImU/ml.
- Children and adolescents:
  <2 years, 85 to 235 ImU/ml;
  2 to 8 years, 65 to 210 ImU/ml;
  9 to 15 years, 60 to 300 ImU/ml (active bone growth); and
  16 to 21 years, 30 to 200 ImU/ml.

Deviations from Normal

- The level is greatly increased in obstructive (both extrahepatic and intrahepatic) biliary disease.
- ALP is also increased in clients with metastatic carcinoma to the liver, infarcted bowel, hyperphosphatasia, hepatoma,

liver abscess, liver granulomas, hyperparathyroidism, Paget's disease, healing fractures, and rheumatoid arthritis.
- Reduced ALP levels may appear in clients with the following: hypothyroidism, hypophosphatemia, excess vitamin B ingestion, scurvy, malnutrition, milk-alkali syndrome, celiac disease, and pernicious anemia.

Indications

- To distinguish between liver and bone disease.

5'-NUCLEOTIDASE

Normal Values

- 0 to 1.6 units.

Deviations from Normal

- Elevation may be an early indication of metastasis, especially if jaundice is absent.

Indications

- To aid in differential diagnosis of liver disease from bone disease and of hepatobiliary disease during pregnancy.

SERUM LEUCINE AMINOPEPTIDASE (LAP)

Normal Values

- Blood: male, 80 to 200 U/ml; female, 75 to 185 U/ml.
- Urine: 2 to 18 U/24 h.

Deviations from Normal

- Elevation may indicate liver metastasis and choledocholithiasis.

Indications

- To diagnose liver disorders.
- To aid in differential diagnosis of increased alkaline phosphatase levels.

SERUM GAMMA-GLUTAMYL TRANSPEPTIDASE (GGTP)

Normal Values

- Male: 8 to 38 U/L.
- Female: <45 yrs, 5 to 27 U/L.

Deviations from Normal

- The level is high in 75% of chronic alcoholics. The level may be increased 4 to 10 days after an acute myocardial infarction.
- Certain medications (e.g., diphenylhydantoin [Dilantin] and phenobarbital) also cause elevations.

Indications

- To detect liver cell dysfunction and alcohol ingestion.
- To help distinguish hepatic disease from skeletal disease when the serum alkaline phosphatase is elevated.
- To aid in differential diagnosis of hepatocellular disease during pregnancy and childhood.

Contraindications

- None.

Procedure

Client preparation

1. Although usually no special preparation is needed, some labs require a 12-hour fast.
2. If abstinence from alcohol is required, the client is instructed accordingly.

Procedure

1. Following the standard procedure for drawing venous blood, approximately 7 to 10 ml of blood are collected in a red-top tube.
2. Pressure or a pressure dressing is applied to the puncture site.

Nursing implications

1. Medications affect many of these liver enzyme tests.
2. Intramuscular injections affect some of the enzymes (AST or SGOT).
3. After the venipuncture, assess the site for bleeding.

SERUM AMYLASE TEST

Normal Values

- 56 to 190 IU/L or 80 to 150 Somogyi units/dl.

Deviations from Normal

- Ongoing inflammation (e.g., severe hemorrhagic pancreatitis), duct obstruction (e.g., cancer), or pancreatic ductal leakage (e.g., pseudocysts) will cause persistently elevated serum amylase levels.
- Disorders affecting salivary glands, liver, intestines, kidneys, and the female genital tract (e.g., parotitis, cholecystitis, perforated bowel, renal infarction, or ectopic pregnancy) will cause a high serum amylase level.
- Decreased levels occur in clients with advanced chronic pancreatitis, chronic alcoholism, and toxic hepatitis.
- A client receiving an IV dextrose solution may have decreased serum amylase levels, causing a false-negative report.

Indications

- To diagnose pancreatitis.
- To aid in diagnosis of conditions listed in "Deviations from Normal" above.

Contraindications

- None.

Procedure

1. Following standard venipuncture procedure, one red-top tube of blood is drawn.
2. Pressure or a pressure dressing is applied to the site after completing the venipuncture.

Nursing implications

1. Observe the puncture site for bleeding.
2. If the client is receiving IV dextrose, note this on the lab slip.

SERUM BILIRUBIN TEST
Normal Values

- Direct bilirubin: 0.1 to 0.3 mg/dl.
- Indirect bilirubin: 0.2 to 0.8 mg/dl.
- Total bilirubin: 0.1 to 1.0 mg/dl.
- Total bilirubin in newborns: 1 to 12 mg/dl.

Deviations from Normal

- The effect of many different drugs (e.g., antibiotics, sulfonamides, allopurinol, diuretics, barbiturates, steroids, and oral contraceptives) may cause elevated serum bilirubin test results.
- Levels of serum bilirubin may be decreased in clients with iron-deficiency anemia and in clients taking penicillin and large amounts of salicylates.
- Obstruction of the biliary ducts (e.g., gallstones) and hepatocellular disease (e.g., hepatitis) may cause conjugated hyperbilirubinemia.
- Accelerated erythrocyte hemolysis in newborns (erythroblastosis fetalis), absence of glucuronyl transferase, and hepatocellular disease cause unconjugated hyperbilirubinemia.

Indications

- See "Deviations from Normal."

Contraindications

- None.

Procedure
Client preparation

1. The client preparation required by the lab is followed.

Procedure

1. Following the standard procedure for drawing venous blood sample, one red-top tube of blood is collected.
2. In infants, a heel puncture is used and two blood microtubes are filled.
3. Pressure or a pressure dressing is applied to the puncture site.

Nursing implications

1. Prevent hemolysis of the blood specimen.
2. The blood specimen should not be exposed to sunlight and artificial light.
3. After the venipuncture, assess the site for bleeding.

SERUM LIPASE TEST

Normal Values

- 0 to 100 units/L or 0 to 1.5 units/ml.

Deviations from Normal

- Levels will be elevated following damage to the pancreas and with pancreatitis.

Indications

- To diagnose pancreatitis.
- To diagnose pancreatic carcinoma.

Contraindications

- None.

Procedure
Client preparation

1. The client's breakfast is withheld until the blood has been drawn.
2. The client is allowed to have water.

Procedure

1. Following standard venipuncture technique, one red-top tube of blood is withdrawn.

2. A pressure dressing or pressure is applied to the venipuncture site.
3. The sample is sent to the lab for analysis.

Nursing implications

1. Observe the venipuncture site for bleeding.
2. Note on the lab slip if narcotics (e.g., morphine, codeine, meperidine) have been given to the client within the 24 hours preceding the test.

SERUM PROTEINS TEST

Normal Values

- Total protein: 6 to 8 g/dl.
- Albumin: 3.2 to 4.5 g/dl.
- Globulin: 2.3 to 3.4 g/dl.

Deviations from Normal

- Low serum albumin may indicate severe liver dysfunction or excessive loss of albumin into the urine (e.g., nephrotic syndrome) or into third-space volumes (e.g., ascites).

Indications

- To aid in diagnosing liver dysfunction.

Contraindications

- None.

Procedure
Client preparation

1. The purpose of the test is explained to the client.
2. Some labs require the client be kept on nothing by mouth except water for the 8 hours before the test.

Procedure

1. Following the standard venipuncture procedure, one red-top tube of blood is collected.
2. Pressure or a pressure dressing is applied to the puncture site.

Nursing implications

1. Observe the venipuncture site for bleeding.

Stool Tests
FECAL FAT TEST
Normal Values

- 5 g/24 h or a fat retention coefficient ≥95%.

Deviations from Normal

- Elevated fecal fat levels indicate cystic fibrosis or a condition affected by malabsorption or maldigestion (e.g., hypermobility, massive bowel resection, and antiobesity surgical procedures).

Indications

- To aid in the diagnosis of cystic fibrosis or other conditions listed under ''Deviations from Normal'' above.

Contraindications

- None.

Procedure
Client preparation

1. The prescribed fat-content diet is explained to the client, and the client is assisted in following the diet for the required time (usually 2 to 3 days before the stool collection and then for the duration of the test).

Procedure

1. The client is told to defecate into a dry, clean bedpan or container.
2. If necessary, the client is given tongue blades to transfer the stool.
3. For an infant, the diapers must be examined for stools and the stools transferred to the stool container.
4. The client is told not to urinate into the stool container or bedpan nor to mix toilet paper with the stool.

Nursing implications

1. Tell the client that diarrheal stools should also be collected.
2. Do not administer laxatives or enemas to the client.

Urine Tests
URINE AMYLASE TEST
Normal Values

- 3 to 35 IU/h, or 60 to 30 Wohlgemuth units/ml, or up to 5000 Somogyi units/24 h.

Deviations from Normal

- See "Serum Amylase Test," p. 74.

Indications

- To diagnose pancreatitis.
- See discussion of "Deviations from Normal" and "Indications" for "Serum Amylase Test," p. 74.

Contraindications

- None.

Procedure

1. The client is given the necessary urine containers.
2. The exact times of the beginning and the end of the collection period are recorded. The collection begins *after* the client empties the bladder and discards that specimen. All subsequent urine is collected, including that at the end of the collection period.

Nursing implications

1. Encourage the client to drink fluids during the collection period unless they are restricted for medical reasons.
2. Keep the specimen on ice or refrigerated until it is sent to the lab.

URINE BILIRUBIN TEST

Normal Values

- None.

Deviations from Normal

- Presence of bilirubin in the urine suggests conjugated hyperbilirubinemia.

Indications

- To determine whether hyperbilirubinemia is unconjugated or conjugated.

Contraindications

- None.

Procedure

1. The client receives the proper urine container.
2. A fresh urine sample is collected from the client and tested as soon as possible (within 1 hour). Bilirubin is not stable in urine, especially when exposed to light.
3. Generally the nurse performs the test with Multistix reagent strips or with Icotest tablets (Ames). Directions are on the bottle.

Nursing implications

1. Immediately after removing the reagent strip or tablets, tightly replace the cap on the bottle to avoid destruction from moisture in the air.
2. Do not use reagent strips or tablets with test mat after the expiration date on the bottle.
3. Many drugs interfere with the bilirubin test results. Phenazopyridine (Pyridium), ethoxazene (Serenium), and chlorpromazine may give false-positive results. Indocin can give either a false-negative or false-positive result. High concentrations of ascorbic acid (vitamin C) are associated with false-negative results.

URINE UROBILINOGEN TEST

Normal Values

- 0.1 to 1.0 Ehrlich units/dl (random specimen).
- 0.3 to 1.0 Ehrlich units/2 h.
- 0.5 to 4.0 Ehrlich units/24 h.

Deviations from Normal

- Urine urobilinogen is increased with hepatocellular disease or with hemolytic anemia.
- The urine urobilinogen will be negative in biliary ductal obstruction or severe liver failure.

Indications

- See "Deviations from Normal."

Contraindications

- None.

Procedure

Client preparation

1. Determine which of the three types of available tests will be used: single or random specimen, 2-hour urine specimen, or 24-hour urine collection.
2. The specific collection procedure is explained to the client:
   a. A *single urine specimen* uses fresh urine and is tested immediately.
   b. The *2-hour urine test* is usually performed between 1 and 3 p.m. or 2 and 4 p.m. because urobilinogen levels are highest then.
   c. Collect the *24-hour urine specimen* as described under the "Creatinine Clearance Test," p. 181. Follow all but "Client Preparation" step 2 and "Procedure" step 3.
   d. Also keep the specimen from light, refrigerate the specimen, and use a preservative.
3. Usually the urine is tested with Multistix reagent strip (see "Urine Bilirubin Test," p. 80).

Nursing implications

1. See "Urine Bilirubin Test," p. 80.

Radiologic Laboratory Tests

X-Ray Tests

ORAL CHOLECYSTOGRAPHY (GALLBLADDER SERIES, GB SERIES, CHOLECYSTOGRAM)

Normal Values

- Visualization of gallbladder, no filling defects, no stones.

Deviations from Normal

- Calculi.
- Gallbladder polyps or tumors.
- Chronically inflamed gallbladder.

Indications

- To aid in the diagnosis of pathologic gallbladder conditions.

Contraindications

- A client who is allergic to iodine dye.
- A client in early pregnancy, because x-ray exposure may be teratogenic (causing congenital abnormalities) to an early fetus.

Procedure

Client preparation

1. The serum bilirubin must be <1.8 mg/dl prior to beginning the test procedure so that visualization is possible.
2. On the evening before the test, the client receives a low-fat or fat-free meal.
3. Before administration of the dye, the client is assessed for allergies to iodine.
4. Approximately 12 hours before the test, the client receives six iopanoic acid tablets. If the client vomits after taking the dye, the physician is notified and will either suggest giving the patient the dye again or postponing the test.
5. The client is told that after taking the dye, no other food can be eaten. Food will stimulate the gallbladder to contract and therefore eliminate the dye from the gallbladder.

Procedure

1. The radiologist takes x-ray films of the right upper quadrant of the abdomen as the client is placed in several positions.
2. After initial x-ray examination the client may be given a fatty meal to test the contractability of the gallbladder.
3. X-ray films are then repeated at intervals until the gallbladder has expelled the dye.
4. The radiologist performs the test in the radiology department in about 1 hour. *Post fatty meal tests,* given to test the contractability of the gallbladder, require another 1 to 2 hours.

Nursing implications

1. After the client takes the dye, assess for side effects (e.g., abdominal cramps, nausea, vomiting, and diarrhea) that can alter dye absorption.
2. If the client will receive a fatty meal to stimulate gallbladder emptying, no other food or fluid is allowed until all follow-up x-ray films are completed.
3. Explain to the client that the dye is eventually excreted in the urine. Some clients report slight dysuria following the test.

Cholangiography Procedures
ENDOSCOPIC RETROGRADE CHOLANGIOPANCREATOGRAPHY OF THE BILIARY DUCT (ERCP)

Normal Values

- Normal biliary ducts.

Deviations from Normal

- Stones, benign strictures, cysts, and malignant tumors can be identified.

Indications

- To determine if obstructive jaundice is intrahepatic or extrahepatic.
- To visualize the biliary tree when the bilirubin level is greater than 3.5 mg/dl.
- To aid in diagnosing conditions listed under ''Deviations from Normal'' above.

Contraindications

- An uncooperative client.
- See discussion of ''Gastroscopy,'' p. 51.

Procedure

Client preparation

1. The client is told that the test takes about 1 hour, during which it is important to lie completely motionless on a hard x-ray table.
2. The client is assured that during the test no discomfort will be felt other than the initial gag when the duodenoscope is passed.
3. The client is kept on nothing by mouth after midnight the day of the test.
4. The premedication is administered as prescribed.

Procedure

1. The client is placed in the supine position.
2. A flat plate of the abdomen (kidney, ureter, and bladder) may be taken prior to the study.
3. A side-viewing fiberoptic duodenoscope is inserted through the oral pharynx and passed through the esophagus and stomach and into the duodenum (Fig. 3-1).
4. The client is given secretin intravenously to paralyze the duodenum so that the ampulla of Vater can be found more easily.
5. Through an accessory lumen within the scope, a small catheter is passed through the ampulla and enters into either the common bile duct or pancreatic duct.
6. Radiographic dye (containing a broad-spectrum antibiotic) is injected, and x-ray films are taken.

7. An endoscopist performs this procedure in the radiology department in approximately 1 hour.

Nursing implications

1. Review "Nursing Implications" for "Gastroscopy," p. 52.
2. Assess the client for signs of bacteremia or septicemia.
3. Occasionally the pressure of the injection into the main pancreatic duct will cause an acute bout of pancreatitis. This condition is best diagnosed by obtaining a serum amylase determination the day following the procedure.

Nurse alert

1. Perforation of the esophagus, stomach, and duodenum are rare complications.
2. Bacteremia, caused when the pressure of the dye pushes infected bile into the bloodstream, is a possible complication.

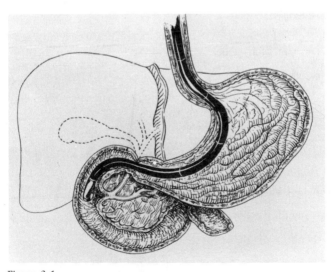

Figure 3-1
Endoscopic retrograde cholangiopancreatogram. The fiberoptic scope is passed into the duodenum. Note a small catheter being advanced into the pancreatic biliary ducts.

ENDOSCOPIC RETROGRADE CHOLANGIOPANCREATOGRAPHY OF THE PANCREATIC DUCT

Normal Values

- Patent pancreatic duct.

Deviations from Normal

- Tumor.
- Chronic pancreatitis.

Indications

- To detect clinically significant degrees of pancreatic dysfunction.

Contraindications

- See "Endoscopic Retrograde Cholangiopancreatography of the Biliary Duct," p. 84.

Procedure

1. See "Endoscopic Retrograde Cholangiopancreatography of the Biliary Duct," p. 84.

Nursing implications

1. See "Endoscopic Retrograde Cholangiopancreatography of the Biliary Duct," p. 85.

INTRAVENOUS CHOLANGIOGRAPHY (INTRAVENOUS CHOLANGIOGRAM, IVC)

Normal Values

- Patent biliary ducts.

Deviations from Normal

- Duct obstruction caused by stones, stricture, or tumor.

Indications

- To demonstrate stone, stricture, or tumor of the hepatic duct, common bile duct, and the gallbladder.

- To study the biliary tree for retained gallstones in cholecystectomized clients.
- To rule out the biliary system as the cause of acute abdominal inflammation.
- To demonstrate passage of the stones into the common bile in clients who have proven gallstones.
- To study clients who cannot tolerate the oral administration of the iopanoic acid tablets used in oral cholecystography.

Contraindications

- A client with an allergy to iodine dye.

Procedure

Client preparation

1. The dye may cause a burning sensation when injected.
2. The client receives a laxative.
3. The client is kept on nothing by mouth after midnight the day of the test and until the test is completed.
4. The bilirubin level must be <3.5 mg/dl so that visualization will be possible.
5. A cleansing enema may be given on the morning of the test.
6. Before the administration of the dye, the client is assessed for allergies to iodine.

Procedure

1. While in the supine position, the client is given an intravenous infusion of iodine dye (Cholografin).
2. X-ray films are taken on the right upper quadrant of the abdomen intermittently for a period of up to 8 hours.
3. A radiologist performs the test in the radiology department in 1 to 8 hours.

Nursing implications

1. After the dye is administered, observe the client for allergic reactions (e.g., dyspnea, tachycardia, sweating, nausea, vomiting, and chills).
2. Explain to the client that the dye is eventually excreted in the urine. Some clients report slight dysuria following IVC.

OPERATIVE CHOLANGIOGRAPHY

Normal Values

- Normal biliary duct.

Deviations from Normal

- Gallstones.
- Tumors.

Indications

- To reduce the possibility of inadvertent common bile duct injury during surgery.
- To reduce the number of unnecessary common bile duct explorations.

PERCUTANEOUS TRANSHEPATIC CHOLANGIOGRAPHY (PTHC)

Normal Values

- Normal gallbladder and biliary ducts.

Deviations from Normal

- Gallstones, benign strictures and cysts, and malignant tumors.

Indications

- To aid in diagnosing conditions of the intrahepatic and extrahepatic biliary ducts and occasionally the gallbladder of jaundiced clients.

Contraindications

- A client with iodine allergy.
- A client with evidence of mild cholangitis; dye injections increase biliary pressure and cause bacteremia, which may lead to septicemia and shock.
- A client who is a poor surgical candidate, since surgical repair of complications may be necessary.
- An uncooperative client.

- A client with prolonged clotting time.
- A client who has had a recent GI contrast study (within the last day); residual barium may obscure radiographic visualization of the bile ducts.

Procedure

Client preparation

1. The client is told that slight discomfort may occur when the abdomen is anesthetized locally, and that a feeling of pressure may occur when the needle is placed into the liver.
2. The client is assessed for allergies to iodine.
3. If recent GI contrast studies were performed for the client, a physician's order for a cathartic to remove any residual barium is obtained.
4. The client is prepared as if for surgery because emergency surgical intervention may become necessary to control hemorrhage or bile leak.
5. The client's blood is typed and cross-matched.
6. The client's platelet count and prothrombin time are checked to be sure they are normal.
7. If ordered, a laxative is administered the evening before the test.
8. If ordered, the client receives a cleansing enema the morning of the test.
9. The premedication is given as ordered.

Procedure

1. Before the client reports to the radiology department, an intravenous infusion is started for venous access and the injection of sedatives.
2. The abdominal wall (over the liver) is anesthetized with lidocaine (Xylocaine).
3. With the use of televised fluoroscopic monitoring, the needle is advanced through the skin and into the liver (Fig. 3-2) as the physician is aspirating.
4. When bile flows freely into the syringe, a catheter is advanced through the needle and well into the biliary system.

5. Dye containing an antibiotic is injected, and x-ray films are taken immediately.
6. If complete obstruction is found, the catheter may be temporarily left in place.
7. If hemorrhage or bile extravasation occurs, the client may have severe right upper quadrant abdominal pain.
8. The radiologist performs the test in the radiology department in approximately 1 hour.

Nursing implications

1. Following the procedure, the client is kept on bed rest and is given nothing by mouth in case surgery becomes necessary to control hemorrhage or significant bile extravasation.
2. If ordered, place a sandbag over the site of needle insertion.

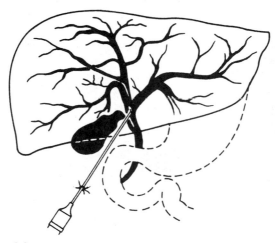

Figure 3-2
Percutaneous transhepatic cholangiogram.
(From Given, B.A., and Simmons, S.J.: Gastroenterology in clinical nursing, ed. 3, St. Louis, 1979, The C.V. Mosby Co.)

3. Observe the site for bile leakage or hemorrhage. A small amount of bleeding is usually present.
4. Assess the vital signs for a decrease in blood pressure or an increase in pulse, either of which would indicate hemorrhage.
5. A hemoglobin and hematocrit determination may be ordered 6 hours after PTHC.
6. If the catheter is left in the biliary tract, establish a sterile closed system of drainage.
7. Withhold pain medications to avoid blunting the abdominal signs associated with hemorrhage or bile extravasation.

Nurse alert

1. Peritonitis, caused by bile extravasation from the liver after the needle is removed, is a potential complication of PTHC.
2. Surgical repair of the bile leak occasionally is necessary.
3. Bleeding, caused by inadvertent puncture of a large hepatic blood vessel, is a potential complication.
4. As with ERCP, bacteremia and sepsis are potential complications, resulting from the pressure of the injection pushing dye into an obstructed bile duct containing infected bile.

T-TUBE CHOLANGIOGRAPHY (POSTOPERATIVE CHOLANGIOGRAPHY)

Normal Values

- No stones.

Deviations from Normal

- Presence of stones.

Indications

- To diagnose retained ductal stones postoperatively in a patient who has had a cholecystectomy and a common bile duct exploration.

Contraindications

- An uncooperative client.
- A client allergic to dyes.

Procedure

Client preparation

1. Assurance is given that no discomfort should occur when the dye is injected through the T-tube.
2. The client receives nothing by mouth after midnight the day of the test.

Procedure

1. In the radiology department, a sterile dye solution containing an antibiotic is attached by a catheter to the T-tube.
2. When the biliary ductal system is filled, x-ray films are taken of the right upper quadrant of the abdomen while the client is placed in the supine, prone, and oblique positions.
3. A radiologist performs the study in approximately 15 minutes.

Nursing implications

1. Observe the client for signs of sepsis.
2. Take vital signs frequently, as ordered, and assess the client for increased temperature, tachycardia, chills, hypertension, and disorientation.
3. If the T-tube is left in place, connect it to a sterile closed drainage system.
4. If the T-tube is removed, keep the T-tube tract site covered with a sterile dressing.
5. Assess the site for drainage and record the amount of drainage.

Nurse alert

1. Sepsis caused by increased ductal pressure with the dye infusion (as in PTHC and ERCP) is a potential complication.
2. Inadvertent removal of the T-tube during the study is a possible complication.

Nuclear Scanning Tests
CHOLESCINTIGRAPHY (HEPATOBILIARY SCINTIGRAPHY, HEPATOBILIARY IMAGING, BILIARY TRACT RADIONUCLIDE SCAN, BILIARY SCINTIGRAPHY, AND DISIDA SCANNING)

Normal Values

- Gallbladder, common bile duct, and duodenum visualization within 60 minutes after radionuclide injection.

Deviations from Normal

- Cystic duct obstruction and acute cholecystitis.

Indications

- To evaluate clients with jaundice, ampullary stenosis, duodenal diverticula, biliary-enteric anastomosis, or biliary leaks.
- To visualize the common bile duct when the serum bilirubin level is elevated.

Contraindications

- None.

Procedure
Client preparation

1. The client is assured that exposure to large amounts of radioactivity will not occur because only tracer doses of radioisotopes are used.
2. The client fasts for 4 hours prior to the test.

Procedure

1. The client is placed in the supine position.
2. After an intravenous injection of iminodiacetic acid derivative Tc 99m (e.g., DISIDA, PIPIDA, HIDA), the right upper quadrant of the abdomen is scanned.
3. If the gallbladder, common bile duct, or duodenum are not visualized within 60 minutes following the injection, de-

layed images up to 4 hours may be obtained. Films are recorded on Polaroid film.

4. The radiologist performs the study in the radiology department in 1 to 4 hours.

LIVER SCANNING

Normal Values

- Normal size, shape, and position of liver.

Deviations from Normal

- Abnormal size, shape, and position of the liver.

Indications

- To outline and detect structural liver changes.
- To differentiate intrahepatic cholestasis from extrahepatic obstruction.
- To detect filling defects.

Contraindications

- An uncooperative client.
- A pregnant client because of potential damage to the fetus from radiation.

Procedure

Client preparation

1. The client is assured that exposure to large amounts of radioactivity will not occur because only tracer doses of isotopes are used.

Procedure

1. Thirty minutes after a peripheral intravenous injection of the radioisotope, a gamma-ray detecting device is slowly passed over the client, who is placed in the supine, lateral, and prone positions to visualize all surfaces of the liver.
2. The radionucleotide uptake is recorded on either x-ray or Polaroid film.
3. A trained technician performs this procedure in the nuclear medicine department in approximately 1 hour.

Computerized Tomography Tests
COMPUTERIZED TOMOGRAPHY OF THE ABDOMEN (CT OF THE ABDOMEN)
Normal Values

- No evidence of tumor or pathologic activity.

Deviations from Normal

- Acute and chronic pancreatitis.
- Pancreatic cancer.
- Peripancreatic cysts.
- Ascites.
- Aneurysms.
- Cirrhosis of the liver.

Indications

- To diagnose pathologic conditions (e.g., inflammation, tumor, and cyst formation).

Contraindications

- An uncooperative client.

Procedure
Client preparation

1. The client is kept on nothing by mouth for the 4 hours preceding the study.

Procedure

1. Sedation is rarely required and is given only to the client who cannot remain still during the length of the procedure.
2. An encircling x-ray camera (body scanner) takes pictures at varying levels (usually 4 cm apart) of the abdomen from the pubic region to the xiphoid process.
3. Television equipment allows for immediate display, and a Polaroid-type camera records the image.
4. Occasionally, radiographic water-soluble dyes are given to the client by mouth. This contrast agent helps to delineate

the pancreatic margins by visually outlining the stomach and the duodenum.

5. A technician or a radiologist performs the examination in the radiology department in approximately 30 minutes.

Nursing implications

1. Because not all hospitals have CT equipment, the nurse may need to make arrangements to transport the client to another facility.

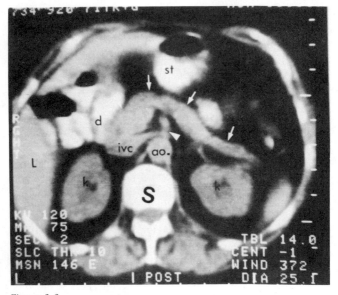

Figure 3-3

Computerized tomogram of the abdomen showing a cross-sectional view of the abdomen at the level of the pancreas. *St,* stomach; *d,* duodenum (both the stomach and the duodenum contain gastrografin); *L,* liver; *k,* kidneys; *ivc,* inferior vena cava; *ao,* aorta; *S,* spine; Arrows indicate pancreas. Arrow indicates superior mesenteric vessels.

Special Studies

Liver Biopsy

Normal Values

- Normal liver histology.

Deviations from Normal

- Abnormal liver histology resulting from disorders listed in "Indications" below.

Indications

- To diagnose liver disorders (e.g., cirrhosis, hepatitis, drug reactions, granuloma, and tumor) in clients.

Contraindications

- An uncooperative client who will not hold his or her breath during sustained exhalation.
- A client with impaired hemostasis.
- A client with profound anemia.
- A client with infection of the right pleural space.
- A client with septic cholangitis.
- A client with obstructive jaundice.

Procedure

Client preparation

1. The client is informed that lying motionless during this procedure is essential. The client is told that he or she will need to hold his or her breath during exhalation when instructed to do so.
2. The results of the client's hemostasis studies (prothrombin time, partial thromboplastin time, and platelet count) are checked to ensure that coagulation disorders do not exist.
3. The client is kept on nothing by mouth after midnight the day of the test in case emergency surgery is needed.
4. If ordered, sedatives are administered 30 to 60 minutes before the study.
5. The client's blood is typed and cross-matched.

Procedure

1. The client is placed in the supine or left lateral position.
2. The skin overlying the area of the liver from which the biopsy specimen is desired is aseptically cleansed and anesthetized.
3. A small incision (about 1 cm) is made in the skin.
4. The client is instructed to exhale and ''hold it.''
5. During a sustained exhalation, the physician rapidly introduces the biopsy needle into the liver, obtains the liver tissue, and then immediately withdraws the needle.
6. The tissue sample is placed in a specimen bottle containing formalin (or saline if a frozen section is requested) and sent to the pathology laboratory.
7. A small dressing is placed over the needle insertion site, and the client is placed on his or her right side to provide pressure on the biopsy site.
8. The physician performs the procedure at the client's bedside in approximately 20 minutes.

Nursing implications

1. Support the client during the procedure.
2. Assist the physician as needed.
3. After the procedure, keep the client on his or her right side for 1 to 2 hours.
4. Keep the client on bed rest for 12 to 24 hours.
5. Assess the client's vital signs frequently for evidence of hemorrhage and peritonitis.
6. Evaluate the client for pain. Be aware that some pain in the right upper quadrant of the abdomen and the top of the right shoulder is common.
7. Report severe pain to the physician immediately.

Nurse alert

1. Complications include:
   a. Hemorrhage caused by inadvertent puncture of a blood vessel within or surrounding the liver.
   b. Peritonitis caused by inadvertent laceration of a bile duct with leakage of bile into the abdominal cavity.

Evaluate the patient for pain and immediately report severe pain to the physician.

c. Pneumothorax caused by improper placement of the biopsy needle up into the adjacent chest cavity.

Secretin-Pancreozymin Test

Normal Values

- Volume: 2 to 4 mg/kg of body weight.
- HCO₃ (bicarbonate): 90 to 130 mEq/L.
- Amylase: 6.6 to 35.2 units/kg of body weight.

Indications

- To confirm the diagnosis of cystic fibrosis and other exocrine pancreatic diseases.

Contraindications

- An uncooperative client.

Procedure

Client preparation

1. The adult patient is kept on nothing by mouth for 12 hours before the study to avoid the presence of food in the duodenum. Food may block the aspirating lumen.

Procedure

1. In the radiology department and with the use of fluoroscopy, a "double lumenal" nasogastric tube is passed through the nose. The distal lumen is to be placed within the duodenum; the proximal lumen lies within the stomach.
2. Both lumens are aspirated separately.
3. The duodenum is aspirated until the contents are clear and the pH is basic.
4. A control specimen is collected for 20 minutes.
5. The client is then tested intradermally for sensitivity to secretin and pancreozymin. If no sensitivity is present, these hormones are administered intravenously. Secretin stimu-

lates pancreatic water and bicarbonate secretions. Pancreozymin stimulates pancreatic enzyme secretion.
6. Four duodenal aspirates are collected at 20-minute intervals and placed in specimen containers.
7. A technician or radiologist performs the test in the laboratory or on the ward in approximately 2 hours.

Nursing implications

1. After the test is completed, clamp and withdraw the nasogastric tube used to aspirate the stomach and duodenum.
2. Give mouth and nose care.

Sweat Electrolytes Test (Iontophoretic Sweat Test)

Normal Values

- Sodium: values in children, normal: <70 mEq/L; equivocal: 70 to 90 mEq/L; abnormal: > 90 mEq/L.
- Chloride: values in children, normal: <50 mEq/L; equivocal: 50 to 60 mEq/L; abnormal: >60 mEq/L.

Deviations from Normal

- Cystic fibrosis in the patient with clinical features sugges-
tive of this disease.

Contraindications

- None.

Procedure
Client preparation

1. Role playing with a doll may help a child understand the
procedure and relieve anxiety.
2. The parents and the child are reassured that the child will
not be shocked by the electrical current.

Procedure

1. The iontophoresis unit contains two electrodes.
2. The electrodes are strapped onto the test area (the thigh in

infants, the forearm in older children), and the iontophoresis unit is turned on for 10 to 12 minutes.
3. The electrodes are then removed, and paper disks are
placed over the test site by the use of dry, clean forceps.
4. After an hour, the paraffin is removed and the paper disks
are transferred immediately by forceps to a weighing jar
and sent for sodium and chloride analysis.
5. A technician performs the test in a laboratory in 1 to 1½
hours.

Nurse alert

1. Take necessary precautions to avoid accidental shock or
electrocution.

Ultrasound Tests
ULTRASOUND EXAMINATION OF THE LIVER AND BILIARY SYSTEM
Normal Values

- Normal gallbladder and biliary duct.

Deviations from Normal

- Tumors, gallstones, cysts.

Indications

- To detect cystic structures of the liver (e.g., benign cysts),
gallstones, and solid intrahepatic tumor (primary and metastatic).

Contraindications

- None.

Procedure
Client preparation

1. If the gallbladder is being studied with ultrasound, the
client is kept on nothing by mouth after midnight the day
of the study to prevent contraction of the gallbladder.
2. If the client has had prior barium contrast studies, an order
for cathartics is requested.

Procedure

1. The ultrasonographer applies a greasy paste to the skin overlying the organ to enhance sound transmission and reception.
2. The transducer is moved along the skin in a vertical and then horizontal line.
3. The combination of horizontal (coronal section) and vertical (sagittal section) views is printed on Polaroid film.
4. The ultrasonographer performs the test in the ultrasound room in approximately 30 minutes.

Nursing implications

1. When the client returns to the floor after the study, cleanse the lubricant from the abdomen.

ULTRASOUND EXAMINATION OF THE PANCREAS (PANCREAS ECHOGRAM)

Normal Values

- Normal size and position of the pancreas.

Deviations from Normal

- Abnormal size and position of pancreas.

Indications

- To diagnose carcinoma, pseudocysts, pancreatitis, and pancreatic abscess.
- To monitor the resolution of pancreatic inflammation.

Contraindications

- None.

Procedure
Client preparation

1. If the client's abdomen appears distended with gas or if the client has recently had a barium study, this study should be cancelled.

Procedure

1. With the client lying in the supine position on an examining table, the ultrasonographer applies mineral oil or glycerine to the skin over the organ to be studied.
2. The transducer is moved along the skin in first a horizontal (cross-sectional) and then a vertical (sagittal) line.
3. The ultrasonographer performs the examination in the radiology department in approximately 1 hour.

Nursing implications

1. When the client returns to the floor, cleanse the gel from the abdomen.

Bibliography

Alfidi, R.J., and others: Computed tomography of the human body, St. Louis, 1977, The C.V. Mosby Co.

Alpert, E., and Jackson, D.: Besides the liver, what does the virus of hepatitis attack? Heart Lung **11**(2):177-180, March/April 1982.

Alyn, I.B.: Disorders of the liver, gallbladder, and pancreas. In Beyers, M., and Dudas, S., editors: The clinical practice of medical-surgical nursing, Boston, 1984, Little, Brown & Co.

Anthony, C.P., and Thibodeau, G.A.: Textbook of anatomy and physiology, ed. 11, St. Louis 1983, The C.V. Mosby Co.

Beeler, M.F., Kao, Y.S., and Scheer, W.D.: Malabsorption, diarrhea, and examination of feces. In Henry, J.B., editor: Todd-Sanford-Davidsohn clinical diagnosis and management of laboratory methods, ed. 16, vol. 1, Philadelphia, 1979, W.B. Saunders Co.

Berner, J.J.: Effects of diseases on laboratory tests, Philadelphia, 1983, J.B. Lippincott Co.

Cassmeyer, V.L., and Greig, J.L.: Problems of the liver and related structures. In Phipps, W.J., Long, B.C., and Woods, N.F., editors: Medical-surgical nursing: concepts and clinical practice, ed. 2, St. Louis, 1983, The C.V. Mosby Co.

Chernesky, M.A., and others: Laboratory diagnosis of hepatitis viruses, Cumitech (American Society of Microbiology) **18**:1-11, Jan. 1984.

Chervu, L.R., Nunn, A.D., and Loberg, M.D.: Radiopharmaceuticals for hepatobiliary imaging, Sem. Nucl. Med. **12**(1):5-17, Jan. 1982.

Czaja, A.J., and Davis, G.L.: Hepatitis non-A, non-B, Mayo Clin. Proc. 57:639, 1982.

Dienstag, J.L.: Serologic testing for hepatitis, Lab. Mgmt. 20:21, 1982.

Dougherty, W.M.: Serum bilirubin, Nurs. '82 12(11):138-139, Nov. 1982.

Doust, B.D., and Maklad, N.F.: Ultrasound B-mode examination of the gallbladder, Radiology 110:643, March 1974.

Elrod, R.: Nursing role in management: problems of the liver, biliary tract, and pancreas. In Lewis, S.M., and Collier, I.C., editors: Medical-surgical nursing: assessment and management of clinical problems, New York, 1983, McGraw-Hill Book Co.

Freitas, J.E.: Cholescintigraphy in acute and chronic cholecystitis, Sem. Nucl. Med. 12(1):18-26, Jan. 1982.

Frey, C.F., and others: Endoscopic retrograde cholangiography, Am. J. Surg. 144(1):109-113, July 1982.

Gannon, R.B., and Pickett, K.: Jaundice, Am. J. Nurs. 83:404-408, March 1983.

Gitnick, G.: Assessment of liver function, Surg. Clin. North Am. 61(1):197-207, Feb. 1982.

Given, B.A., and Simmons, S.J.: Gastroenterology in clinical nursing, ed. 4, St. Louis, 1984, The C.V. Mosby Co.

Gliedman, M.L., and Wilk, P.J.: A surgeon's view of hepatobiliary scintigraphy, Sem. Nucl. Med. 12(1):2-4, Jan. 1982.

Gracie, W.A., and Ransohoff, D.F.: The natural history of silent gallstones, N. Engl. J. Med. 307(13):798-800, Sept. 1982.

King, J.W.: A clinical approach to hepatitis B, Arch. Intern. Med. 142:925-928, May 1982.

Krebs, C.A., and Carson, J.C.: Gallbladder examinations: a comparison between sonography and radiography, Radiol. Tech. 54(3):181-188, Jan./Feb. 1983.

Micozzi, M.S., and London, W.T.: The clinical laboratory diagnosis of viral hepatitis, Lab. Mgmt. 21:18, 1983.

Pagana, T.J., and Stahlgren, L.H.: Indications and accuracy of operative cholangiography, Arch. Surg. 115:1214, 1980.

Petersdorf, R.G., editor: Harrison's principles of internal medicine, ed. 10, New York, 1983, McGraw-Hill Book Co.

Serafini, A.N.: Biliary scintigraphy: comparison with other modern techniques for evaluation of biliary tract disease, Postgrad. Med. 72(4):157-162, Oct. 1982.

Stiklorius, C.: Two diagnostic procedures that demand your all-out care, RN **42**(8):64-65, Aug. 1982.

Thomas, M.J., Pellegrini, C.A., and Way, L.W.: Usefulness of diagnostic tests for biliary obstruction, Am. J. Surg. **144**(1):102-106, July 1982.

West, K.H.: The dilemma—hepatitis B, what is it all about? J. Operating Room Res. Inst. **2**(12):8-12, Dec. 1982.

Zimmon, D.S.: Endoscopic management of biliary colic, Hosp. Pract. **13**:103, Dec. 1978.

Pulmonary System

4

Clinical Laboratory Tests

Blood Tests

ACID-FAST BACILLI

See "Sputum Studies," p. 128.

ANGIOGRAPHY

See "Pulmonary Angiography," p. 114.

ARTERIAL BLOOD GAS STUDIES

Normal Values

- pH, P_{CO_2}, HCO_3^-: see Table 4-1.
- P_{O_2}: 80 to 100 torr.
- Oxygen saturation: 95% to 100%.

Deviations from Normal

- Measurements for pH, P_{CO_2}, and HCO_3^- may indicate acidosis or alkalosis, as Table 4-1 shows.
- A lowered P_{O_2} level may indicate pneumonia, shock lung, congenital heart disease, Pickwickian syndrome, or pulmonary embolus.
- See Table 4-1.

Indications

- To assess and monitor the client's respiratory and metabolic status.

Contraindications

- None.

Procedure

Client preparation

1. The lab is notified before the sample is drawn.
2. A site of easily palpable pulse (e.g., radial, brachial, or femoral artery) is chosen.

Procedure

1. The artery is punctured and 3 to 5 ml of blood are withdrawn into a heparinized syringe.
2. The needle is removed and pressure firmly applied to the site for 5 minutes.
3. Any bubbles are expelled from the syringe immediately.
4. The syringe is capped and gently rotated to mix blood with heparin.
5. The sample is placed in an iced container and sent immediately to the lab for study.

Nursing implications

1. Maintain pressure at puncture site as needed to prevent hematoma formation.
2. Be sure no active subcutaneous bleeding is occurring before leaving the client.
3. Instruct the client not to flex the wrist or elbow joint for 10 to 15 minutes.

Nurse alert

1. Arterial puncture is more painful than venous puncture.
2. Be familiar with the arterial site anatomy to prevent nerve damage.
3. If using the radial artery, perform the Allen test first to confirm the presence of ulnar artery (obliterate radial and ulnar pulses, release pressure over ulnar artery, confirm ulnar flow by observing flushing).
4. Be sure all equipment is prepared before beginning the procedure, including an iced container for transport to the lab.

Table 4-1 Normal values for arterial blood gases and abnormal values in uncompensated acid-base disturbances

Acid-Base Disturbance	pH	P_{CO_2} (torr)	HCO_3^- mEq/L	Common Cause
None (normal values)	7.35-7.45	35-45	22-26	
Respiratory acidosis	Decreased	Increased	Normal	Respiratory depression (drugs, central nervous system trauma) Pulmonary disease (pneumonia, COPD, respirator underventilation)
Respiratory alkalosis	Increased	Decreased	Normal	Hyperventilation (emotions, pain, respirator overventilation)
Metabolic acidosis	Decreased	Normal	Decreased	Diabetes, shock, renal failure, intestinal fistula
Metabolic alkalosis	Increased	Normal	Increased	Sodium bicarbonate overdose, prolonged vomiting, or nasogastric drainage

ALPHA$_1$-ANTITRYPSIN DETERMINATION

Normal Values

- \>250 mg/dl.

Deviations from Normal

- Deficient or absent serum levels indicate the early onset of emphysema.

Indications

- To diagnose emphysema.

Contraindications

- None.

Procedure

1. Following standard venipuncture procedure, approximately 1 tube of blood is collected as specified by the lab.
2. Pressure or a pressure dressing is applied to puncture site.

Nursing implications

1. Observe the venipuncture site for bleeding or hematoma formation.
2. If the test results show that the client is at risk for developing emphysema, appropriate client teaching is begun.

Radiologic Laboratory Tests

X-Ray Tests

BRONCHOGRAPHY (BRONCHOGRAM; LARYNOGRAPHY)

Normal Values

- Normal tracheobronchial tree.

Deviations from Normal

- Bronchial malformations, obstructions, or bronchiectasis.

Indications

- To diagnose bronchiectasis.
- To identify obstruction in the distal bronchi.
- To detect congenital or acquired forms of tracheobronchial malformation.
- To evaluate clients for possible surgery (bronchopulmonary segment resection).

Contraindications

- A pregnant client.
- An uncooperative client.
- A client allergic to iodine dye.
- A client with acute infections.
- A client with respiratory insufficiency.

Procedure

Client preparation

1. The client is instructed not to swallow the local anesthetic the radiologist will spray into the client's throat. An emesis basin is provided for expectoration of the lidocaine.
2. The client is told to make a great effort to suppress coughing during the procedure. Rapid, shallow breathing will help to suppress the cough reflex.
3. The client is kept on nothing by mouth after midnight on the day of the study.
4. Ensure that the client performs thorough mouth care the night before and the morning of the test.
5. Perform postural drainage, if ordered, prior to this procedure.
6. The client's dentures, glasses, or contact lenses are removed and safely stored before the preprocedure medication is administered.
7. The preprocedure medications are administered as ordered.

Procedure

1. For this procedure the client is placed in a sitting position.
2. After the client's nose or mouth is sprayed with a local anesthetic to suppress the gag reflex, a catheter or bronchoscope is passed into the trachea.

3. The pharynx, larynx, and major bronchi are anesthetized prior to introduction of the radiopaque dye.
4. The client's position and the placing of the catheter allow the radiologist to selectively fill regions of interest with radiopaque material. These positions are usually the reverse of those used in postural drainage.
5. Multiple x-ray views are then obtained.
6. A radiologist performs the test in the radiology department in approximately 45 minutes.

Nursing implications

1. After the procedure, perform postural drainage if ordered.
2. After the procedure, do not allow the client to eat or drink anything until the gag reflex returns (usually about 2 hours).
3. Monitor the vital signs frequently, as ordered.
4. Observe postanesthesia precautions for the client until the effect of the sedative medications no longer exist.
5. After the procedure, coughing is usually encouraged to help clear the tracheobronchial tree.
6. A slight temperature elevation is common for 2 to 3 days after the test.
7. After the procedure, a sore throat is often common.
8. Follow-up x-ray films may be taken at a later date to ascertain if any dye remains in the tracheobronchial tree.
9. The client may usually resume normal activities 24 hours after completion of this study.

Nurse alert

1. Following the study, observe the client closely for evidence of impaired respiration or laryngospasm. The vocal cords may go into spasms after intubation. Emergency resuscitation equipment should be readily available.
2. Anaphylaxis induced by the iodine dye is a potential complication.

CHEST X-RAY STUDY (CHEST ROENTGENOGRAM)
Normal Values

- Normal lungs and surrounding structures.

Deviations from Normal

- Tumors of the lung, heart, chest wall, and bony thorax.
- Pneumonia, pleuritis, pericarditis.
- Pleural effusion.
- Pericardial effusion.
- Pulmonary edema.
- COPD.
- Pneumothorax.
- Fractures of the bones of the thorax.
- Diaphragmatic hernia.

Indications

- To assist in the diagnosis of pulmonary and cardiac disease.

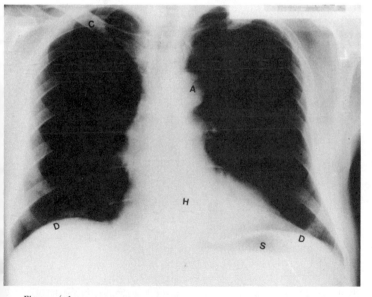

Figure 4-1
Normal chest x-ray film. *H,* heart; *D,* diaphragm; *A,* aortic arch; *S,* stomach bubble; *C,* clavicle.

Contraindications

■ A pregnant client. If study is needed, a lead shield is placed over the uterus.

Procedure
Client preparation

1. The following aspects of the procedure are explained to the client: he or she will need to remove clothing above the waist and will receive a gown to wear; he or she will need to remove any metal objects because they block the body structures they cover and will appear on the x-ray film.

Procedure

1. Men should cover their testes and women their ovaries with a lead shield to prevent radiation-induced abnormalities that may result in congenital abnormalities in future children.
2. Most chest x-ray films are taken at a distance of 6 feet, with the client standing. The sitting or supine position may also be used.
3. After the client is correctly positioned, he or she is told to take a deep breath and hold it until the film is taken.
4. A technician takes the x-ray films, preferably in the radiology department, in several minutes.

PULMONARY ANGIOGRAPHY
Normal Values

■ Normal pulmonary vasculature.

Deviations from Normal

■ Pulmonary embolism.

Indications

■ To detect and locate pulmonary embolism.
■ To detect congenital and acquired lesions of the pulmonary vessels.

Contraindications

- An uncooperative client.
- An unstable client who cannot safely tolerate the absence of monitoring and nursing care the test requires.
- A client allergic to dyes.

Procedure

Client preparation

1. Tell the client where the catheter will be inserted (usually the femoral vein). The client is informed that he or she will feel a warm flush when the dye is injected.
2. The client is assessed for allergies to the iodine dye.
3. The client is kept on nothing by mouth after midnight on the day of the study.
4. The preprocedure medications are administered as ordered.

Procedure

1. The client is placed on an x-ray table and the groin is prepared and draped in a sterile manner.
2. A catheter is placed into the femoral vein and passed into the inferior vena cava.
3. With fluoroscopic visualization, the catheter is advanced to the right atrium and the right ventricle and then into the main pulmonary artery, where dye is injected via the catheter.
4. X-ray films of the chest are immediately taken in timed sequence, allowing all vessels visualized by the injection to be photographed.
5. Usually an angiographer performs this study in the angiography room of the radiology department in about 1 hour.

Nursing implications

1. After the procedure, observe the catheter insertion site for inflammation, hemorrhage, hematoma, or absence of peripheral pulse.
2. Assess the involved extremity for numbness, tingling, pain, or loss of function.
3. Assess the vital signs for evidence of bleeding.

Nurse alert

1. The complications associated with this test are:
   a. *Cardiac arrhythmia*. Premature ventricular contractions (PVCs) during right-sided heart catheterization may lead to ventricular tachycardia and ventricular fibrillation.
   b. *Anaphylaxis*. The dye used in this test can produce anaphylaxis in patients with dye allergies.
   c. *Risk of death*. Without the close monitoring provided in the intensive care unit, unstable patients can develop severe problems that can go unrecognized and lead to death.

TOMOGRAPHY OF THE LUNG (LAMINOGRAPHY; PLANIGRAPHY)

Normal Values

- Normal lungs and surrounding structures.

Deviations from Normal

- Abnormal lungs and surrounding structures indicating, for example, tumor.

Indications

- To augment a routine chest x-ray study.

Contraindications

- A pregnant client.

Procedure

1. With the client remaining completely still, an x-ray tube is rapidly moved back and forth while the film is rapidly moved in the opposite directions.
2. Prone, supine, and lateral positions may be required.
3. Usually a radiologist performs the study in approximately 15 minutes in the radiology department.

Nursing implications

1. The client is unaware of any movement of the x-ray equipment.

Nuclear Scanning Tests
LUNG SCANNING (PULMONARY SCINTIPHOTOGRAPHY)
Normal Values

■ Diffuse and homogeneous uptake of nuclear material by the lungs.

Deviations from Normal

■ Pulmonary embolism, pneumonia, tuberculosis, and emphysema.

Indications

■ To rule out pulmonary embolism.

Contraindications

■ A client with pulmonary parenchymal problems (e.g., pneumonia, emphysema, pleural effusion, and tumors) who will give a false-positive result.
■ A pregnant client because of possible radiation damage to the fetus.

Procedure
Client preparation

1. If ^{131}I will be used, a physician's order is obtained for 10 drops of Lugol's solution, which is administered several hours before the test to block the thyroid gland uptake of the iodine.

Procedure

1. A peripheral intravenous injection of radionucleotide-tagged albumin aggregate is given.

2. A gamma-ray detecting device is passed over the client, which records nucleotide uptake on either x-ray or Polaroid film. This is performed with the client in the supine, prone, and lateral positions.
3. A technician or radiologist performs the study in the nuclear medicine department in approximately 30 minutes.

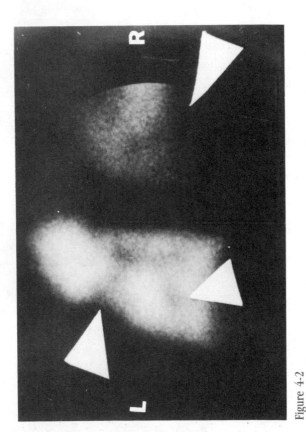

Figure 4-2
Lung scan (posterior view). Arrows indicate areas of decreased blood perfusion. There are more areas of decreased perfusion on the right side, indicative of embolic occlusion of the pulmonary vessels.

Computerized Tomography Tests
COMPUTERIZED TOMOGRAPHY OF THE CHEST
(CT OF THE CHEST OR LUNG)

Normal Values

- No evidence of tumor or pathology.

Deviations from Normal

- Tumors, nodules, coin lesions, cysts, pleural effusion, and enlarged lymph nodes.

Contraindications

- A pregnant client.
- A client allergic to iodine dye.

Procedure
Client preparation

1. Assurance is given that CT scanning of the lungs is a safe and painless x-ray method that incurs no more radiation than a series of regular x-ray films. The client is informed that he or she will be required to lie motionless during the study. If possible, show the client a picture of the donut-like x-ray scanner. Inform the client that he or she will hear clicking noises from the scanner.
2. The client is kept on nothing by mouth for 4 hours prior to the test. One does not usually know before the test whether enhanced visualization by the dye injection will be indicated.
3. The client is assessed for allergies to iodinated dye.

Procedure

1. The client is asked to remain motionless in the supine position.
2. An encircling x-ray camera (body scanner) takes pictures at varying intervals (usually 4 cm apart).
3. Television equipment allows for immediate display, and Polaroid-type cameras record the image.

4. A technician performs the study in the radiology department in approximately 30 to 45 minutes.
5. Occasionally, intravenous dye is administered to the client and the x-ray films are repeated.

Nursing implications

1. Encourage the client who receives the dye injection to increase fluid intake.

Nurse alert

1. Observe the client for signs of anaphylaxis (such as respiratory distress, palpitations, blood pressure drop, itching, urticaria [hives], or diaphoresis). Always keep emergency drugs available to counteract any severe allergic reaction.

Special Studies

Biopsy
LUNG BIOPSY
Normal Values

- No evidence of pathology.

Deviations from Normal

- Pulmonary disease or lesion, carcinomas, granulomas, and sarcoidosis.

Indications

- To identify the cause of a parenchymal pulmonary disease or lesion.
- To diagnose carcinomas, granulomas, and sarcoidosis.

Contraindications

- A client with bullae or lung cysts.
- A client with suspected vascular anomalies.
- A client with bleeding abnormalities.
- A client with pulmonary hypertension.
- A client with severe respiratory insufficiency.

Procedure
Client preparation

1. Usually the client is kept on nothing by mouth after midnight on the day of the test.
2. The preprocedure medications are administered as ordered 30 to 60 minutes prior to the test.

Procedure

1. A surgeon performs this procedure using one of the approaches explained below.
2. A *transbronchial lung biopsy* is performed via a flexible fiberoptic bronchoscopy using cutting forceps.
3. A *transbronchial needle aspiration biopsy* provides a specimen via a fiberoptic bronchoscope using a needle.
4. A *transcatheter bronchial brushing* is also performed via a fiberoptic bronchoscope.
5. *Percutaneous needle biopsy* provides the specimen after x-ray film determination of the desired site.
6. An *open-lung biopsy* requires that the client be taken to the operating room and a general anesthesia used.

Nursing implications

1. During the lung biopsy, instruct the client to remain still.
2. After the specimens are obtained, place them in the appropriate jars for histologic and microbiologic examinations.
3. After the lung biopsy procedure, take vital signs frequently.
4. Evaluate vital signs for signs of bleeding.
5. The client's breath sounds should be evaluated, and any decrease noted on the biopsy side reported immediately.
6. After the lung biopsy, a chest x-ray film is usually ordered to check for complications such as pneumothorax. Observe the client for signs of pneumothorax.

Nurse alert

1. During the procedure, observe the client carefully for signs of respiratory distress. The most common complications of lung biopsy include pneumothorax, pulmonary hemorrhage, and empyema.

PLEURAL BIOPSY

Normal Values

- No evidence of pathology.

Deviations from Normal

- Evidence of pathology such as neoplasms or tuberculosis.

Indications

- To distinguish between neoplasm and inflammation (such as tuberculosis) after a thoracentesis (see p. 131) shows the presence of exudative fluid.

Contraindications

- A client with prolonged bleeding or clotting times.

Procedure

1. The nonfasting, unsedated client is placed in the sitting position with shoulders and arms elevated and supported on a padded overbed table.
2. After thoracentesis has determined the presence of fluid, the skin overlying the biopsy site is anesthetized and pierced, usually with a no. 11 scalpel blade.
3. The no. 13-gauge needle usually is inserted within the cannula until fluid is removed.
4. The inner needle is then removed, and a blunt-tipped hooked biopsy trocar, attached to a three-way stopcock, is substituted in the cannula.
5. The client is instructed to expire all air and then to perform Valsalva's maneuver.
6. The cannula and the biopsy trocar are then withdrawn while the hook catches the parietal wall and takes a biopsy with its cutting edge.
7. Usually three biopsy specimens are taken from different sites at the same session. The specimens are placed in a fixative solution (e.g., formaldehyde) and sent immediately to the lab.
8. After the biopsies are taken, additional parietal fluid can be removed.

9. An adhesive bandage is applied to the site.
10. A chest x-ray film is usually performed after the study to detect the potential complication of pneumothorax.
11. A physician performs this procedure at the bedside or in the physician's office in approximately 30 minutes.

Nursing implications

1. After the test, observe the patient for signs of respiratory distress.
2. Make sure the chest x-ray film is repeated as ordered.
3. After the test, check the vital signs frequently.

Nurse alert

1. The major risk of this procedure is bleeding and injury to the lung, which can produce a pneumothorax.
2. Instruct the client to remain still and to refrain from talking during the procedure.

Bronchoscopy
Normal Values

- Normal larynx, trachea, bronchi, and aveoli.

Deviations from Normal

- Visualization of foreign bodies, retained secretions, bleeding, or abnormal findings on specimen analysis.

Indications

- To visualize tumors, inflammation, or strictures.
- To remove or biopsy specimens.
- To aspirate "deep" sputum.
- To aspirate retained secretions.
- To control bleeding within the bronchus.
- To remove small aspirated foreign bodies.
- To place radiation beads for therapy for lung tumors.

Contraindications

- A client on high-flow oxygen who cannot tolerate interruption.

Procedure

Client preparation

1. The client is kept on nothing by mouth after midnight the day of the test.
2. Preprocedure medications are administered as ordered.
3. The client's dentures, glasses, or contact lenses are removed.
4. The client is instructed not to swallow the local anesthetic that will be sprayed in the throat.

Procedure

1. When the *flexible fiberoptic scope* is used, the client's nasopharynx and oropharynx are anesthetized topically with lidocaine (Xylocaine) spray before the insertion of the bronchoscope.
   a. The client is placed in the sitting or supine position, and the tube is inserted through the nose and into the bronchi and the first- and second-generation bronchioles for systematic examination of the bronchial tree.
   b. Biopsy specimens and washings are taken if a pathologic condition is seen or strongly suspected.
2. For rigid bronchoscopy, the client is placed in the supine position with the neck hyperextended.
   a. The tube is inserted through the mouth and larynx and then into the trachea.
3. A surgeon or pulmonary specialist usually performs the procedure, often at the bedside, with the flexible fiberoptic scope or in the operating room under general anesthesia with the rigid bronchoscope.

Nursing implications

1. If biopsy specimens are removed, observe the client's sputum for signs of hemorrhage. A small amount of blood streaking is normal.
2. Monitor vital signs frequently throughout the procedure, and observe the client closely for evidence of impaired respiration of laryngospasm.

3. Continue postanesthesia precautions until the sedative medication effects have worn off.
4. If a tumor is suspected, collect sputum samples for cytology after the procedure (see "Sputum Studies," p. 129).

Nurse alert

1. Potential complications include hypoxemia, laryngospasm, bronchospasm, pneumothorax, and hemorrhage if a biopsy specimen is removed.
2. Because of the potential complication of pulmonary cardiac arrest, a full "code cart" must be immediately available.

Mediastinoscopy

Normal Values

- No abnormal mediastinal lymph node tissues.

Deviations from Normal

- Carcinoma, granulomatous infections, and sarcoidosis.

Indications

- To establish the diagnosis of several intrathoracic diseases (see "Deviations from Normal" above).
- To "stage" clients with lung cancer.
- To assess the operability of a lung cancer.

Contraindications

- A client in whom the risk involved in receiving anesthesia is high.

Procedure
Client preparation

1. The client is kept on nothing by mouth after midnight the day of the test.
2. The nurse ensures that the client's blood has been typed and cross-matched, that several units of blood are available, and that the client is ready for thoracotomy if necessary.

3. The same preoperative care is provided as for any other surgical procedure.

Procedure

1. With the client under general anesthesia, an incision is made in the suprasternal notch, and the mediastinoscope is passed through this neck incision into the superior mediastinum.
2. After the lymph nodes are examined and biopsy specimens removed, the scope is withdrawn and the incision sutured closed.
3. A surgeon performs this procedure in approximately 1 hour in the operating room.

Nursing implications

1. Perform postoperative care as for any surgical procedure.

Nurse alert

1. The possibility of inadvertent puncture of the esophagus, trachea, or central vessels exists. If a puncture occurs, immediate thoracotomy is necessary (see "Client Preparation," no. 2).

Pulmonary Function Studies
Normal Values

- Vary with the age, sex, height, and weight.
- Predicted values can be obtained from tables correlated for these factors.

Deviations from Normal

- Values less than 50% of the predicted norm indicate poor pulmonary function.
- Forced vital capacity (FVC) is decreased below the expected norm in obstructive and restrictive pulmonary disease.
- Forced expiratory volume in 1 second (FEV_1) is decreased (80% of the expected norm) in restrictive lung disease.

FEV_1 is decreased below 80% of the expected norm in obstructive lung disease.

- Maximal midexpiratory flow (MMEF) is reduced below the expected norm in obstructive disease, but normal in restrictive disease.
- Maximal voluntary ventilation (MVV) is decreased below the expected value in both restrictive and obstructive pulmonary diseases.
- A comprehensive pulmonary function study may also include evaluation of the following lung volumes and lung capacities: tidal volume, inspiratory reserve volume, expiratory reserve volume, residual volume, inspiratory capacity, functional residual volume, vital capacity, total lung capacity, minute volume, dead space, diffusing capacity (the diffusing capacity of carbon monoxide (D_1CO) may be altered in interstitial fibrosis, emphysema, and pneumonectomy), and inhalation tests (e.g., metacholine or histamine challenge test).

Indications

- To contribute to preoperative evaluation.
- To evaluate the response of clients with COPD to bronchodilator therapy.
- To differentiate between restrictive forms of chronic pulmonary disease (pulmonary fibrosis) and obstructive forms (emphysema, bronchitis, asthma).
- To determine the severity of the disease and to follow its process and the effect of therapy by assessing diffusing capacity.

Contraindications

- Clients in pain because they will be unable to cooperate by deep inspiration and expiration.
- An uncooperative client.

Procedure
Client preparation

1. The client's cooperation is needed to obtain accurate results. Assure the client that air supply will not become inadequate during this procedure.

2. The client is instructed not to use any bronchodilators nor to smoke for 6 hours before this study.
3. The client's height and weight are measured and recorded before this study to determine the predicted values.
4. Intermittent positive pressure breathing (IPPB) is not given 2 to 4 hours prior to this test. The time of the last IPPB treatment is indicated on the request form.

Procedure

1. The client breathes into a sterile cylinder that is connected to a computerized machine that measures and records the desired volumes.
2. The diffusing capacity of carbon monoxide (D_1CO) is usually measured by having the client inhale a carbon dioxide mixture. The D_1CO is then calculated by analysis of the amount of carbon monoxide exhaled compared with the amount inhaled.
3. An inhalation therapist or a technician usually performs these studies in the pulmonary function laboratory in about 10 minutes.

Nursing implications

1. Occasionally clients with severe respiratory problems are exhausted after the testing and need planned periods of rest.

Sputum Studies
Normal Values

- Culture and sensitivity (C & S): normal throat flora.
- Acid-fast bacilli (AFB): no bacilli seen.
- Cytology: normal epithelial cells.

Deviations from Normal

- Pneumonia.
- Active tuberculosis.
- Cancer.

Indications

- To aid in diagnosing pneumonia.
- To aid in the diagnosis of active tuberculosis.
- To aid in the diagnosis of malignancy.

Contraindications

- None.

Procedure
Client preparation

1. The client is reminded that the sputum must be coughed up from the lungs and that saliva is not sputum.
2. The client is given a sterile sputum container the night before the sputum is to be collected so that the morning specimen can be obtained upon the client's arising.
3. The client is instructed to rinse out the mouth with water before the sputum collection.
4. The client should not use toothpaste or mouthwash before the collection.
5. If an aerosol treatment is necessary to stimulate coughing and sputum expectoration, the procedure is explained to the client.

Procedure

1. Only sputum that has come from deep within the lungs should be collected.
2. At least 1 tsp of sputum must be collected in a sterile, widemouth sputum container.
3. For cytology or AFB determinations, sputum is usually collected on three separate occasions.

Nursing implications

1. Provide the client with an ample supply of tissues with which to wipe the mouth after expectorating the sputum.
2. For aesthetic reasons, wrap the sputum container in paper towels so that the contents cannot be seen.

Thoracentesis and Pleural Fluid Analysis (Pleural Tap)

Normal Values

- Normal pleural fluid.

Deviations from Normal

- Gross appearance: a foul odor and thick, pus-like fluid characterize empyema. An opalescent, pearly fluid characterizes chylothorax (chyle in the pleural cavity).
- Cell counts (white blood cell [WBC] and differential): a WBC over $1000/m^3$ suggests an exudate. The predominance of polymorphonuclear leukocytes (PMNs) usually indicates an acute inflammatory condition (e.g., pneumonia, pulmonary infarction, or early tuberculosis effusion). When more than one half of the white cells are small lymphocytes, tuberculosis or tumor usually causes the effusion.
- Specific gravity: *transudate* fluid (specific gravity <1.015) suggests congestive heart failure, cirrhosis, nephronic syndrome, myedema, peritoneal dialysis, or acute glomerulonephritis. *Exudate* fluid (specific gravity >1.016) commonly indicates infectious disease or neoplastic conditions. Exudates also occur with collagen vascular disease, pulmonary infarction, gastrointestinal diseases, trauma, and drug hypersensitivities.
- Protein content: levels greater than 3 g/dl characterize exudates, while transudates usually have a protein content of less than 3 g/dl.
- Lactic dehydrogenase (LDH): a pleural fluid to serum LDH ratio of >0.6 is typical of an exudate. Comparing the pleural fluid determination of protein and the LDH is a better method of identifying a transudate or an exudate than either is separately.
- Glucose: values <60 mg/dl are occasionally seen in tuberculosis or in malignancy. Very low values (<20 mg/dl) are seen in rheumatoid effusions, and extremely low values (<10 mg/dl) are seen in empyema.
- Amylase: the amylase concentration is slightly elevated in

a malignant effusion. Very high amylase levels occur with pancreatitis or rupture of the esophagus with leakage of salivary amylase.

- Gram stain and bacteriologic culture: the presence of bacteria indicates bacterial pneumonia or empyema.
- Cultures for Mycobacterium tuberculosis and fungus: the presence of mycobacterium tuberculosis indicates tuberculosis. Fungus may be a cause of pulmonary effusion in clients with compromised immunologic defense.
- Cytology: tumor cells are detected in about 50% to 60% of clients with malignant effusions.
- Carcinoembryonic antigen (CEA): pleural fluid CEA levels are elevated in various malignant and some benign conditions.
- Special tests: the *ph of pleural fluids* is commonly <7.20 with empyema. The pH may be between 7.2 and 7.4 in tuberculosis or malignancy. An abnormal *total lipid* and *cholesterol count* may confirm chylothorax.

Indications

- To relieve pain, dyspnea, and other symptoms of pleural pressure.
- To permit better radiographic visualization of the lungs.
- To diagnose pleural effusion.

Contraindications

- An uncooperative client.
- A client with clinically significant thrombocytopenia.
- A client who is fully anticoagulated with heparin or coumadin presents a risk of bleeding.

Procedure
Client preparation

1. If ordered, a cough suppressant is administered.
2. Prior to the procedure, a sterile thoracentesis tray is obtained from central supply.
3. The client's chest x-ray film or ultrasound scan are made available at the procedure site prior to thoracentesis.

Procedure

1. A physician performs this study under strict sterile technique at the client's bedside, in a procedure room, or in the physician's office.
2. The client is usually placed in an upright position with arms and shoulders raised and supported on a padded overbed table. Clients who cannot sit are placed in a side lying position on the unaffected side with the side to be tapped uppermost.
3. The needle insertion site is aseptically cleansed and anesthetized with a local anesthetic.
4. The needle is positioned in the pleural space and fluid is withdrawn with a syringe and a three-way stopcock. A short polyethylene catheter (Intracath) may be inserted into the pleural space for fluid aspiration.
5. After the fluid is obtained, the needle is removed and a small bandage is placed over the site.
6. The client is then usually turned on the unaffected side for 1 hour to allow the pleural puncture site to heal.

Nursing implications

1. Help position the client appropriately (usually sitting) to make the client comfortable and to allow the fluid to pool in the base of the pleural space.
2. During the procedure the nurse should monitor the pulse for reflex bradycardia and evaluate the client for diaphoresis and feelings of faintness.
3. Record the exact location of the thoracentesis, the quantity of the fluid obtained, and the gross appearance of the fluid.
4. After the study, monitor the vital signs frequently as ordered.
5. Observe the client for coughing or for the expectoration of blood.
6. Evaluate the client for signs and symptoms of pneumothorax, tension pneumothorax, subcutaneous emphysema, and pyogenic infection.
7. Observe the client for pulmonary edema or cardiac distress if a large amount of fluid was aspirated.

8. After the test, obtain a chest x-ray film as ordered to check for the complications of pneumothorax.
9. After the procedure, listen to the client's lungs for diminished breath sounds, which could be a sign of pneumothorax.
10. The client with no complaints of dyspnea can usually resume normal activity 1 hour after the procedure.

Nurse alert

1. The most common complication of thoracentesis is pneumothorax caused by puncture of the visceral pleura or entry of air into the pleural space with the aspirating needle.
2. Other complications include intrapleural bleeding caused by puncture of tissue (e.g., lung, liver, spleen) or a blood vessel; hemoptysis caused by needle puncture of a pulmonary vessel or an area of inflammation; reflex bradycardia and hypertension; pulmonary edema; pain (shoulder top pain on the affected side); and seeding of the needle track with tumor.
3. Be certain the client knows not to move or cough during the procedure to avoid inadvertent needle damage to the lung or pleura.

Bibliography

Anthony, C.P., and Thibodeau, G.A.: Textbook of anatomy and physiology, ed. 11, St. Louis, 1983, The C.V. Mosby Co.

Braunwald, E.: Approach to the patient with disease of the respiratory system. In Petersdorf, R.G., and others, editors: Harrison's principles of internal medicine, ed. 10, New York, 1983, McGraw-Hill Book Co.

Brunner, L.S., and Suddarth, D.S.: Textbook of medical-surgical nursing, ed. 5, Philadelphia, 1984, J.B. Lippincott Co.

Chalon, J., and others: Routine cytodiagnosis of pulmonary malignancies, Arch. Path. Lab. Med. **105**(1):11-14, Jan. 1981.

Corsella, B.F., and others: Flexible fiberoptic bronchoscopy: its role in diagnosis of lung lesions, Postgrad. Med. **72**:95, 1982.

Fuller, B.: Normal structure and function of the respiratory system. In Hudak, C.M., and others, editors: Critical care nursing, ed. 3, Philadelphia, 1982, J.B. Lippincott Co.

Kozier, B., and Erb, G.: Fundamentals of nursing: concepts and procedures, ed. 2, Menlo Park, Calif., 1983, Addison-Wesley Publishing Co., Inc.

Moser, K.M.: Fiberoptic bronchoscopy and other diagnostic procedures. In Petersdorf, R.G., and others, editors: Harrison's principles of internal medicine, ed. 10, New York, 1983, McGraw-Hill Book Co.

Murray, J.F.: Bronchiectasis and broncholithiasis. In Petersdorf, R.G., and others, editors: Harrison's principles of internal medicine, ed. 10, New York, 1983, McGraw-Hill Book Co.

Petty, T.L.: Pulmonary diagnostic techniques, Philadelphia, 1975, Lea & Febiger.

Phipps, W.J., and Daly, B.J.: Problems of the lower airway. In Phipps, W.J., Long, B.C., and Woods, N.F., editors: Medical-surgical nursing: concepts and clinical practice, ed. 2, St. Louis, 1983, The C.V. Mosby Co.

Programmed instruction: Pulmonary function tests in patient care, Am. J. Nurs. **80**(6):1135-1161, June 1980.

Rogers, P.A.: Percutaneous needle aspiration biopsy of pulmonary lesions, Rad. Tech. **55**(1):527-531, Sept./Oct. 1983.

Sackner, M.A., editor: Diagnostic techniques in pulmonary medicine, New York, 1981, Marcel Dekker, Inc.

Sahn, S.A.: Pleural manifestations of pulmonary disease, Hosp. Pract. **16**(3):73-89, March 1981.

Sinner, W.N., editor: Needle biopsy and transbronchial biopsy, New York, 1982, Thieme-Stratton, Inc.

Stevens, R.P., and others: Fiberoptic bronchoscopy in the intensive care unit, Heart Lung **10**(6):1037-1045, Nov./Dec. 1981.

Weaver, T.E.: Helping your patient through thoracentesis and pleural biopsy, RN **46**(1):64, Jan. 1983.

Weaver, T.E.: Quick reminders on pulmonary function tests . . . and terminology, RN **46**(2):64, Feb. 1983.

Weaver, T.E.: ABGs: taking the sample, interpreting the results, RN **46**(3):64, March 1983.

West, J.B.: Disturbances of respiratory function. In Petersdorf, R.G., and others, editors: Harrison's principles of internal medicine, ed. 10, New York, 1983, McGraw-Hill Book Co.

Wyper, M.A., Daly, B.J., and Norman, A.: Assessment of the respiratory system. In Phipps, W.J., Long, B.C., and Woods, N.F., editors: Medical-surgical nursing: concepts and clinical practice, ed. 2, St. Louis, 1983, The C.V. Mosby Co.

Nervous System 5

Clinical laboratory tests
  Blood tests
  Anti-acetylcholine receptor antibody tests
Radiologic laboratory tests
  X-ray tests
    Cerebral angiography (cerebral arteriography)
    Lumbosacral spinal x-ray study (LS spine)
    Myelography
    Pneumoencephalography (PEG)
    Skull x-ray study
    Ventriculography (ventriculogram)
  Nuclear scanning test
    Brain scanning
  Computerized tomography tests
    CAT scanning (computerized axial tomography, computerized
      tomography—CT scan of the brain; computerized axial trans-
      verse tomography—CATT; electronic musical instrument
      scanning—EMI scanning)
Special studies
  Caloric study
  Cisternal puncture
  Echoencephalography (brain echogram; ultrasound of the brain)
  Electroencephalography (EEG)
  Electromyography
  Evoked potentials (EP)
  Lumbar puncture and cerebrospinal fluid examination (LP, spinal
    tap, spinal puncture)
  Nerve conduction studies (electroneurography)

Clinical Laboratory Tests

Blood Tests

ANTI-ACETYLCHOLINE RECEPTOR ANTIBODY TESTS

Normal Values

- Absent.

Deviations from Normal

- Myasthenia gravis.

Indications

- To assist in evaluation of muscle weakness and the diagnosis of myasthenia gravis.

Contraindications

- None.

Procedure

Client preparation

1. The purpose and procedure are explained.

Procedure

1. Following standard venipuncture procedure, a red-top tube of blood is drawn.
2. Pressure is applied to the venipuncture site.

Nursing implications

1. Observe the site for bleeding.

Radiologic Laboratory Tests

X-Ray Tests

CEREBRAL ANGIOGRAPHY (CEREBRAL ARTERIOGRAPHY)

Normal Values

- Normal cerebral vessels.

Deviations from Normal

- Vascular tumors appear as masses containing multiple small AV fistulas.
- Nonvascular tumors, abscesses, and hematomas present an avascular mass, distorting the normal vascular location.

Indications

- Conventional angiography: to detect abnormalities of the cerebral circulation (e.g., aneurysms, occlusion, or AV malformations [Fig. 5-1]).
- Digital subtraction angiography: to evaluate clients before and after vascular and tumor surgery.

Contraindications

- An unstable client.
- A client with dye allergies.

Procedure

Client preparation

1. The client is told where the catheter will be inserted (usually into the femoral artery). Inform the client that an uncomfortably warm flush will occur during dye insertion.
2. The client is assessed for allergies to iodine dye.
3. Prior to the study, baseline data is obtained. Baseline data should include vital signs, level of consciousness, pupil reaction, facial symmetry, strength and motion of the extremities, and distal pulses (if the femoral artery approach is to be used).
4. The client is kept from having solid foods after midnight on the day of the test. Liquids are usually allowed because the client should be well hydrated.

Procedure

1. The clinical problem under investigation and the personal preference of the physician performing the test determine puncture site location.
2. The catheter is followed under fluoroscopy as it passes into the desired artery.

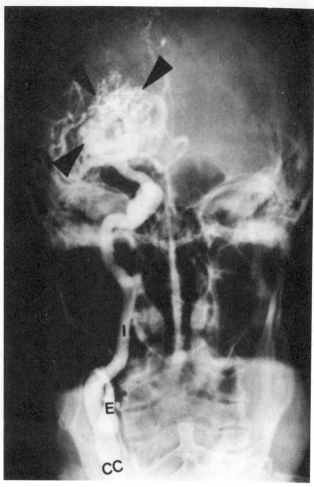

Figure 5-1
Cerebral angiogram. Black arrows indicate large
arteriovenous malformation. *CC,* common carotid artery;
E, external carotid artery; *I,* internal carotid artery.

3. Radiopaque contrast material is then injected, and the flow of blood through the cranial cavity is seen.
4. Serial x-ray films are taken in timed sequence to show the arterial and venous phases of the cerebral circulation.
5. After the x-ray films are completed, the catheter is removed and a pressure dressing applied to the puncture site.
6. For *digital subtraction angiography,* an image ''mask'' is made of the area of clinical interest and then stored in the computer.
   a. After the intravenous injection of the contrast material, subsequent images are made.
   b. The computer then subtracts the preinjection ''mask'' image from the postinjection image, removing all undesired tissue images (e.g., bone) and leaving an arterial image of high contrast and high quality.
7. An angiographer (radiologist) usually performs the study in the angiography room in approximately 1 hour.

Nursing implications

1. After the procedure, monitor vital signs and perform a neurologic evaluation frequently (every 15 minutes for four times, then every 30 minutes for four times, then every hour for four times, and then every 4 hours) and compare these findings with the preprocedure data base. An increase in pulse and a decrease in blood pressure may indicate bleeding.
2. Assess the catheter insertion site for hemorrhage, hematoma, and inflammation each time the vital signs are taken. If the neck arteries were used for arterial access, assess the neck region for swelling or hematoma that could compromise respiration. If the brachial or femoral arteries were cannulated, assess the involved extremity for peripheral pulses, numbness, tingling, pain, color, temperature, and loss of function.
3. Keep the client on bed rest for 12 to 24 hours after the procedure. During this time the involved extremity should be extended and immobilized to prevent kinking of the vessel and clot formations.

4. Apply an ice bag to the puncture site to reduce swelling and pain.
5. The client can usually resume a regular diet after the procedure. Unless contraindicated for medical purposes, force fluids to promote dye excretion by the kidneys.

Nurse alert

1. Anaphylaxis caused by an allergic reaction to the iodinated contrast material may occur.
2. Hemorrhage or hematomas at the puncture site used for arterial access may occur. Assess the client for anticoagulant therapy prior to the study.
3. Neurologic deficits can result if the angiocatheter dislodges an atherosclerotic plaque that then travels to the brain.

LUMBOSACRAL SPINAL X-RAY STUDY (LS SPINE)
Normal Values

- Normal lumbar anatomy.

Deviations from Normal

- Degenerative arthritic changes of the spine.
- Traumatic fractures, spondylosis (stress fracture of the vertebrae), and spondylolisthesis (slipping of one vertebral body on the other).
- Metastatic tumor invasion of the spine (e.g., from breast cancer, melanoma, or colorectal cancer).

Indications

- To diagnose the cause of low back pain.
- To detect traumatic fractures, spondylosis (stress fracture of the vertebrae), and spondylolisthesis (slipping of one vertebral body on another).

Contraindications

- An uncooperative client.
- A pregnant client.

Procedure
Client preparation

1. The client is told that he or she must remove all clothing above and below the waist.
2. Unnecessarily moving the client is avoided until the extent of damage has been determined.

Procedure

1. All of the client's clothing is removed, and a long x-ray gown is placed on the client.
2. Metal objects (e.g., sanitary belts) must be removed.
3. Anterior, posterior, lateral, and oblique x-ray films are taken of the lumbar and sacral areas.
4. Any area of the spine (cervical, thoracic, lumbar, sacral, or coccygeal) can be studied in a similar manner and can reveal the same information as described above.
5. Usually a radiology technician or a radiologist performs this study in the radiology department in a few minutes.

Nursing implications

1. Assess the client's menstrual status, being sure that the client is not pregnant at the time of the study.

MYELOGRAPHY
Normal Values

- Normal spinal canal.

Deviations from Normal

- Cord tumors, meningeal tumors, metastatic spinal tumors, herniated intravertebral discs, and arthritic bone spurs present as canal narrowing or as varying degrees of obstruction to the flow of the dye column within the canal.

Indications

- To diagnose the cause of severe back pain.
- To aid in interpreting neurologic signs incriminating the canal as the location of injury or disease.

Contraindications

- See "Lumbar Puncture," p. 165.

Procedure

See "Lumbar Puncture," p. 165.

Client preparation

1. Usually, food and fluid to the client are stopped approximately 4 hours before the study to avoid the client's vomiting during the study.
2. Inform the client that he or she will be tilted into an up-and-down position on a table so that the dye can properly fill the spinal canal and provide adequate visualization of the desired area.

Procedure

1. A lumbar puncture (or cisternal puncture) (see pp. 165-167) is performed on the unsedated client.
2. Fifteen ml of cerebrospinal fluid is withdrawn, and 15 cc or more of radiographic dye or air is injected into the spinal canal.
3. With the needle in place, the client is placed in the prone position on a tilt table with the head tilted down.
4. The lights are turned off, and the column of dye is followed cephalad under fluoroscopy.
5. Representative x-ray films are taken.
6. Different types of contrast material can be used for myelography.
   a. An oil-based dye (e.g., Pantopaque) must be aspirated as much as possible after the procedure before removing the spinal needle. The client's head is then kept elevated above the level of the spine to prevent upward dispersion of the dye, which could cause irritative meningitis.
   b. A new water-soluble contrast material, metrizamide (Amipaque) does not need to be removed at the end of the procedure, since it is water soluble and will be completely reabsorbed. Because metrizamide may pre-

cipitate seizure activity after the procedure, the client should be well hydrated and should avoid medications that could decrease the seizure threshold (e.g., phenothiazines, tricyclics, antidepressants, C & S stimulants, and amphetamines).

c. To avoid some of the side effects associated with radiopaque substances, some neurosurgeons prefer to perform an air myelography.

7. After myelography is performed (using an oil-based medium, water-based medium, or air), the needle is removed and a dressing applied.

8. The client returns to the unit on a stretcher and is placed on bed rest.

9. A radiologist or a neurologist usually performs this study in the radiology department in approximately 45 minutes.

Nursing implications

1. If the oil-based dye has been completely removed, keep the client flat in bed for at least 12 hours and then allow resumption of normal activity.

2. If the water-soluble dye has not been removed, keep the client's head elevated (30 to 50 degrees) for 6 to 8 hours to prevent an upward dispersion of the dye.

3. After myelography using air, the client is positioned (for about 48 hours) with the head lower than the trunk to prevent air from gravitating to the cerebral space and causing headaches.

4. Observe the client for signs and symptoms of meningeal irritations (e.g., fever, stiff neck, occipital headache, or photophobia).

5. Monitor the client's vital signs and ability to void.

Nurse alert

1. See "Lumbar Puncture," p. 167.

PNEUMOENCEPHALOGRAPHY (PEG)
Normal Values

- No cerebral abnormalities.

Deviations from Normal

■ Cerebral abnormalities indicating, for example, hydrocephalus, mass lesions, or atrophy of the cerebrum or cerebellum.

Indications

■ To detect hydrocephalus, mass lesions (which deform or displace the ventricles), and atrophy of the cerebrum or cerebellum.

Contraindications

■ See "Lumbar Puncture," p. 165.

Procedure

Client preparation

1. The client is informed that he or she will be able to feel the inserted air rising up the spinal cord to the ventricles. The client may hear a sloshing sound as the air moves through the ventricles. These noises will disappear when the gas is absorbed into the cerebrospinal fluid.
2. The client is instructed to remove all items from the hair.

Procedure

1. Some neurologists require that the client's legs be Ace-wrapped from toes to groin bilaterally to mobilize venous return.
2. The client is placed in the sitting position on a specially designed chair with an opening in the back.
3. The physician then performs a lumbar puncture (p. 165) or cisternal puncture (p. 155). Approximately 8 cc of room air or oxygen is injected.
4. Posteroanterior and lateral skull x-ray films are taken.
5. Then a small amount of cerebrospinal fluid is usually removed and more air (25 to 30 cc) is gradually introduced into the spinal fluid space.
6. The needle is removed, and the client is assisted onto a table or a specially designed chair that allows the head to be tilted downward.

7. During the procedure the vital signs are monitored frequently, and the client is assessed for headache, nausea, and vomiting.
8. Immediate surgery (craniotomy) may be necessary if an intracranial tumor is detected or if the procedure itself causes dangerous intracranial pressure shifts.
9. A neurologist or radiologist performs this study in the radiology department in approximately 60 minutes.

Nursing implications

1. After the procedure, keep the client on bed rest for 24 to 48 hours.
2. The client should turn the head from side to side at least every 2 hours to hasten the absorption of air.
3. The client will often complain of a severe headache. The headache usually disappears in 24 to 48 hours after the intracranial air is absorbed in the cerebrospinal fluid. An ice bag may be applied to the head, and the client may require analgesics and antiemetics.
4. Encourage fluids to replace the cerebrospinal fluid lost during this study.
5. After 48 hours the head of the bed is progressively elevated over several hours, during which time the client is evaluated for headache and nausea. If headache and nausea do occur, lowering the head of the bed usually relieves them.
6. After the procedure, evaluate the client frequently (every 15 minutes for four times, then every 30 minutes for four times, then every hour for four times, and then every 4 hours) for changes from baseline vital signs and neurologic status (which were established before the study). Fever and chills are often noted and treated symptomatically.
7. The client may resume a normal diet after the nausea subsides. The client usually resumes normal diet and routine activity by the second day.

Nurse alert

1. Possible complications include herniation of the brain, seizures, severe headache, nausea, vomiting, chills, fever, and other complications, including those associated with lumbar puncture (see p. 167).

SKULL X-RAY STUDY

Normal Values

- Normal skull and surrounding structures.

Deviations from Normal

- Skull fractures.
- Primary or metastatic tumors of the skull.
- Opacification of the nasal sinuses may indicate sinusitis, hemorrhage, or tumor.
- Conditions such as unilateral hematoma or tumor will cause a shift of midline structures.
- Tumors of the pituitary gland.

Indications

- To diagnose pathologic conditions (see "Deviations from Normal" above) in the skull and surrounding structures.

Contraindications

- An uncooperative client who cannot remain still.

Procedure

Client preparation

1. The client is instructed to remove all objects above the neck because metal objects and dentures will prevent x-ray visualization of the covered part. Note is made on the x-ray request form if the client has a glass eye.
2. As in all clients with head trauma, sedation solely for the purpose of completing the test should be avoided.

Procedure

1. The unsedated client is placed on the x-ray table.
2. Metal objects and dentures are removed.
3. The technician usually takes posteroanterior, axial (submentovertical) and half-axial (Towne), and lateral views of the skull.
4. A radiologic technician takes the films in a few minutes in the radiology department. A radiologist interprets them.

Nursing implications

1. If the client is unstable or unconscious, provide constant nursing supervision during transportation to and from the radiology department and also while x-ray films are being taken.
2. Hyperextension and manipulation of the head should not be permitted until cervical injuries are ruled out.

VENTRICULOGRAPHY (VENTRICULOGRAM)

Normal Values

- No ventricular anomalies.

Deviations from Normal

- Presence of ventricular anomalies indicating lesions (e.g., brain tumor) or cerebral anomalies.

Indications

- To identify lesions or cerebral anomalies.
- To determine the patency of the ventricular system.

Contraindications

- See "Lumbar Puncture," p. 165.

Procedure

Client preparation

1. The usual preoperative routine (e.g., remove dentures, void) is followed. The client is told that a hole will be drilled into the skull and then a special needle will be inserted into the ventricle of the brain.
2. Craniotomy may be necessary to prevent brain stem compression.

Procedure

1. The fasting client is taken to the operating room and placed sitting in a special chair.
2. After using either general or local anesthesia, the neurosurgeon makes trephines (burr holes) through scalp inci-

sions and then punctures the ventricles with a special needle or catheter.

3. After removing cerebrospinal fluid, either air or contrast material is injected into the ventricles.

4. The client is repositioned during the x-ray study that follows to ensure adequate visualization of the ventricular structures.

5. Immediate surgery (craniotomy) may be necessary if an intracranial tumor is detected or if the procedure itself causes dangerous intracranial pressure shifts.

6. If the results of this test are normal, the needle is removed and the skin over the burr holes is sutured closed.

7. The scalp wounds are covered with a sterile dressing. The sutures are usually removed within 4 to 5 days.

8. A neurosurgeon performs this procedure in the operating room.

Nursing implications

1. After the procedure, monitor the client's vital signs and the neurologic signs frequently (every 15 to 60 minutes for the first 12 to 24 hours).

2. Elevate the head of the client's bed 10 to 15 degrees for the first 24 hours and then as tolerated.

3. Usually allow the client out of bed on the second or third day after the procedure.

4. Use side rails as indicated.

5. After the procedure, check the scalp dressing for drainage. Reinforce it as necessary to keep the dressing dry and to prevent the entrance of microorganisms.

6. After the procedure, encourage fluids (when the client is conscious) to replace the cerebrospinal fluid lost during the procedure.

7. Most clients have a headache after this procedure, which will usually disappear within 24 to 48 hours after the intracranial air is absorbed in the cerebrospinal fluid. An ice bag may help relieve the headache.

8. Administer analgesics as ordered and as necessary to relieve severe discomfort.

Nuclear Scanning Test
BRAIN SCANNING
Normal Values

- No areas of increased radionucleotide uptake within the brain.

Deviations from Normal

- Cerebral neoplasms, brain abscess, acute infarction, cerebral hemorrhage, acute hematoma, or arteriovenous (AV) malformation.
- Tumors (Fig. 5-2).
- Subdural hematomas.
- Brain abscess.

Indications

- To provide a (nonspecific) indicator of the pathologic process (see ''Deviations from Normal'' above) by providing information about the size, location, and shape of the abnormality.
- To detect changes in the dynamics of cerebral blood flow.

Contraindications

- A pregnant client.
- An uncooperative client.

Procedure
Client preparation

1. The client is assured that the body will excrete radioactive material within 24 hours.
2. The potassium chloride capsule is administered as ordered 2 hours before scanning. The potassium chloride prevents excessive uptake of technetium by the choroid plexus, which would simulate a pathologic condition.

Procedure

1. Shortly after the technetium injection, the client is placed in the supine, lateral, and prone positions while a counter is passed over the patient's head.

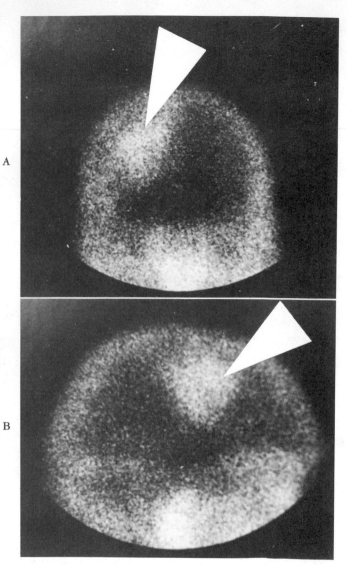

Figure 5-2
Brain scans. **A,** Anteroposterior view. **B,** Lateral view. White arrows indicate tumor seen in both views.

2. The radioisotope counts are anatomically displayed and photographed while the client remains still.
3. When cerebral flow studies are performed, the client is placed in the supine position and injected with isotopes, and the counter is immediately placed over the head.
4. The counts are anatomically recorded in timed sequence to follow the isotope during its first flow through the brain.
5. A technician in the nuclear medicine department performs this study in 35 to 45 minutes.

Computerized Tomography Tests
CAT SCANNING (COMPUTERIZED AXIAL TOMOGRAPHY, COMPUTERIZED TOMOGRAPHY— CT SCAN OF THE BRAIN; COMPUTERIZED AXIAL TRANSVERSE TOMOGRAPHY—CATT; ELECTRONIC MUSICAL INSTRUMENT SCANNING—EMI SCANNING)

Normal Values

- No evidence of pathologic condition.

Deviations from Normal

- Neoplasms, infarction, ventricular displacement or enlargement, cortical atrophy, cerebral aneurysm, intracranial hemorrhage and hematoma, and AV malformation.

Indications

- To diagnose pathologic conditions listed under ''Deviations from Normal'' above.
- To monitor the progress of the disease.
- To monitor the healing process of the disease.

Contraindications

- An uncooperative client.
- A client with an iodine dye allergy.

Procedure
Client preparation

1. The client is informed that he must lie motionless during the study. Even talking or sighing may cause artifacts on the computer image.
2. The client is told that during the procedure the scanner machine will make audible clicking noises as it moves around the head. The client will not be able to feel the scanner rotate.
3. If possible, the client is shown a picture of the scanning machine.
4. The client is kept on nothing by mouth for 4 hours before the study because the iodine dye may cause nausea.
5. The client is instructed to remove wigs, hairpins, or clips before this procedure.
6. The client is assessed for allergies to iodinated dye to prevent dye-induced anaphylaxis. The client is observed for signs of anaphylaxis (e.g., respiratory distress, palpitations, or diaphoresis).
7. Sedation is restricted to the client who cannot lie still during the procedure.

Procedure

1. The client lies in the supine position on an examining table with the head resting in a snug-fitting rubber cap within a water-filled box.
2. The client's head is enclosed only to the hair line (as in a hair dryer).
3. The face is not covered, and the client can see out of the machine at all times.
4. Sponges are placed along the side of the head to ensure that the client's head does not move during this study. Any movement will cause computer-generated artifacts on the image produced. The client is instructed not to talk or sigh during the scanning.
5. The scanner passes a small x-ray beam through the brain from one side to the other.
6. Usually an iodinated dye will then be used. A peripheral IV line is started, and the iodine dye is then administered through it.

7. The entire scanning process is repeated.
8. The data is immediately available in the form of an x-ray film or as a Polaroid print.
9. A technician performs this study in the radiology department in approximately 45 to 60 minutes.

Nursing implications

1. No special postprocedure care is required.
2. The client can resume all activities after the study.
3. Encourage clients who received a dye injection to increase their fluid intake, because the dye is excreted by the kidneys and causes diuresis.

Nurse alert

1. If the client receives an intravenous dye injection to enhance CAT scanning visualization, anaphylaxis is a possible complication if allergies to iodine dye exist.

Special Studies

Caloric Study
Normal Values

■ Nystagmus with irrigation.

Deviations from Normal

■ Lack of nystagmus with irrigation suggests a disease labyrinth or a tumor of the eighth cranial nerve.

Indications

■ To aid in the differential diagnosis of lesions in the brainstem and cerebellum.

Contraindications

■ A client with a perforated eardrum (however, cold air may be used as a substitute for the fluid).
■ A client with an acute disease of the labyrinth (e.g., Meniere's syndrome). The test can be performed when the acute attack subsides.

Procedure
Client preparation

1. Solid foods are withheld prior to the test to reduce the incidence of vomiting.
2. Sedatives are not usually given because they may alter the client's response.

Procedure

1. The client is usually taken to a treatment room. The exact procedure for caloric studies varies with different hospitals and physicians.
2. Before the test is performed, the client is examined for the presence of nystagmus and Romberg's sign and for the presence of past-pointing.
3. The ear on the affected side is irrigated first, since the client's response may be minimal. After placing an emesis under the ear, the examiner directs irrigation solution into the external auditory canal until the client complains of nausea or dizziness or until nystagmus is observed (usually within 20 to 30 seconds). If after 3 minutes no symptoms occur, the irrigation is stopped.
4. The client is tested for nystagmus, past-pointing, and Romberg's sign (postural deviation).
5. After approximately 5 minutes, the procedure is repeated on the other ear.
6. When the test is over, the client is usually taken back to bed via wheelchair.

Nursing implications

1. Keep the client on bed rest until the nausea and vomiting subside after the test. Usually these last approximately 30 to 60 minutes. After that time the client may resume fluid, food, and normal activities.

Cisternal Puncture
Normal Values

■ See "Lumbar Puncture" and "CF Examination," p. 163.

Deviations from Normal

- See ''Lumbar Puncture'' and ''CF Examination,'' p. 163.

Indications

- To obtain cerebrospinal fluid for examination when it cannot be obtained at the lumbar level.
- To demonstrate a subarachnoid block by performing a cisternal puncture simultaneously with a lumbar puncture.
- To provide drainage of cerebrospinal fluid when a lumbar puncture is contraindicated.
- To introduce contrast material or air for myelography.
- To perform encephalography.

Contraindications

- See ''Lumbar Puncture,'' p. 165.
- This procedure should also be avoided if a lesion may be in the cisternal magna or if suspicion exists of a developmental anomaly at the foramen magnum level.

Procedure

See ''Lumbar Puncture,'' p. 165.

Client preparation

1. A cisternal puncture is often more frightening than a lumbar puncture, since the needle insertion is closer to the brain.
2. If requested, the occipital area at the back of the client's head is shaved and cleansed with an antiseptic.

Procedure

1. Strict sterile technique must be maintained throughout this procedure to avoid problems such as brain abscess and meningitis.
2. The client is placed on his or her side with a pillow under the head to keep the head and spine aligned. The chin rests on the chest, and a nurse or an assistant holds it in place to prevent rotation.
3. The needle is inserted about 4 to 5 cm between the first cervical vertebra and the rim of the foramen magnum.

4. The rest of this procedure is the same as that of "Lumbar Puncture," p. 165.

5. A neurologic specialist usually performs this procedure in 20 to 60 minutes in a treatment room.

Nursing implications

1. Hold the client's head still with the client's chin resting on his or her own chest during the procedure.

2. After the procedure, observe the client for cyanosis, dyspnea, apnea, and irregularities of the heart rate, which could indicate injury to the medulla. Headaches do not usually follow this procedure.

3. Maintain the client on bed rest as ordered, usually for several hours.

Echoencephalography (Brain Echogram; Ultrasound of the Brain)

Normal Values

- Normal position and size of the cerebral midline structures and ventricles.

Deviations from Normal

- Subdural hematoma, intracerebral hemorrhage, cerebral infarction, or tumor,

Indications

- To aid in diagnosing conditions listed under "Deviations from Normal" above.

Contraindications

- An uncooperative client.

Procedure

Client preparation

1. Assurance is given that the study is painless.

2. The client is told that a gel will be applied to several areas of the head to enhance transmission of the echo waves.

Procedure

1. All objects are removed from the client's hair.
2. The ultrasonographer (usually a trained technician) applies mineral oil or glycerine to several areas on the head to enhance transmission and reception of the sound waves by the hand-held transducer.
3. The ultrasonographer (usually a trained technician) performs the study in the ultrasonography lab in approximately 10 minutes.

Nursing implications

1. After the procedure, remove the gel from the client's head.

Electroencephalography (EEG)

Normal Values

- Normal frequency, amplitude, and characteristics of brain waves.

Deviations from Normal

- Seizure activity.
- Cerebral lesions (e.g., hemorrhage, abscess, neoplasm, or infarction).

Indications

- To investigate epileptic states.
- To diagnose cerebral lesions.
- To determine cerebral death in comatose clients.
- To monitor cerebral blood flow during a surgical procedure.

Contraindications

- None.

Procedure
Client preparation

1. Many clients fear that the EEG can "read the mind" or detect senility. Some clients fear that the EEG is a form of electric shock therapy. They should be reassured that these ideas are false.

2. The client should be assured that the flow of electrical current is *from* the client and that this study causes no discomfort.
3. The client is instructed to wash his or her hair on the night before the study. Also, hair oils, sprays, or lotions should not be used.
4. If so desired, the physician should specify discontinuation of medications before the study.
5. Preferably, the client's sleep time is shortened on the night before the test. Adults should not sleep more than 4 to 5 hours and children not more than 5 to 7 hours. Less sleep allows the client to relax and possibly fall asleep during the study.
6. The sedatives or hypnotics are administered before the study, as indicated for the sleep EEG, if one is to be performed. Otherwise sedatives or hypnotics should not be given because they cause abnormally low-voltage, fast waves to appear on the EEG.
7. The client is told that during the recording of the EEG, his or her activity should be minimal, if any. Movement, including opening the eyes, will create interference and alter the EEG recording.
8. The client should *not* fast before the study. Fasting may cause hypoglycemia, which could modify the EEG pattern. Coffee, tea, and cola are omitted on the morning of the study because of their stimulating effect.

Procedure

1. The client is placed in a supine position on a bed or reclining in a chair.
2. Sixteen or more electrodes are applied to the scalp with electrode paste in a uniform pattern over both sides of the head, covering the prefrontal, frontal, temporal, parietal, and occipital areas. One electrode may be applied to each earlobe for grounding.
3. After the electrodes are applied, the client is instructed to lie still with eyes closed.
4. Approximately every 5 minutes the recording is interrupted to permit the client to move if desired.

5. In addition to the resting EEG, a number of "activating" procedures can be performed.

   a. The client is hyperventilated to induce alkalosis and cerebral vasoconstriction, which may activate abnormalities.

   b. By flashing a light over the client's face with the eyes closed and opened, photostimulation is performed. Photostimulated seizure activity may be seen on EEG.

   c. A sleep EEG may be performed to aid in the detection of abnormal brain waves that are seen only if the client is sleeping (e.g., frontal lobe epilepsy). A recording is performed while the client is asleep and while waking up.

6. After the study the electrodes and the paste are removed.

7. EEG is usually performed in a specially constructed room that is shielded from outside disturbances (electrical, auditory, and visual). EEG can be performed at the bedside if the client is too ill to be moved.

8. An EEG technician usually performs this study in 45 minutes to 2 hours.

Nursing implications

1. After the study the electrical paste the technician applied can be removed with acetone or witch hazel and then shampooing.

2. Ensure safety precautions (side rails up) after the test until the effects of the sedatives have worn off.

3. If the client is having the study done as an outpatient, an adult should accompany the client and provide transportation home after the study.

Electromyography
Normal Values

- No evidence of neuromuscular abnormalities.

Deviations from Normal

- Fibrillation and fasciculation.
- Primary muscle disorder (e.g., polymyositis, muscular dystrophies, and various myopathies).

- Myasthenia gravis.
- Peripheral nerve damage.

Indications

- To detect primary muscular disorders or muscular abnormalities caused by other system diseases (e.g., nerve dysfunction, sarcoidosis, and paraneoplastic syndrome).

Contraindications

- An uncooperative client.
- A client on anticoagulant therapy.
- A client with extensive skin infection.

Procedure
Client preparation

1. The client is assured that the needle will not electrocute him or her.
2. Premedication or sedation is usually avoided because the client's cooperation is necessary.

Procedure

1. The client is positioned according to the muscle being studied.
2. A needle that acts as a recording electrode is inserted into the muscle being examined.
3. A reference electrode is placed nearby on the skin surface.
4. The client is asked to keep the muscle at rest.
5. The oscilloscope display is viewed for any evidence of spontaneous electrical activity, such as fasciculation or fibrillation.
6. Next the client is asked to contract the muscle slowly and progressively.
7. The electrical waves produced are examined for their number and form.
8. A physical therapist, a physiatrist, or a neurologist performs the study at the client's bedside or in the electromyography lab in approximately 20 minutes.

Nursing implications

1. After the procedure, observe the needle site for hematoma or inflammation.

Evoked Potentials (EP)

Evoked potentials are divided by sensory modality into visual evoked responses (VER), auditory brain stem evoked potentials (ABEP), and somatosensory evoked responses (SEP).

Normal Values

- Vary according to the lab performing the test.

Deviations from Normal
VER

- Multiple sclerosis.
- Other neurologic disorders (e.g., Parkinson's disease).
- Lesions of the optic nerve, optic tract, visual center, and the eye.

ABEP

- In low birth weight newborns, an abnormal latency may indicate an auditory disorder. An abnormal latency may indicate posterior fossa tumor.

SEP

- Abnormal latency may indicate brain dysfunction or early tumor.

Indications
VER

- To aid in diagnosing multiple sclerosis, neurologic disorders, and lesions of the optic nerve, optic tract, visual center, and the eye.
- To detect and evaluate the absence of binocularity in infants.

ABEP

- To screen low birth weight newborns for auditory disorders.
- To detect early posterior fossa tumors.

SEP

- To evaluate clients with spinal cord injuries.
- To monitor spinal cord functioning during surgery or during treatment of diseases (such as multiple sclerosis).
- To evaluate the location and extent of areas of brain dysfunction after head injury.
- To pinpoint tumors at an early stage.

Contraindications

- None.

Procedure
Client preparation

1. Many clients fear the diagnosis that the studies may substantiate.
2. The client is instructed to shampoo his or her hair prior to the test.
3. No fasting or sedation is required.

Procedure

1. The evoked potential to be performed determines the electrode position.
   a. For visual evoked potentials, electrodes are placed on the scalp along the vertex and cortex lobes. Stimulation occurs by using strobe light, checkerboard patterns, or retinal stimuli.
   b. For auditory brain stem evoked potentials, scalp electrodes are placed on the vertex and on each ear lobe. Stimulation occurs by clicking noises or tone bursts delivered via earphones.
   c. For somatosensory evoked potentials, electrodes are placed over the sensory cortex of the opposite hemisphere or the scalp. Electrical stimuli are applied to nerves at the wrist (medial nerve) or the knee (peroneal).

2. A neurologist performs the study in 30 minutes in a physician's office.

Nursing implications

1. After the test, remove the gel used for adherence of the electrodes.

Lumbar Puncture and Cerebrospinal Fluid Examination (LP, Spinal Tap, Spinal Puncture)
Normal Values and Deviations from Normal

- Pressure

  Normal values: <200 mm H_2O.

  Deviations from normal: Tumor, hemorrhage, hematoma, tissue edema, scarring, foreign body, or intervertebral disc.

- Color

  Normal values: None.

  Deviations from normal: Blood either from subarachnoid bleeding or from the lumbar needle puncture penetrating a blood vessel.

- Blood

  Normal values: None.

  Deviations from normal: Blood in the cerebrospinal fluid indicates cerebral hemorrhage into the subarachnoid space or a traumatic tap.

- Cells

  Normal values: No red blood cells; <5 lymphocytes/mm^3.

  Deviations from normal: The presence of polymorphonuclear leukocytes (neutrophils) in the cerebrospinal fluid indicates bacterial meningitis or cerebral abscess. The presence of mononuclear leukocytes indicates viral or tubercular meningitis or encephalitis.

- Culture and sensitivity

  Normal values: No organisms present.

  Deviations from normal: Cultured organisms may include atypical bacterial, fungi, or *Bacterium tuberculosis*.

- Protein

  Normal values: 15 to 45 mg/dl cerebrospinal fluid.

  Deviations from normal: Infectious or inflammatory processes such as meningitis, encephalitis, or myelitis (inflammation of the spinal cord). Tumors may also cause an increase in protein count. Clients with multiple sclerosis, neurosyphilis, or degenerative cord or brain disease will have an elevation of the globulin fraction of total protein.

- Glucose

  Normal values: 50 to 75 mg/dl or >40% of blood glucose level.

  Deviations from normal: A cerebrospinal fluid glucose level of less than 40% of the blood glucose level may indicate meningitis or neoplasm.

- Chloride

  Normal values: 700 to 750 mg/100 dl.

  Deviations from normal: The chloride concentration in the cerebrospinal fluid may be decreased in clients with meningeal infections, tubercular meningitis, and conditions of low blood chloride levels.

- Lactic dehydrogenase (LDH)

  Normal values: 2.0 to 7.2 U/ml.

  Deviations from normal: Elevated LDH levels indicate infection or inflammation (e.g., bacterial meningitis).

- Cytology

  Normal values: No malignant cells.

  Deviations from normal: The presence of tumor cells indicates neoplasm.

- Serology for syphilis

  Normal value: Negative.

  Deviations from normal: Positive results on Wassermann, Venereal Disease Research Laboratory (VDRL), or fluorescent treponemal antibody (FTA) tests indicate neurosyphilis.

Indications

- To diagnose brain or spinal cord neoplasm, cerebral hemorrhage, meningitis, encephalitis, and degenerative brain disease.

Contraindications

- An uncooperative client.
- A client with increased intracranial pressure, because the lumbar puncture may induce cerebral or cerebellar herniation.
- A client who has severe degenerative spinal joint disease because the physician is almost always unsuccessful in placing the needle through the degenerated interspinal space.
- A client prone to psychosomatic illness because such a client may occasionally associate a lumbar puncture with the potential of paraplegia.
- A client with infections near the lumbar puncture site because meningitis can result from contamination with the infected material.

Procedure
Client preparation

1. The client is assured that insertion of the needle into the spine will not cause paralysis because the needle is inserted into the area below the spinal cord.
2. The necessary lumbar puncture tray is ordered from the central supply department of the hospital.
3. If possible, the client should empty the bladder and bowels before the procedure. A misdirected needle may puncture these organs if they are distended with urine or feces.
4. The client is told to lie still throughout this procedure because movement may cause traumatic injury.

Procedure

1. The client is placed in the lateral decubitus position (fetal position). The client should clasp his or her hands on the knees to maintain this position. The lumbar area must be flexed as much as possible to assure maximum bowing of the spine and allow as much space as possible between the vertebrae.
2. A vertebral interspace anywhere between L2 and S1 is chosen for the puncture, because the spinal cord ends around L2.

3. A local anesthetic (usually 1% lidocaine) is injected into the skin and subcutaneous tissues after the site has been aseptically cleansed.

4. Next a spinal needle containing an inner obturator is placed through the skin and into the spinal canal.

5. The subarachnoid space is entered.

6. The insert (obturator) is removed, and cerebrospinal fluid can be seen slowly dripping from the needle.

7. The needle is then attached to a sterile manometer and the pressure is recorded.

8. Next three sterile test tubes are filled with about 5 to 10 ml of the cerebrospinal fluid and sent for appropriate testing.

9. Finally, the pressure is again measured (i.e., the closing pressure).

10. If blockage in cerebrospinal fluid circulation in the spinal (subarachnoid) space is suspected, a *Queckenstedt test* is performed.

    a. The jugular veins are occluded either manually by digital pressure or by a medium-sized blood pressure cuff inflated to approximately 20 torr.

    b. Within 10 seconds after jugular vein occlusion, cerebrospinal fluid pressure should increase from 150 to 400 mm H_2O and then promptly return to normal within 10 seconds after release of the pressure.

11. After the procedure the spinal needle is removed, and digital pressure is placed over the area of needle insertion.

12. An adhesive bandage can be placed over the puncture site.

13. The client is then placed in the prone position with a pillow under the abdomen to increase the intraabdominal pressure, thus indirectly increasing pressure on the tissues surrounding the spinal canal and retarding continued cerebrospinal fluid flow from the spinal canal.

14. A physician performs the lumbar puncture in 20 to 60 minutes under sterile conditions at the client's bedside.

Nursing implications

1. Assist the client in assuming the fetal position. The nurse may place a pillow between the client's legs to prevent the upper part of the legs from rolling forward.
2. The nurse may be required to assist the physician by holding the manometer straight.
3. Label the specimen jars appropriately.
4. After the procedure, keep the client on bed rest with the head flat. Most physicians order bed rest for 12 hours.
5. The client may turn from side to side.
6. Encourage increased fluids taken with a straw.
7. After the procedure, assess the client for movement of the extremities, pain at the injection site, blood or cerebrospinal fluid drainage at the injection site, and the ability to void.

Nurse alert

1. Complications of lumbar puncture include the following:
   a. Persistent cerebrospinal fluid leak, causing severe headache.
   b. Introduction of bacteria into the cerebrospinal fluid, causing suppurative meningitis.
   c. Herniation of the brain through the tentorium cerebelli or herniation of the cerebellum through the foramen magnum. In clients with increased intracranial pressure, lumbar puncture may induce herniation of the brain, causing compression of the brainstem. Deterioration of the client's neurologic status and death will result.
   d. Inadvertent puncture of the spinal cord, caused by an inappropriately high puncture of the spinal canal.
   e. Puncture of the aorta or the vena cava, causing serious retroperitoneal hemorrhage. Puncture is the result of a misdirected spinal needle probe.

Nerve Conduction Studies (Electroneurography)
Normal Values

- No evidence of peripheral nerve injury or disease.

Deviations from Normal

- Traumatic transection or contusion of a nerve.
- Neuropathies.

Indications

- To detect and locate peripheral nerve injury or disease.

Contraindications

- None.

Procedure
Client preparation

1. The client is encouraged to verbalize fears regarding the electric stimulation (shock) necessary for this study.

Procedure

1. The area of specific suspected peripheral nerve injury or disease determines the position in which the client is placed.
2. A recording electrode is placed on the skin overlying a muscle innervated solely by the relevant nerve.
3. A reference electrode is placed nearby.
4. All skin-to-electrode connections are assured by using electrical paste.
5. A shock-emitter device at an adjacent location stimulates the nerve.
6. The time between nerve impulse and muscular contraction (distal latency) is measured in milliseconds on a cathode-ray oscilloscope (electromyograph). Next the nerve is similarly stimulated at a location proximal (i.e., more central) to the area of suspected injury or disease.
7. The time required for the impulse to travel from the site of initiation to muscle contraction (total latency) is recorded in milliseconds.
8. Usually a neurologist, a physiatrist, or a physical therapist performs this study in the nerve conduction lab, the clinician's office, the physical rehabilitation department, or at the patient's bedside. The test requires approximately 15 minutes to complete. A physician interprets the results.

Nursing implications

1. After the nerve conduction study is performed, remove the electrode gel from the client's skin.

Bibliography

Adams, R.D., Chiappa, K.H., Martin, J.B., and Young, R.R.: Diagnostic methods in neurology. In Petersdorf, R.G., and others, editors: Harrison's principles of internal medicine, ed. 10, New York, 1983, McGraw-Hill Book Co.

Adams, R.D., and Victor M.: Principles of neurology, ed. 2, New York, 1981, McGraw-Hill Book Co.

Beyers, M., and Dudas, S.: The clinical practice of medical-surgical nursing, ed. 2, Boston, 1984, Little, Brown & Co.

Brunner, L.S., and Suddarth, D.S.: Textbook of medical-surgical nursing, ed. 5, Philadelphia, 1984, J.B. Lippincott Co.

Budd, D.: Neurodiagnostic studies: pre- and post-procedure care, RN **44**(11):64-65, Nov. 1981.

Collins, R.: Illustrated manual of neurological diagnosis, ed. 2, Philadelphia, 1982, J.B. Lippincott Co.

Conway-Rutkowski, B.L.: Carini and Owens' neurological and neurosurgical nursing, ed. 8, St. Louis, 1982, The C.V.Mosby Co.

Goodgold, J.: Anatomical correlates with clinical electromyography, Baltimore, 1974, The Williams & Wilkins Co.

Greenberg, R.P., and Ducker, T.B.: Evoked potentials in the clinical neurosciences, J. Neurosurg. **56**(1):1-18, Jan. 1982.

Kolb, D.: Understanding aphasia and the aphasic. J. Neurosurg. Nurs. **9**:15-18, 1977.

Lamb, S.A.: The nurse's changing role in water soluble myelography. J. Neurosurg. Nurs. **10**(4):189-191, 1978.

Mahoney, E.K.: Alterations in cognitive functioning in the brain-damaged patient, Nurs. Clin. North Am. **15**:283-292, 1980.

Malasanos, L., and others: Health assessment, ed. 2, St. Louis, 1981, The C.V. Mosby Co.

Mitchell, P.H., and Irvin, N.J.: Neurological examination: nursing assessment for nursing purposes, J. Neurosurg. Nurs. **9**:23-28, 1977.

Mohr, J.P., Kase, C.S., and Adams, R.D.: Cerebrovascular disorders. In Petersdorf, R.G., and others, editors: Harrison's principles of internal medicine, ed. 10, New York, 1983, McGraw-Hill Book Co.

Nebe, D.E.: Diagnostic studies. In Snyder, M., editor: A guide to neurological and neurosurgical nursing, New York, 1983, John Wiley & Sons.

Nosse, E.S., and Kinney, M.: Assessment of the nervous system. In Phipps. W.J., Long, B.C., and Woods, N.F., editors: Medical-surgical nursing: concepts and clinical practice, St. Louis, 1983, The C.V. Mosby Co.

Ozuna, J.: Nursing assessment—nervous system. In Lewis, S.M., and Collier, I.C., editors: Medical-surgical nursing: assessment and management of clinical problems, New York, 1983, McGraw-Hill Book Co.

Ross, A.J., and others: Neuromuscular diagnostic procedures, Nurs. Clin. North Am. **14**:107-121, 1979.

Rudy, E.G.: Advanced neurological and neurosurgical nursing, St. Louis, 1984, The C.V. Mosby Co.

Schottelius, B.A., and Schottelius, D.D.: Textbook of physiology, ed. 19, St. Louis, 1982, The C.V. Mosby Co.

Tilkian, S.M., Conover, M.B., and Tilkian, A.G.: Clinical implications of laboratory tests, ed. 3, St. Louis, 1983, The C.V. Mosby Co.

Ziporyn, T.: Evoked potential emerging as valuable medical tool. JAMA **246**(12):1287-1291, Sept. 18, 1981.

Urinary System

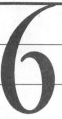

6

Clinical laboratory tests
  Blood tests
    Acid phosphate (prostatic acid phosphate [PAP])
    Aldosterone
    Angiotensin-converting enzyme (ACE; serum angiotensin-con-
      verting enzyme [SACE])
    Antistreptolysin O titer (ASO titer)
    Blood urea nitrogen and creatinine test
    Plasma renin activity
  Urine tests
    Creatinine clearance test
    Twenty-four-hour urine test for vanillylmandelic acid and cate-
      cholamines
    Urinalysis
Radiologic laboratory tests
  X-ray tests
    Nephrotomography
    Pyelography
      Antegrade pyelography
      Intravenous pyelography (IVP, excretory urography)
      Retrograde pyelography
    Renal angiography (renal arteriography)
    Voiding cystourethrography (voiding cystogram)
    X-ray study of the kidneys, ureters, and bladder (KUB)
  Nuclear scanning
    Renal scanning (kidney scan, radiorenography, radionucleotide
      renal imaging, nuclear imaging of the kidney)
  Computerized tomography tests
    Computerized tomography of the kidney (CT of the kidney)
Special studies
  Cystometry
  Cystoscopy

Endourology
Pelvic floor sphincter electromyography (pelvic floor sphincter EMG)
Renal biopsy
Renal ultrasonography (kidney sonogram)
Renal vein assays for renin
Split renal function studies
Ultrasound-guided cyst aspiration study
Urethral pressure measurements (urethral pressure profile)
Urine flow studies (uroflometry)

Clinical Laboratory Tests

Blood Tests

ACID PHOSPHATE (PROSTATIC ACID PHOSPHATE [PAP])

Normal Values

- Adults: 0.10 to 0.63 U/ml (Bessey-Lowry), 0.5 to 2.0 U/ml (Bodansky), 1.0 to 4.0 U/ml (King-Armstrong), 0.0 to 0.8 U/L at 37° C (SI units).
- Children: 6.4 to 15.2 U/L.

Deviations from Normal

- For the client being treated for prostatic carcinoma, rising levels of acid phosphate may indicate a poor prognosis.
- Elevated levels of acid phosphatase also occur in clients with the following conditions: multiple myeloma, Paget's disease, hyperparathyroidism, sickle cell crisis, Gaucher's disease, renal impairment, cancer of the breast and bone, cirrhosis, hepatitis, obstructive jaundice, thrombocytosis, and any cancer metastasis to the bone.
- False high levels of acid phosphatase may occur after a rectal examination and after instrumentation of the prostate gland (such as cystoscopy) because of prostatic stimulation.
- Drugs that may cause elevations of this enzyme include androgens (in females) and clofibrate (Atromid-S).
- Fluorides, phosphates, oxalates, and alcohol may cause decreased levels.

Indications

- To diagnose prostatic carcinoma.
- To monitor the efficacy of treatment for prostatic carcinoma.
- To investigate alleged rape because phosphate occurs in high concentrations in seminal fluid.

Contraindications

- None.

Procedure

1. Following standard peripheral venipuncture technique, 5 to 10 ml blood in a red-top tube is collected.
2. Pressure or a pressure dressing is applied to the puncture site.
3. The sample is sent immediately to the lab. If the test is not performed immediately, the sample should be frozen.

Nursing implications

1. Note on the lab slip if the client has had a prostatic exam or instrumentation of the prostate gland (such as cystoscopy) within 24 hours.
2. The activity of the enzyme in the specimen will be decreased if the specimen is left at room temperature for 1 hour because the enzyme is heat and pH sensitive.

ALDOSTERONE

Normal Values

- Serum: 1 to 21 ng/dl (morning, standing, peripheral vein); 7.4 $\pm$ 4.2 ng/dl (morning, supine for 2 hours, peripheral vein).
- Urine: 2 to 16 μg/24 h.

Deviations from Normal

- Increased aldosterone and decreased renin level (see p. 179) occur in primary aldosteronism (Conn's syndrome).

- Aldosterone may be elevated in certain nonadrenal conditions (secondary aldosteronism), for example, hyponatremia, hyperkalemia, stress, Cushing's syndrome, malignant hypertension, generalized edema (from congestive heart failure, nephrotic syndrome, cirrhosis), renal ischemia, and Bartter's syndrome (a renin-producing renal tumor).
- Pregnancy and oral contraceptives can also increase aldosterone levels.
- Diuretics and steroids promote sodium excretion and may raise aldosterone levels.
- Decreased aldosterone levels are seen in clients consuming a high sodium diet and in clients with hypokalemia.
- They may also indicate Addison's disease or toxemia of pregnancy.
- Antihypertensives may reduce aldosterone levels because they promote sodium and water retention.

Indications

- To aid in diagnosing pathologic conditions listed under "Deviations from Normal" above.

Contraindications

- None.

Procedure

Client preparation

1. The client maintains a normal sodium diet (approximately 3 g/day) for at least 2 weeks before the test.
2. For the two weeks before the study, drugs that alter sodium, potassium, and fluid balance (e.g., diuretics, antihypertensives, steroids, oral contraceptives) are withheld.
3. For 1 week before the test, renin inhibitors (e.g., propranolol) are withheld.
4. For 2 weeks before the test, licorice is withheld because of its aldosterone-like effect.

Procedure

1. Blood collection

   a. One red-top tube of blood is collected following standard peripheral venipuncture technique.

   b. Pressure or a pressure dressing is applied to the venipuncture site.

   c. The sample is sent to the lab immediately for analysis. (Whether the client was supine or standing during the venipuncture is indicated on the lab slip.)

   d. If ordered, a second sample is drawn 4 hours later (after the client has been up and moving) with the client in the standing position.

2. Urine collection

   a. The client is instructed to avoid strenuous exercise and stressful situations during the 24-hour collection period. Both can increase aldosterone levels.

   b. The procedure for collecting a 24-hour urine sample for a creatinine clearance test is followed (p. 181), except for the client preparation step no. 2 and procedure no. 3.

   c. A preservative is used in the 24-hour collection.

   d. The urine is kept on ice or refrigerated for the 24 hours.

   e. The sample is sent to the lab at the end of the 24 hours.

Nursing implications

1. Give the client written dietary and medication restriction instructions.

2. After the urine or blood test is completed, the client may resume a normal diet and may have restricted medications reordered.

3. Blood collection

   a. Handle the blood sample gently. Rough handling may cause hemolysis and alter the test results.

ANGIOTENSIN-CONVERTING ENZYME (ACE; SERUM ANGIOTENSIN-CONVERTING ENZYME [SACE])

Normal Values

- 23 to 57 U/ml (units = nanomoles/min).

Deviations from Normal

- Elevated levels of ACE occur in a high percentage of clients with sarcoidosis.
- Other conditions that result in elevation of ACE include Gaucher's disease (a rare familial disorder of fat metabolism), leprosy, alcoholic cirrhosis, active histoplasmosis, tuberculosis. Hodgkin's disease, myeloma, scleroderma, pulmonary embolism, and idiopathic pulmonary fibrosis. Levels may be decreased in persons with sarcoidosis who are treated with prednisone.

Indications

- To evaluate the severity of diagnosed sarcoidosis.
- To evaluate the patient's response to therapy for sarcoidosis.

Contraindications

- A client under 20 years of age, because young people normally have high levels.

Procedure

1. Using standard peripheral venipuncture technique, approximately 2 to 5 ml of blood is withdrawn.
2. Pressure or a pressure dressing is applied to the puncture site.
3. The sample is sent to the lab for analysis.

Nursing implications

1. Assess the venipuncture site for bleeding or hematoma.
2. Note on the lab slip if the patient is taking steroid drugs. These drugs usually cause decreased SACE levels.

ANTISTREPTOLYSIN O TITER (ASO TITER)
Normal Values

- Adults: ≤160 Todd units/ml.
- Children: newborn, similar to mother's value; 6 mos to 2 yrs: ≤50 Todd units/ml; 2 to 4 yrs: ≤160 Todd units/ml; 5 to 12 yrs: ≤200 Todd units/ml.

Deviations from Normal

- ASO elevation in a patient with glomerulonephritis or endocarditis indicates that streptococcal infection caused the disease.

Indications

- To assist in making the differential diagnosis of poststreptococcal disease (e.g., glomerulonephritis, rheumatic fever, bacterial endocarditis, and scarlet fever).

Contraindications

- None.

Procedure

1. Following standard peripheral venipuncture technique, one red-top tube of blood is withdrawn.
2. Pressure or a pressure dressing is applied to the puncture site.
3. The sample is sent to the lab for analysis.

Nursing implications

1. Observe puncture site for bleeding or hematoma formation.

BLOOD UREA NITROGEN AND CREATININE TEST

The *blood urea nitrogen (BUN) test,* the *creatinine test,* and the *creatinine clearance test* (p. 181) compose the *renal function studies.*

Blood Urea Nitrogen (BUN)
Normal values

- 5 to 20 mg/dl.

Deviations from normal

- Elevated BUN levels indicate primary renal disease (e.g., glomerulonephritis, pyelonephritis, acute tubular necrosis, and urinary obstruction from tumor or stones). The level may also be elevated when the kidneys are overwhelmed by the presence of excessive amounts of protein for hepatic catabolism and so are unable to excrete the sudden load of urea. BUN levels may also increase in gastrointestinal (GI) bleeding disorders.

- Decreased BUN levels occur from toxins (e.g., gentamicin, tobramycin, myoglobin, and free hemoglobin).
- Dehydration, shock, and congestive heart failure lower BUN levels.
- Decreased BUN levels may also occur with overhydration, liver failure, negative nitrogen balance, and pregnancy.

Creatinine
Normal values

- 0.7 to 1.5 mg/dl.

Deviations from normal

- Renal disorders (e.g., glomerulonephritis, pyelonephritis, acute tubular necrosis, and urinary obstructions) cause elevated creatinine levels.

Bun-Creatinine Ratio
Normal values

- 20:1 (some sources use 15:1).

Deviations from normal

- A BUN level risen out of proportion to the creatinine level indicates dehydration, gastrointestinal bleeding, or malnutrition.
- A BUN level decreased out of proportion to the creatinine level suggests low protein intake, overhydration, or severe liver failure.
- Elevation of both levels suggests kidney failure or disease.

Indications

- To assess kidney function and aid in diagnosing conditions listed under ''Deviations from Normal'' above.

Contraindications

- None.

Procedure

1. Following standard venipuncture technique, one or two red-top tubes of blood is drawn.
2. A pressure or pressure dressing is applied to the puncture site.

Nursing implications

1. Observe the puncture site for bleeding or hematoma.

PLASMA RENIN ACTIVITY

Normal Values

- Adults (upright position); sodium depleted; peripheral vein: ages 20 to 39, 2.9 to 24 ng/ml/h; >40, 2.9 to 10.8 ng/ml/h.
- Adults (upright position); sodium replete; peripheral vein: ages 20 to 39, 0.1 to 4.3 ng/ml/h; >40, 0.1 to 3 ng/ml/h.

Deviations from Normal

- An increased aldosterone level with a decreased renin activity occurs with primary hyperaldosteronism.
- Pregnancy and several drugs (e.g., oral contraceptives, antihypertensives, vasodilators) and certain foods (e.g., licorice) affect renin levels.
- Elevated renin levels may occur in essential hypertension, malignant and renovascular hypertension, Addison's disease, cirrhosis, hypokalemia, hemorrhage, and renin-producing renal tumors (Bartter's syndrome).
- Decreased levels are associated with salt-retaining steroid therapy and antidiuretic hormone therapy.

Indications

- To use with a measurement of plasma aldosterone level (p. 173) in the differential diagnosis of primary versus secondary hyperaldosteronism.
- To detect essential, renal, or renovascular hypertension.

Contraindications

- A pregnant client (pregnancy affects renin levels).
- A client using drugs that affect renin levels (e.g., antihy-

pertensives, L-dopa, estrogens, diuretics, and vasodilators) because the results will be inaccurate.

Procedure
Client preparation

1. The client is kept on the prescribed pretest diet, usually a normal diet with a restricted amount of sodium (approximately 3 g/day) for 3 days prior to the test. A high sodium diet causes a renin decrease.
2. The client must discontinue diuretics or oral contraceptives, antihypertensives, vasodilators, and licorice as ordered. These can all affect the plasma renin levels.
3. Prior to the test the client is positioned as ordered. The upright position is usually ordered; for this have the client stand or sit upright for the 2 hours before the test.
4. If a recumbent sample is ordered, have the client remain in bed until the blood sample is collected. A change from the recumbent to the upright position increases renin secretion.

Procedure

1. Usually a fasting blood sample is drawn because renin values are higher in the morning.
2. The lavender-top collection tube (containing EDTA) is chilled prior to withdrawing the blood sample to prevent renin breakdown.
3. Pressure or a pressure dressing is applied to the venipuncture site.
4. After the blood is drawn, the tube is gently inverted and then placed on ice.
5. Record the client's position and the time of the day on the lab slip. Note any medications that the client may be currently taking.

Nursing implications

1. Usually allow the client to resume a normal diet after the test.
2. Usually reorder medications discontinued prior to the test.
3. After puncture, assess the site for bleeding or hematoma.

Urine Tests
CREATININE CLEARANCE TEST

Normal Values

- Men: 95 to 104 ml/min.
- Women: 95 to 125 ml/min.

Deviations from Normal

- The level may be decreased in renal artery atherosclerosis, dehydration, or shock.
- Most primary renal diseases (e.g., glomerulonephritis and acute tubular necrosis) cause a decreased creatinine clearance level.
- Long-standing obstruction to urinary outflow causes decreased levels.

Indications

- To assess renal function and aid in diagnosing the conditions listed under "Deviations from Normal" above.

Contraindications

- None.

Procedure
Client preparation

1. The client is told to collect the urine for an entire 24-hour period. The client is shown where to store the urine specimen.
2. The 24-hour urine specimen for creatinine does not need refrigeration.

Procedure

1. The 24-hour collection period begins after the client urinates.
2. The starting time is indicated on the urine container or lab slip. The first sample is discarded.
3. The nurse makes sure that all urine the client passes during the next 24 hours is collected. Test results are calculated

on the basis of a 24-hour output, and results will be inaccurate if any specimens are missed. If one voided specimen is accidentally discarded, the 24-hour collection usually must begin again.

4. A venous blood sample is drawn in a red-top tube during the 24-hour collection period for a serum creatinine level test (see p. 181).

5. The last specimen is collected as close as possible to the end of the 24-hour period. The client is reminded when the last sample is needed.

6. The time of the last specimen is indicated on the lab slip or urine container.

Nursing implications

1. Post the hours for the urine collection on the client's door, bedpan hopper, and in the utility room to prevent accidental discarding of a specimen.

2. Remind the client to void before defecating so that the urine is not contaminated by feces. Remind him or her also not to place toilet paper in the collection container.

3. Encourage the client to drink fluids during the 24-hour period unless this is contraindicated for medical purposes.

TWENTY-FOUR-HOUR URINE TEST FOR VANILLYLMANDELIC ACID AND CATECHOLAMINES

Normal Values

VMA

- 1 to 9 mg/24 h.

Catecholamines

- Epinephrine: 5 to 40 µg/24 h.
- Norepinephrine: 10 to 80 µg/24 h.
- Metanephrine: 24 to 96 µg/24 h.
- Normetanephrine: 75 to 375 µg/24 h.

Deviations from Normal

- In clients with pheochromocytoma, one or all of the above substances will be present in excessive quantities in a 24-hour collection of urine.

- Elevated VMA and catecholamine levels also appear in neuroblastomas, ganglioneuromas, and ganglioblastomas.
- Severe stress, strenuous exercise, and acute anxiety can cause elevated catecholamine levels.

Indications

- To diagnose hypertension secondary to pheochromocytoma.

Contraindications

- None.

Procedure
Client preparation

1. When VMA levels are being measured, the client is kept on a VMA restricted diet for 2 or 3 days before the 24-hour urine collection. Although dietary restrictions may vary with labs, the restricted foods usually include coffee, tea, bananas, chocolate, cocoa, licorice, citrus fruits, all foods and fluids containing vanilla, and aspirin. (Note: catecholamine levels require no dietary preparation.)
2. As ordered, the client is kept off antihypertensive medications (or all medications) for 2 to 3 days prior to the collection.
3. The procedure is explained to the client. The client is shown where to store the urine specimen. The 24-hour urine specimen for VMA requires a preservative.

Procedure

1. See "Procedure" for 24-hour urine collection under the "Creatinine Clearance Test" (p. 181), except for "Client Preparation" step no. 2 and "Procedure" step no. 3.

Nursing implications

1. After the 24-hour collection for VMA is completed, allow the client to have the foods and drugs that had been restricted in preparation for the test.
2. Excessive physical exercise and emotion can alter catecholamine test results by causing an increased secretion of epinephrine and norepinephrine. Therefore identify and minimize factors contributing to client stress and anxiety.

URINALYSIS

pH: indicates the acid-base balance.

Appearance: normally clear.

Color: indicates the concentration of the urine and varies with the specific gravity.

Odor: normally aromatic from the presence of volatile acids.

Specific gravity: measure of the concentration of particles in the urine; high specific gravity indicates concentrated urine; low specific gravity indicates dilute urine.

Protein: normally not present in the urine because it is too large to pass through spaces in the glomerular filter membrane.

Blood: enters the urine upon the disruption of the blood-urine barrier.

Casts: clumps of material or cells.

Crystals: indicate imminent renal stone formation.

pH
Normal values

- 4.6 to 8.0 (6.0 average).

Deviations from normal

- Alkademia (alkaline pH) results from bacteruria, urinary tract infection (caused by *Pseudomonas* or *Proteus* organisms), or a diet high in fruits and vegetables.
- Acidemia (acid urine) results from metabolic or respiratory acidosis, starvation, diarrhea, or a diet high in meat protein or cranberries.

Appearance
Normal values

- Clear.

Deviations from normal

- The presence of pus, red blood cells, or bacteria may cause cloudy urine as may the ingestion of certain foods (e.g., large amounts of fat), urates, or phosphates.

Color
Normal values

- Amber yellow.

Deviations from normal

- Abnormally colored urine can result from a pathologic condition (e.g., bleeding from the kidneys produces dark red urine; bleeding from the urinary tract produces bright red urine). Dark yellow urine may indicate the presence of urobilinogen or bilirubin. *Pseudomonas* organisms usually produce a green urine. Certain foods and medicines alter urine color (e.g., beets can cause a red urine; rhubarb can cause the urine to be brown colored). Many commonly used drugs can affect the urine color (see Table 6-1).

Odor
Normal values

- Aromatic.

Deviations from normal

- The urine of clients in diabetic ketosis has a severe smell of acetone. Infected urine has an unpleasant odor.

Specific Gravity
Normal values

- 1.005 to 1.030 (usually 1.010 to 1.025).

Deviations from normal

- The specific gravity is *increased* in clients with the following conditions: dehydration, pituitary tumor that causes the release of excessive amounts of ADH, a decrease in renal blood flow, glucosuria, and proteinuria.
- The specific gravity is *decreased* in clients with the following conditions: overhydration, diabetes insipidus, and chronic renal failure.

Protein (Albumin)
Normal values

- Up to 8 mg/dl.

Table 6-1 Commonly used drugs that can affect urine color

Generic Drug Name (Brand Name)	Drug Classification	Urine Color
Anisindione (Miradon)	Oral anticoagulant	Red-orange in alkaline urine
Cascara	Stimulant laxative	Red in alkaline urine
		Yellow-brown in acid urine
Chloroquine (Aralen)	Antimalarial	Rusty yellow or brown
Chlorzoxazone (Paraflex)	Skeletal muscle relaxant	Orange or purple-red
Danthron (Modane)	Stimulant laxative	Pink or red in alkaline urine
Dioctyl Calcium	Laxative	Pink to red to red-brown
Sulfosuccinate (Doxidan, Surfak)		
Furazolidone (Furoxone)	Anit-infective, antiprotozoal	Brown
Iron preparations (Ferotran, Imferon)	Hematinic	Dark brown or black on standing
Levodopa	Antiparkinsonian	Dark brown on standing
Methylene blue (Urolene blue)	Antimethemoglobinemic	Blue-green
Nitrofurantoin (Macrodantin, Nitrodan)	Antibacterial	Brown
Phenazopyridine (Pyridium)	Urinary tract analgesic	Orange to red
Phenindione (Eridione)	Anticoagulant	Red-orange in alkaline urine
Phenolphthalein (Ex-Lax)	Contact laxative	Red or purplish pink in alkaline urine
Phenothiazines (example: Compazine)	Antipsychotic, neuroleptic, antiemetic	Red-brown
Phenytoin (Dilantin)	Anticonvulsant	Pink, red, red-brown
Riboflavin (vitamin B)	Vitamin	Intense yellow
Rifampin	Antibiotic	Red-orange
Sulfasalazine (Azulfidine)	Antibacterial	Orange-yellow in alkaline urine
Triamterene (Dyrenium)	Diuretic	Pale blue fluorescence

Deviations from normal

- The presence of protein in the urine can indicate glomerulonephritis or preeclampsia in pregnant women.

Glucose
Normal values

- None.

Deviations from normal

- Elevated glucose levels occur in diabetic clients who are not
well controlled with hypoglycemic agents.
- Intravenous (IV) administration of dextrose-containing
fluids produce artificially high glucose levels.
- Central nervous system disorders (e.g., stroke), Cushing's
syndrome, severe stress, infection, and certain drugs (e.g.,
ascorbic acid, aspirin, keflin, epinephrine, and streptomy-
cin) can cause elevated glucose levels.

Ketones
Normal values

- None.

Deviations from normal

- Elevated ketone levels occur in poorly controlled diabetes
(most often in juvenile diabetes). Nondiabetic clients suf-
fering from dehydration, starvation, and excessive aspirin
ingestion may also have elevated levels.

Blood
Normal values

- Up to 2 red blood cells (RBC).

Deviations from normal

- Blood cells enter the urine with glomerulonephritis, renal
trauma, or tumor. Pathologic conditions involving the mucosa of the collecting system (e.g., tumor or infection) will
cause hematuria (blood in the urine).

Microscopic examination

- Normal values: RBC, 1 to 2 at low-power field; WBC, 0 to 4 at low-power field; casts, negative or occasional hyaline; crystals, negative; bacteria, none.

Deviations from normal

- Red blood cells (RBCs): 5 cells indicate microscopic hematuria.
- White blood cells (WBCs): 5 cells indicate a urinary tract infection.
- Casts: White blood cell casts (clumps of WBCs indicate pyelonephritis). Red blood cell casts indicate glomerulonephritis. Hyaline casts are conglomerations of protein and signal proteinuria.

Crystals

- Urate crystals occur in clients with high serum acid levels (gout).
- Phosphate and calcium oxalate crystals occur in the urine of clients with hyperparathyroidism or malabsorption states.

Bacteria

- The presence of bacteria indicates urinary tract infection.

Indications

- To provide a tentative diagnosis.
- To indicate the need for further studies.
- To monitor the progression of a disorder (e.g., diabetes mellitus).

Contraindications

- None.

Procedure

Client preparation

1. If relevant, the client is given the proper specimen jars and necessary cleaning agents. Most hospitals use commercial kits for a clean-catch specimen; these contain all the necessary equipment and provide directions for obtaining the specimen.

2. For collecting a specimen for culture, the nurse determines if the client is capable of obtaining the urine specimen himself or herself. If not, assistance is given.

Procedure

1. If possible, the first voided specimen of the day is obtained because it is usually more concentrated than other specimens.
2. The client or nurse should wash the client's perianal area if it is soiled with feces.
3. Collection methods:
   a. Routine urinalysis specimen: The client voids into a clean bedpan, urinal, or urine container.
   b. Clean catch or midstream specimen: (1) The client (or nurse) meticulously cleans the perineal area or penis with an iodine preparation to reduce specimen contamination by external organisms; (2) the cleaning agent is completely removed to avoid contaminating the specimen; (3) the client begins to urinate and then stops—this urine is discarded; (4) the client voids 3 to 4 oz of urine into a sterile urine container; (5) the container is capped, and the client finishes voiding.
   c. Indwelling urinary catheter: Clients unable to void may require urinary catheterization, although because of the risk of infection and the client's discomfort, this procedure is rarely performed. (1) The nurse attaches a small-gauge needle to a syringe and aseptically inserts the needle into the catheter at a point distal to the sleeve leading to the balloon; (2) the nurse aspirates urine and places it in the urine container; (3) usually 15 to 30 minutes before aspiration the nurse clamps the catheter tubing distal to the puncture site to allow urine to fill the tubing. After collection, the nurse removes the clamp.
   d. U-bag collection: used for collecting urine specimens from infants and small children. (1) The nurse or parent attaches the bag, which has an adhesive backing, to the child.
   e. Suprapubic aspiration in neonates and infants: (1) The nurse prepares the child's abdomen with an antiseptic;

(2) the nurse then inserts a no. 25-gauge needle (attached to a 5 cc syringe) into the suprapubic area, 1 inch above the symphysis pubis; (3) next the nurse aspirates urine into the syringe and transfers it to a sterile urine container.

   f. Composite urine specimens: collected over 2 to 24 hours and used to examine for specific components (e.g., electrolytes). (1) To begin the test the client voids and discards the urine; (2) the client saves all subsequent urine for the designated time; (3) at the end of the time the client urinates and adds this urine to the collection container.

4. If the specimen cannot be tested immediately, cover and refrigerate it. Refrigeration may reduce the bacterial cell proliferation and retard deterioration of casts and cells. The pH of uncovered specimens will become alkaline because CO_2 will diffuse into the air.

5. If the client is menstruating, indicate this on the lab slip. Hematuria will then be discounted.

6. Typically the nurse analyzes the urine for pH, protein, glucose, ketones, and blood by using a Multistix reagent strip. The nurse should read the directions on the bottle or package insert and follow the directions precisely. The color reaction must be compared with the manufacturer's color chart at the *exact* time specified.

Test	When to Read Results	Range of Results
pH	Anytime	5-9
Protein	Anytime	Negative- +4 (>2000 mg/dl)
Glucose	10 sec (qualitative)	Negative- +4
	30 sec (quantitative)	Negative- +4 (2%)
Ketones	15 sec	Negative- +3 (large)
Blood	25 sec	Negative- +3 (large)

7. After removing the dipstick from the bottle, close the bottle tightly to prevent the stick's absorbing moisture and altering future results. Check the expiration date on the bottle before use.

Nursing implications

1. Inform the client that toilet paper or feces should not be placed in the urine container. This would contaminate the specimen.

Radiologic Laboratory Tests

X-Ray Tests
NEPHROTOMOGRAPHY
Normal Values

- Diffusely normal kidney.

Deviations from Normal

- The presence of solid renal and adrenal tumors.

Indications

- To differentiate solid renal and adrenal tumors from benign renal cysts.

Contraindications

- See "IVP," p. 193.

Procedure

1. See "IVP" (p. 193) and "Computerized Tomography of the Kidney" (p. 205).

PYELOGRAPHY
Antegrade Pyelography
Normal values

- Normal outline, size, and position of the ureters and bladder.

Deviations from normal

- See "Retrograde Pyelography," p. 196.

Indications

- To localize ureteral obstruction caused by stricture, non-opaque stone, or tumor.
- To evaluate ureteral obstruction after a urinary diversion operation.
- Ureteropelvic and ureterovesical obstruction in a child with hydronephrosis who has poor opaque excretion.

Contraindications

- None.

Procedure

1. The client is placed in a prone position. The renal pelvis is localized by ultrasound or by fluoroscopy.
2. Skin overlying the desired site is marked and prepared.
3. Under local anesthesia the skin is incised, and a 1.5-inch no. 14-gauge needle with a stylet is inserted its full length toward the renal pelvis.
4. With the client suspending respiration, a no. 20-gauge thin-walled biopsy needle with a stylet is advanced through the needle into the lumen of the renal pelvis.
5. Contrast medium is injected to outline the upper collecting system to the point of obstruction below.
6. Posteroanterior, oblique, and anteroposterior x-ray films are taken.
7. Antibiotic drugs are usually recommended for several days afterward because of the instrumentation above the ureteral obstructed area.
8. A radiologist or urologist performs this study in less than 1 hour in the radiology department.

Nursing implications

1. After the test, apply a small pressure dressing to the incisional site. Assess the site for bleeding.
2. Because the kidney is a highly vascular area, check the vital signs frequently, as ordered.

Intravenous Pyelography (IVP; Excretory Urography)
Normal values

- Normal size, shape, and position of the kidneys, renal pelvis, ureters, and bladder.

Deviations from normal

- Glomerulonephritis.
- Tumors (benign or malignant) or benign renal cyst.
- Intrinsic tumors (Fig. 6-1) or stones.
- Retroperitoneal and pelvic tumors, aneurysms, and enlarged lymph nodes can also produce extrinsic compression.
- Renal hematomas.
- Renal artery laceration.
- Lacerations of the kidney, pelvis, ureters, and bladder.

Indications

- To assess the effects of trauma to the urinary system.
- To assess congenital absence or malposition of kidneys.
- To aid in diagnosing conditions listed under ''Deviations from Normal'' above.

Contraindications

- A client allergic to shellfish or iodinated dyes and not properly prepared beforehand with prednisone and diphenhydramine (see ''Nurse Alert'' and ''Procedure'').
- A severely dehydrated client, unless appropriate measures have been taken (see ''Nurse Alert'').

Procedure
Client preparation

1. The client is told that the dye injection often causes flushing of the face, a feeling of warmth, and a salty taste in the mouth. The effects are transitory.
2. The client is given cathartics or strong laxatives (e.g., castor oil), as ordered, on the evening before the test.
3. If ordered, a suppository or enema is given the morning of the study.

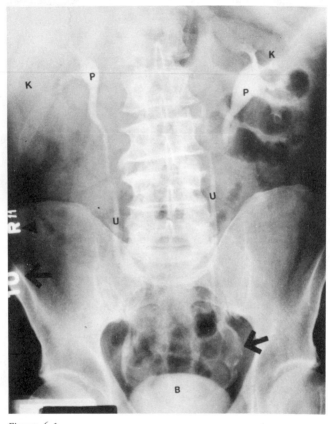

Figure 6-1
Intravenous pyelogram. Black arrow at right indicates a left
ureteral tumor. *K,* kidney; *P,* renal pelvis; *U,* ureter; *B,*
bladder. Note black arrow at left indicating that x-ray film
was taken 10 minutes after injection of dye. The *R* on left
side of picture indicates right side of patient.

4. The client is kept on nothing by mouth after midnight the day of the test. Moderate dehydration is necessary for the concentration of the contrast dye within the urinary system. The oral fasting time in infants and children will vary and will be ordered specifically for each child. The oral fasting time for elderly and debilitated clients will also vary according to the client.

5. Before the study the client is assessed for allergy to iodine dye. If the client has a history of allergy to iodine dye, administer, as ordered, the prednisone (5 mg, four times a day) and diphenhydramine (25 mg, four times a day), as ordered, for 3 days before and 3 days after the study.

Procedure

1. A plain x-ray film of the client's abdomen is taken to ensure that no residual stool exists that may obscure visualization of the renal system.

2. Skin testing for iodine allergy is often performed.

3. A peripheral IV line (scalp vein in an infant) is started of contrast dye (Hypaque or Renografin).

4. Larger doses of dye can be given by an IV infusion drip (called *infusion drip pyelography* or *drip-infusion IVP*).

5. X-ray films are taken at specified times, usually at 1, 5, 10, 15, 20, and 30 minutes, and sometimes longer. The films follow the dye course from the cortex of the kidney to the bladder. Tomograms may be taken to identify a mass.

6. The client is then taken to the bathroom and asked to void.

7. A postvoiding film is taken to assess bladder emptying.

8. Occasionally occluding the ureters temporarily is necessary to achieve a better fill of the collective system and the upper part of the ureters. This is done by compressing the abdomen with an inflatable rubber tube wrapped tightly around the abdomen slightly below the umbilicus.

9. The radiologist performs this study in the radiology department in approximately 45 minutes.

Nursing implications

1. Assess the IV site for infiltration by the contrast agent.
2. After the dye injection, look for signs and symptoms of anaphylaxis (e.g., respiratory distress, shock, and drop in blood pressure). Have emergency drugs (diphenhydramine, steroids, epinephrine) and equipment (oxygen and endotracheal equipment) on hand for immediate use in the event of anaphylaxis.
3. After the procedure, allow the client to resume a normal diet. Encourage fluids to counteract the fluid depletion caused by the preparation for this test.
4. After the study, assess the elderly and debilitated client for fasting-induced weakness. Encourage bed rest and ambulation only with assistance.

Nurse alert

1. Complications of IVP include the following:
   a. Allergic reaction varying from mild flush and urticaria to severe, life-threatening anaphylaxis. The reaction is treated with diphenhydramine (Benadryl), steroids, and epinephrine.
   b. Infiltration of the contrast agent. Being certain of the patency of the IV line avoids this complication. The treatment of this infiltration is elevation of the extremity and warm soaks.
   c. Renal shutdown and failure. This occurs most frequently in the elderly client who is dehydrated before the dye injection. The treatment is supportive care. Assuring adequate hydration in these clients prevents this occurrence.

Retrograde Pyelography
Normal values

- Normal outline and size of the ureters and bladder.

Deviations from normal

- Tumors, benign strictures, stones, and extrinsic compression.

Indications

- To examine the ureters in clients for whom IVP visualization is inadequate.
- To rule out ureteral obstruction as a cause of unilateral kidney disease.
- To demonstrate ureter lesions more adequately than IVP can.

Contraindications

- None.

Procedure
Client preparation

1. See "Cystoscopy," p. 208.

Procedure

1. See "Cystoscopy," p. 209.
2. The urologist performs the study in the radiology department in approximately 1 hour.

Nursing implications

1. See "Cystoscopy," p. 209.
2. The necessity for catheterization to inject the dye makes the study uncomfortable for the client.

RENAL ANGIOGRAPHY (RENAL ARTERIOGRAPHY)
Normal Values

- Normal renal vasculature.

Deviations from Normal

- Abnormal renal vasculature.
- Transection of the renal artery.

Indications

- To evaluate renal blood flow dynamics.
- To demonstrate abnormal blood vessels.
- To differentiate primary renal cysts from tumors.

■ To demonstrate the angiographic location of stenosis of the renal artery when vascular surgery is being considered.

Contraindications

■ A client with dye allergies.
■ A client with atherosclerosis.
■ An unstable client.
■ A pregnant client.
■ A client with a bleeding disorder.

Procedure

Client preparation

1. The client is told where the catheter will be inserted (usually the femoral artery). The client is informed that he or she will feel a warm flush when the dye is injected. Verbalization of the client's feelings regarding angiography is encouraged. This test is frightening for most clients.
2. The client is assessed for allergies to iodine dye. If allergies exist, the physician is notified, who may order an antiallergy regimen (see "Cardiac Catheterization," p. 13).
3. The client is kept on nothing by mouth after midnight on the day of the study.
4. Cathartics are administered as ordered.
5. The preprocedure medications are administered as ordered (usually meperidine and atropine).
6. The client voids before this study because the dye acts as an osmotic diuretic.

Procedure

1. The client is placed in the supine position on an x-ray table.
2. Access to the renal arteries is usually achieved through the femoral artery.
3. The catheter is passed into the femoral artery and advanced into the aorta.
4. With fluoroscopic visualization (motion picture x-ray images displayed on a television monitor), the catheter is manipulated into the renal artery.

5. Dye is injected and x-ray films are taken in timed sequence over several seconds. This allows all portions of the injection to be photographed.
6. Delayed films may be taken to visualize subsequent filling of the renal vein.
7. After the x-ray films are taken, the catheter is removed and a pressure dressing is applied to the puncture site.
8. An angiographer performs this study in the radiology department in approximately 1 hour.

Nursing implications

1. After the procedure, observe the arterial puncture site frequently for hematoma, hemorrhage, or absence of pulse.
2. Assess the extremity for signs of ischemia (numbness, tingling, pain, absence of peripheral pulses, and loss of function).
3. Compare the color and temperature of the extremity with those of the uninvolved extremity.
4. Assess the pulses and vital signs frequently (every 15 minutes for four times, then every 30 minutes for four times, then every hour for four times, and then every 4 hours) because embolism or bleeding requires immediate intervention. Notify the physician of any abnormalities.
5. Keep the client on bed rest for 12 to 24 hours after the procedure.
6. Apply cold compresses to the puncture site if these are needed to reduce discomfort and swelling.
7. Force fluids after the study to prevent diuretic-induced dehydration caused by the dye.

Nurse alert

1. An anaphylactic reaction to the iodine dye is a potential complication (see ''Cardiac Catheterization,'' p. 15).
2. An atherosclerotic plaque may be dislodged from the aorta and travel to any abdominal organ or to the legs. Organ ischemia and infarction may be the result.
3. Persistent hemorrhage from the puncture site used for arterial access may occur.

VOIDING CYSTOURETHROGRAPHY (VOIDING CYSTOGRAM)

Normal Values

- Normal bladder structure and function.

Deviations from Normal

- Bladder tumors.
- Extrinsic compression or distortion of the bladder occurs with pelvic tumors.
- Hematomas.
- Traumatic rupture of the bladder.
- Vesicoureteral reflux.

Indications

- To diagnose conditions listed in ''Deviations from Normal'' above.
- To allow study of the urinary tract in children and adults with recurrent urinary tract infections.

Contraindications

- An unstable or uncooperative client.
- A client with urethral or bladder infection or injury.

Procedure
Client preparation

1. Because embarrassment may inhibit the client's ability to urinate on command, the client is assured that draping will prevent unnecessary exposure.
2. The client receives clear liquids for breakfast on the day of the examination.
3. If the client has a large amount of residual urine, the client voids or is catheterized to avoid bladder distention.

Procedure

1. The client is placed in the lithotomy or supine position.
2. Unless one is already in place, a catheter is placed through the urethra and into the bladder.

3. Through the catheter, approximately 300 cc of air or radi-opaque dye (much less for children) is injected into the bladder and the catheter clamped.
4. X-ray films are taken.
5. If the client is able to void, the catheter is removed and the client is asked to void.
6. Further x-ray films are then taken.
7. The radiologist performs this study in the radiology department in 15 to 30 minutes.

Nursing implications

1. Following the study, assess the client for signs of urinary tract infection.

X-RAY STUDY OF THE KIDNEYS, URETERS, AND BLADDER (KUB)

Normal Values

- No evidence of abnormality.

Deviations from Normal

- Tumor, malformations, and calculi (Fig. 6-2).

Indications

- To demonstrate the size, shape, and location of the kidneys, bladder, and ureters.
- To aid in diagnosing tumors, malformations, and calculi in these organs.

Contraindications

- A pregnant client.

Procedure

1. The client is placed in the supine position with the arms extended overhead.
2. X-ray films are taken of the client's lower abdomen.
3. An upright KUB film may be ordered if better visualization is needed.

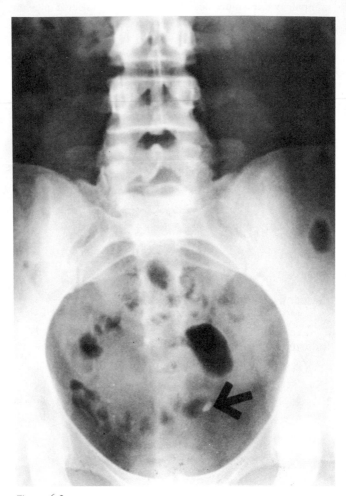

Figure 6-2
KUB. Plain film of the abdomen demonstrating abnormalities
in the kidneys, ureters, and bladder. Arrow indicates
radiopaque calcified stone in the left ureter.

4. Usually a technician takes the x-ray in the radiology department in a matter of minutes.

Nursing implications

1. The KUB should be taken before IVP or GI studies.
2. The technician should place a lead shield over the male client's gonads to prevent irradiation of the testes. The female ovaries cannot be shielded because of their proximity to the organs being studied.

Nuclear Scanning
RENAL SCANNING (KIDNEY SCAN, RADIORENOGRAPHY, RADIONUCLEOTIDE RENAL IMAGING, NUCLEAR IMAGING OF THE KIDNEY)

Normal Values

- Normal size, shape, and kidney function.

Deviations from Normal

- Renal infarction.
- Renal arterial atherosclerosis.
- Trauma.
- Kidney transplant rejection.
- Glomerulonephritis or acute tubular necrosis.
- Tumors, abscesses, or cysts.

Indications

- To detect renal infarctions, renal arterial atherosclerosis, or renal trauma.
- To monitor rejection of a transplanted kidney.
- To detect primary renal disease, tumors, abscesses, or cysts.
- To detect pathologic renal conditions in patients who cannot have IVP because of dye allergies.

Contraindications

- A pregnant client.

Procedure
Client preparation

1. The client is assured that he or she will not be exposed to large amounts of radioactivity because only tracer doses of isotopes are used. The radioactive substance is usually excreted from the body within 6 to 24 hours.

Procedure

1. A peripheral IV injection of a radionucleotide is given.
2. While the client assumes a supine, prone, or sitting position, a gamma-ray detecting device is passed over the kidney area. It records the radioactive uptake on either x-ray or Polaroid film.
3. The client must lie still during the study.
4. A nuclear medicine technologist performs the study in the nuclear medicine department in 1 to 4 hours, depending on the information required.

Nursing implications

1. Unless contraindicated, fluids are encouraged to aid in the dye excretion from the body via the urine.

Computerized Tomography Tests
COMPUTERIZED TOMOGRAPHY OF THE KIDNEY (CT OF THE KIDNEY)
Normal Values

■ No evidence of abnormality.

Deviations from Normal

■ Tumors, cysts, obstructions, calculi, and congenital anomalies.

Indications

■ To diagnose pathologic renal conditions.

Procedure
Client preparation

1. See "CT of the Abdomen," p. 95.
2. The client receiving a dye administration is kept on nothing by mouth for 4 hours before the test.

Procedure

1. See "CT of the Abdomen," p. 95.

Nursing implications

1. See "CT of the Abdomen," p. 96.

Nurse alert

1. Acute renal failure can be a complication of dye infusion. Adequate hydration before the procedure may reduce the chances of this occurring.

Special Studies

Cystometry
Normal Values

- Maximum cystometric capacity: men range from 350 to 750 ml; women range from 250 to 550 ml.
- Intravesical pressure when bladder is empty usually <40 cm H_2O.
- Detrusor pressure <10 cm H_2O.

Deviations from Normal

- Abnormalities as listed below under "Indications."

Indications

- To elucidate the cause (neurologic, infectious, obstructive disease) for frequency and urgency, especially before surgery on the outflow tract of the kidney.
- To evaluate for the following: incontinence, persistent residual urine, vesico-ureteric reflex, neurologic disorders, sensory disorders, and the effect of certain drugs on bladder function.

Contraindications

- A client with urinary tract infection because false readings may result and because of the potential for pyelonephritis and septic shock.

Procedure
Client preparation

1. Many clients are embarrassed by this procedure. Nursing personnel should assure them that they will be draped to ensure privacy. The client is told that throughout the study any sensations such as pain, flushing, sweating, nausea, bladder filling, and an urgency to void should be reported.
2. The client is assessed for signs and symptoms of urinary tract infection, which would make the examination contraindicated because of possibility of false results and the potential for the spread of infection.
3. The client is instructed not to strain while voiding because this might cause the results to be skewed.
4. If the client has a spinal cord injury, he or she should be transported to the test on a stretcher. The test will then be performed with the client on the stretcher.

Procedure

1. The test begins with the client being asked to void.
2. The following are recorded: the amount of time required to initiate voiding; the size, force, and continuity of the urinary stream; the amount of urine; the time of voiding; and the presence of any straining, hesitancy, and terminal urine dribbling.
3. The client is then placed in a lithotomy or supine position.
4. A retention catheter is inserted through the urethra and into the bladder. (The catheter can also be inserted suprapubically.)
5. Residual urine volume is measured and recorded.
6. Thermal sensation is evaluated by the installation of approximately 30 ml of room temperature sterile saline or water into the bladder followed by an equal amount of

warm water. The client reports any sensations experienced.

7. This fluid is then withdrawn from the bladder.
8. Usually with the client sitting, the urethral catheter is connected to a cystometer (a tube used to monitor bladder pressure), and sterile water, normal saline, or carbon dioxide gas is slowly introduced into the bladder at a controlled rate.
9. The client is then asked to indicate the first urge to void and the feeling when voiding is necessary.
10. The pressures and volumes are plotted on a graph.
11. The client is then asked to void, and the maximal intravesical voiding pressure is recorded.
12. The bladder is then drained for any residual urine.
13. A urologist performs the test in the urologist's office or in a special procedure room.

Nursing implications

1. After the test, a warm sitz bath or tub bath may be comforting to the client.
2. After the cystometry, observe the client for any manifestations of infection (such as elevated temperature or chills) that could indicate sepsis.
3. After the test, examine the urine for hematuria. Notify the physician if the hematuria persists after several voidings.

Cystoscopy

Normal Values

- Normal structure and function of the urethra, bladder, prostate, and ureters.

Indications

- Diagnostically to allow (1) direct inspection and removal of biopsy specimens of the prostate, bladder, and urethra for tumor determination; and (2) collection of separate urine specimens directly from each kidney by the placement of ureteral catheters.

- Measurement of bladder capacity and evidence of ureteral reflux (1) for identification of bladder and ureteral calculi; (2) for placement of urethral catheters for the performance of retrograde pyelography (see p. 197); and for identification of the source of hematuria.
- Therapeutically to permit resection of small tumors, removal of foreign bodies and stones, dilatation of the urethra and ureters, placement of catheters to drain urine from the renal pelvis, coagulation of bleeding areas, and implantation of radium seeds into a tumor.

Contraindications

- An unstable client.

Procedure
Client preparation

1. The client is told that the cystoscope is inserted into the bladder in the same manner as a Foley catheter. The client is encouraged to verbalize fears, and emotional support is provided. The study is uncomfortable under local anesthesia.
2. If enemas are ordered to clear the bowel, the client is assisted as needed and the results are recorded.
3. If the procedure will be performed with the client under *local anesthesia*, a liquid breakfast may be given. Fluids are encouraged to provide urine samples as needed and to prevent stasis of urine in the event that bacteria are introduced during cystoscopy.
4. If the procedure will be performed with the client under *general anesthesia* (usually children and uncooperative or overly anxious adults), routine anesthesia precautions are followed.
5. The client is kept on nothing by mouth after midnight. Fluids may be given intravenously.
6. The preprocedure medications (usually diazepam [Valium] or meperidine) are administered, as ordered, 1 hour before the study. In addition to reducing anxiety, the sedatives decrease the spasm of the bladder sphincter, thus decreasing the client's discomfort. Deep-breathing exercises can also minimize spasms.

Procedure

1. The client is placed in the lithotomy position with his or her feet in the stirrups.
2. The client is instructed to lie still during the procedure to avoid urinary tract trauma.
3. The external genitalia are cleaned with an antiseptic solution (e.g., povidone-iodine [Betadine]).
4. Local anesthetic is instilled into the urethra.
5. The client will have the desire to void as the cystoscope passes the bladder neck.
6. When the procedure is completed, the client remains on bed rest for a short time.
7. The urologist performs the study in the hospital cystography room or in the urologist's office. The procedure requires about 25 minutes.

Nursing implications

1. Do not allow the client to stand or walk alone immediately after the legs are removed from the stirrups.
2. Assess the client's ability to void for at least 24 hours after the procedure. Urinary retention may be secondary to edema caused by instrumentation. If urinary retention does occur, an indwelling catheter may need to be inserted.
3. Record the urine color and test the urine for blood. Pink-tinged urine is common. Report the presence of bright-red blood and clots to the physician.
4. The client may complain of back pain, bladder spasms, urinary frequency, and burning upon urination. Warm sitz baths and mild analgesics may be ordered and given. Sometimes belladonna and opium (B & O) suppositories are given to relieve bladder spasms. Warm, moist heat to the lower abdomen may help relieve pain and promote muscle relaxation.
5. Encourage increased intake of fluids.
6. Check and record the client's vital signs as ordered.
7. Observe for signs and symptoms of sepsis (elevated temperature, flush, chills, decreased blood pressure, and increased pulse).
8. Occasionally antibiotics are ordered 1 day before and 3 days following the procedure.

Nurse alert

1. Complications of cystoscopy include hematuria, perforation of the bladder, and sepsis by seeding the bloodstream with bacteria from infected urine.
2. Following the study, monitor clients for a decrease in blood pressure indicating hemorrhage.
3. Observe for signs of sepsis (elevated temperature, flush, chills, decreased blood pressure, and increased pulse).

Endourology
Normal Values

- No abnormalities of the bladder and urethra.

Deviations from Normal

- Infection.
- Stricture, neoplasia, and prostatic hypertrophy.

Indications

- To evaluate hematuria, chronic infection, suspected stone, and radiographic filling defects.

Contraindications

- See "Cystoscopy," p. 208.

Procedure

1. See "Cystoscopy," p. 208.

Pelvic Floor Sphincter Electromyography (Pelvic Floor Sphincter EMG)
Normal Values

- Increased EMG signal during bladder filling.
- Silent EMG signal on voluntary micturition.
- Increased EMG signal at end of voiding.

Deviations from Normal

- Voiding disturbances.

Indications

- To evaluate external sphincter (skeletal muscle) activity during voiding.
- To evaluate the bulbocavernous reflex and voluntary control of external sphincter or pelvic floor muscles.
- To aid in investigating "functional" or psychologic voiding disturbances.

Contraindications

- An uncooperative client.

Procedure

Client preparation

1. If the client's perianal area is soiled, it is washed before the electrodes are placed.

Procedure

1. Two electrodes (possibly pediatric surface electrocardiographic electrodes) are placed at the 2 and 10 o'clock positions on the perianal skin. These electrodes monitor the pelvic floor muscular activity during voiding.
2. The third electrode is placed on the thigh as a grounding plate.
3. The electrical activity is recorded with the bladder empty and the client relaxed.
4. Reflex activity is recorded by having the client cough and by stimulating the urethra and trigone by gentle tugging of the Foley catheter.
5. Voluntary activity is recorded by having the client contract and relax the sphincter muscle.
6. The client's bladder is filled with sterile room temperature water at 100 ml per minute. EMG responses to filling and detrusor hyperflexia (if present) are recorded.
7. With the client in the voiding position with a full bladder, the filling catheter is removed and the client voids. Electrical waves are recorded.

Nursing implications

1. If needle electrodes were used, after the test observe the needle site for hematoma or inflammation.

Renal Biopsy
Normal Values

- No pathologic conditions found.

Deviations from Normal

- Glomerulonephritis or malignancy.

Indications

- To diagnose the cause of glomerulonephritis (e.g., post-streptococcal, Goodpasture's syndrome, lupus nephritis).
- To diagnose or rule out primary and metastatic malignancy of the kidneys in clients who are not surgical candidates.
- To evaluate the amount of rejection occurring after kidney transplant.

Contraindications

- A client with coagulation disorders.
- A client with operable kidney tumors.
- A client with hydronephrosis.
- A client with infections.

Procedure
Client preparation

1. The client is kept on nothing by mouth after midnight on the day of the biopsy in the event that bleeding necessitates surgical intervention.
2. The results of the client's coagulation studies (prothrombin time and partial thromboplastin time) are checked.
3. The client's hemoglobin and hematocrit values are checked.
4. The client may also be typed and cross-matched for blood in the event of severe hemorrhage requiring transfusions.

Procedure

1. The client is placed in the prone position with a sandbag or pillow under the abdomen to straighten the spine.
2. Under sterile conditions the skin overlying the kidney is infiltrated with a local anesthetic (lidocaine).
3. While the client holds his or her breath to stop kidney movement, the physician inserts the biopsy needle (the type that he or she is most comfortable using) into the kidney and takes a specimen.
4. After this procedure is completed, the needle is removed and pressure is applied to the site for approximately 20 minutes.
5. A pressure dressing is then applied, and the client is turned on his or her back and remains on bed rest for 24 hours.
6. The biopsy specimen is placed in a container filled with a fixative solution and sent to the pathology department for appropriate staining and microscopic review.
7. After the removal of the biopsy specimen, pressure is applied to the site of the needle stick.
8. The physician performs the needle biopsy at the client's bedside in about 10 minutes. If fluoroscopic or ultrasound guidance is used, the surgeon performs the biopsy in the ultrasound or radiology department.

Nursing implications

1. After the biopsy the client is usually kept in the prone position for 20 to 30 minutes. The client is then kept on bed rest for 24 hours. Advise the client to avoid any activity that increases abdominal venous pressure (e.g., coughing).
2. Check the vital signs and puncture site every 15 minutes for the first hour after the needle stick and then with decreasing frequency, as ordered.
3. Assess the client for signs and symptoms of hemorrhage.
4. Evaluate the abdomen for signs of bowel or liver penetration (e.g., abdominal pain and tenderness, abdominal muscle guarding and rigidity, and decreased bowel sounds).

5. Inspect all urine specimens for gross hematuria. Usually the client's urine will contain blood initially, but typically not after the first 24 hours. Place the samples in consecutive chronological order to facilitate comparison for evaluation of hematuria.

6. Encourage the client to drink large amounts of fluid to prevent clot formation and urine retention. (However, an oliguric client in renal failure could develop pulmonary edema with increased fluid intake.)

7. Frequently the nurse will need to draw peripheral venous blood for a hemoglobin and hematocrit determination 8 hours after removal of the biopsy specimen to assess for active bleeding.

8. Instruct the client to avoid, for at least 2 weeks, strenuous activities.

9. Teach the client the signs and symptoms of renal bleeding and instruct him or her to call the nurse or physician if any of these symptoms occur.

10. Instruct the client to report burning on urination or temperature elevation that could indicate a urinary tract infection.

Renal Ultrasonography (Kidney Sonogram)
Normal Values

- Normal size, shape, and position of the kidneys.

Deviations from Normal

- Tumors and pelvic calculi.

Indications

- To locate renal cysts.
- To differentiate renal cysts from solid renal tumors.
- To demonstrate renal or pelvic calculi.
- To guide a percutaneously inserted needle for cyst aspiration or removal of a biopsy specimen.

Contraindications

- A client who has recently had barium contrast studies unless he or she has received adequate cathartics.

Procedure

1. The nonfasting, unsedated client is placed on the ultrasonography table in a prone position.
2. The ultrasonographer (usually a radiologist) applies a greasy conductive paste to the client's back to enhance sound transmission and reception.
3. A transducer is then passed over the skin, and pictures are taken of the reflections.
4. The ultrasonographer, usually a radiologist, performs this study in the ultrasound or radiology department in about 20 minutes.

Nursing implications

1. If the client's abdomen appears distended or if the client has recently had a barium study, this test should be cancelled.
2. After the procedure, remove the coupling agent (grease) from the client's back. The ultrasonographer applies it to aid conduction.

Renal Vein Assays for Renin
Normal Values

- Renin ratio of involved kidney to uninvolved kidney <1.4.

Deviations from Normal

- Renal artery stenosis.

Indications

- To diagnose renovascular hypertension.

Contraindications

- A client allergic to iodine dye.

Procedure
Client preparation

1. See "Renal Angiography," p. 198.
2. The client is assessed for allergies to iodine.
3. If ordered, the client is kept on a "no added salt" diet and diuretics for 3 days prior to the examination.
4. The client is kept in the upright position for 2 hours before the test because the renin level is at its maximum when the client is in this position.
5. The preprocedure medications (meperidine and atropine) are administered as ordered, usually 1 hour before the procedure.

Procedure

1. The client is placed on the fluoroscopy table in the supine position.
2. The client's groin is prepared and draped in a sterile manner and then anesthetized.
3. The femoral vein is punctured, and a catheter is placed into the vein and advanced into the inferior vena cava.
4. Fluoroscopy is used to monitor the catheter placement.
5. Dye is injected and the renal veins are identified.
6. The catheter is placed into one renal vein at a time, and separate blood specimens are withdrawn.
7. Usually a radiologist performs this procedure in the radiology department in approximately 1 hour.

Nursing implications

1. After the procedure, assess the client for bleeding. Check the client's urine for blood.
2. Assess the client for renal vein thrombosis, which may occur 1 to 7 days after the procedure. This will be manifested by costovertebral angle (CVA) tenderness, hematuria, and elevated creatinine levels.
3. Be sure that the blood specimens, obtained via catheter from each renal vein, are correctly labeled.

Split Renal Function Studies
Normal Values

- Equal volume, osmolality, and concentrations of sodium and creatinine in both kidneys.

Deviations from Normal

- Renal artery stenosis.

Indications

- To diagnose renal artery stenosis.

Contraindications

- See "Cystoscopy," p. 208.

Procedure
Client preparation

1. See "Cystoscopy," p. 208.

Procedure

1. See "Cystoscopy," p. 209.
2. The urine catheters and specimens must be correctly labeled.
3. The specimens are transported to the lab as soon as the test is completed.

Nursing implications

1. See "Cystoscopy," p. 209.

Ultrasound-Guided Cyst Aspiration Study
Normal Values

- No evidence of abnormality.

Deviations from Normal

- Evidence of abnormality indicating tumor.

Indications

- To diagnose a cystic tumor.

Contraindications

- None.

Procedure
Client preparation

1. See "Renal Ultrasonography," p. 215.

Procedure

1. The ultrasonographer and urologist perform this procedure in approximately 30 minutes in the ultrasound or radiology department.

Nursing implications

1. See "Renal Ultrasonography," p. 215.

Urethral Pressure Measurements (Urethral Pressure Profile)
Normal Values

- Maximum urethral pressures in normal patients (cm H_2O):

Age	Male	Female
<25	37-126	55-103
25-44	35-113	31-115
45-64	40-123	40-100
>64	35-105	35-75

Deviations from Normal

- Abnormal pressure measurements resulting from prostatic obstruction, stress incontinence, incompetent external sphincter, and drug therapy.

Indications

- To assess prostatic obstruction and postprostatectomy problems.
- To assess stress incontinence in females.
- To assess the adequacy of external sphincterotomy and the adequacy of implanted artificial urethral sphincter devices.

- To analyze the effects of drugs on the urethra and the effects of stimulation on urethral flow.

Contraindications

- A client with a urinary tract infection.

Procedure
Client preparation

1. Many clients are embarrassed by this procedure and are reassured when told they will be draped to ensure privacy.

Procedure

1. A catheter is passed into the bladder and withdrawn slowly through the urethra.
2. Fluids (or gas) are instilled through the catheter that is withdrawn while the pressures along the urethral wall are obtained.
3. A motorized pump maintains a constant infusion of the fluids or gas.
4. The catheter is removed and the test is completed in fewer than 15 minutes.
5. A urologist performs this study in about 15 minutes in the urologist's office or special study room.

Nursing implications

1. After the study a warm bath or sitz bath may be comforting to the client.

Urine Flow Studies (Uroflometry)
Normal Values

- Depend on the patient's age, sex, and volume voided.

Age	Minimum vol (ml)	Male (ml/sec)	Female (ml/sec)
4-13	100	>10-12	>10-15
14-45	200	>21	>18
46-65	200	>12	>15
66-80	200	>9	>10

Deviations from Normal

- Abnormalities as listed under "Indications."

Indications

- To investigate dysfunctional voiding.
- To investigate suspicious outflow tract obstruction.
- To assess the outflow tract of the kidney before and after any procedure designed to modify its function.

Contraindications

- None.

Procedure

Client preparation

1. The nurse ensures that the client knows how to void into the urine flowmeter and that the client has privacy during voiding.
2. The nurse determines the number of flow rates that will be needed. If a series of flow rates will be needed, this procedure is explained to the client.

Procedure

1. The test is performed when the client has a normal desire to void and the bladder is adequately full (200 to 400 ml).
2. The client's position, the method of filling the bladder (preferably natural), and whether this study is part of another evaluation are recorded. Uroflometry is usually the first of the urodynamic investigations performed.

Nursing implications

1. If urine samples are needed for another test, the client should void separately for them.
2. If the flow rates are abnormally low, the test should be repeated to check for accuracy.
3. If flowmeters are not available, the client can time the urinary stream with a stopwatch and record the voided volume. From this the average flow is calculated.

Bibliography

Abrams, P., Feneley, R., and Torrens, M.: Urodynamics, New York, 1983, Springer-Verlag.

Abvelo, J.G.: Proteinuria: diagnostic principles and procedures, Ann. Intern. Med. **98:**186, 1983.

Aiken, C., Sokeland, J., and Engel, R.: Urology: guide for diagnosis and therapy, New York, 1982, Georg Thieme Verlag.

Anthony, C.P., and Thibodeau, G.A.: Textbook of anatomy and physiology, ed. 11, St. Louis, 1983, The C.V. Mosby Co.

Barrett, D.M., and Wein, A.J.: Flow evaluation and simultaneous external sphincter electromyography in clinical urodynamics, J. Urol. **125:**538-541, 1981.

Boh, D.M., and VanSon, A.R.: The water-load test, Am. J. Nurs. **82**(1):112-113, Jan. 1982.

Brenner, B.M., Humes, H.D., and Milford, E.L.: Urinary tract obstruction. In Petersdorf, R.G., and others, editors: Harrison's principles of internal medicine, ed. 10, New York, 1983, McGraw-Hill Book Co.

Brunner, L.S., and Suddarth, D.S.: Textbook of medical-surgical nursing, ed. 5, Philadelphia, 1984, J.B. Lippincott Co.

Fischbach, F.: A manual of laboratory diagnostic testing, ed. 2, Philadelphia, 1984, J.B. Lippincott Co.

Govoni, L.E., and Hayes, J.E.: Drugs and nursing implications, ed. 4, Norwalk, Conn., 1982, Appleton-Century-Crofts.

Hargiss, C.O., and Larson, E.: How to collect specimens and evaluate results, AJN **81**(12):2166-2174, Dec. 1981.

Jamison, R.L., and Oliver, R.E.: Disorders of urinary concentration and dilution, Am. J. Med. **72:**308, 1982.

Larson, E., Lindbloom, L., and Davis, K.B.: Development of the clinical nephrology practitioner, St. Louis, 1982, The C.V. Mosby Co.

Malseed, R.T.: Pharmacology: drug therapy and nursing considerations, Philadelphia, 1982, J.B. Lippincott Co.

Marie, S.M.: Assessing the excretory system, AORN J. **33**(4):734-756, March 1981.

Mayo, M.E.: Value of sphincter electromyography in urodynamics, J. Urol. **122:**357-360, 1979.

McConnell, E.A.: Urinalysis: a common test, but never routine, Nursing '82 **12**(2):108-111, Feb. 1982.

Mellins, H.Z.: Radiology of the urinary tract: urography and cystourethrography. In Harrison, J.H., and others, editors: Campbell's urology, ed. 4, vol. 1, Philadelphia, 1978, W.B. Saunders Co.

Phipps, W.J., Long, B.C., and Woods, N.F., editors: Medical-surgical nursing: concepts and clinical practice, St. Louis, 1983, The C.V. Mosby Co.

Rakel, R.E.: Conn's current therapy, Philadelphia, 1984, W.B. Saunders Co.

Schottelius, B.A., and Schottelius, D.D.: Textbook of physiology, ed. 19, St. Louis, 1983, The C.V. Mosby Co.

Schulman, C.C.: Advances in diagnostic urology, New York, 1981, Springer-Verlag.

Sherman, R.A., and Byun, K.J.: Nuclear medicine in acute and chronic renal failure, Semin. Nucl. Med. **12:**265, 1982.

Shovlin, M.: Radionuclide screening for renovascular hypertension, J. Nucl. Med. **21:**104, 1980.

Smeltzer, S.C.: Disorders of the urinary system. In Beyers, M., and Dudas, J., editors: The clinical practice of medical-surgical nursing, Boston, 1984, Little, Brown & Co.

Endocrine System

7

Clinical laboratory tests
  Blood tests
    Antithyroglobulin antibody test (thyroid-auto-antibody)
    Antithyroid microsomal antibodies (antimicrosomal antibody test, microsomal antibody)
    Cortisone administration test (Dent test)
    Free thyroxine index (FTI)
    Growth hormone stimulation tests
    Growth hormone suppression test
    Long-acting thyroid stimulation (LATS)
    Serum calcium test (total serum calcium)
    Serum growth hormone (GH), RIA
    Serum parathyroid hormone (PTH, parathormone test)
    Serum thyroxine (T_4) test
    Serum triiodothyronine (T_3) test
    T_3 resin uptake (RT_3U) test
    Thyroid-stimulating hormone (TSH) test (thyroid stimulation test)
    TSH stimulation test (thyroid stimulation test)
    TSH suppression test (thyroid suppression test)
    Thyrotropin-releasing hormone test (TRH test)
    Thyroxine-binding globulin (TBG) test
    Water deprivation tests
  Urine tests
    Urine calcium
Radiologic laboratory tests
  Nuclear scanning tests
    Prolactin RIA (PRL, lactogenic hormone, luteotrophin, mammotropin)
    Radioactive iodine uptake (RAIU) test
    Thyroid scanning (thyroid scintiscan)

Special studies
  Ultrasound examination of the thyroid (thyroid echogram)
Adrenal glands
  Clinical laboratory tests
    Blood tests
      Adrenocorticotropic hormone stimulation test (ACTH stimu-
        lation test)
      Dexamethasone suppression test (prolonged/rapid)
      Metyrapone test
      Serum adrenocorticotropic hormone (ACTH) test
      Plasma cortisol test
    Urine tests
      Urine tests for 17-hydroxycorticosteroids and 17-ketosteroids
  Radiologic laboratory tests
    X-ray tests
      Adrenal angiography
      Adrenal venography
      X-ray study of the sella turcica
    Computerized tomography tests
      Computerized tomography of the adrenal glands (CT scan of
        the adrenals)
Endocrine glands
  Clinical laboratory tests
    Blood tests
      Glucose tolerance test (GTT, oral glucose tolerance test,
        OGTT)
      Glycosylated hemoglobin (HbA$_{1c}$, glycohemoglobin)
      Plasma insulin assay
      Serum glucose test
      Serum osmolality test
      Two-hour postprandial glucose test (2-hour PPG, 2-hour post-
        prandial blood sugar, 2-hour PPBS)
    Urine tests
      Urine test for glucose and acetone (urine S & A; fractional
        urine)
      Serum phosphate (phosphorus) concentration test

Clinical Laboratory Tests

Blood Tests
ANTITHYROGLOBULIN ANTIBODY TEST (THYROID-AUTO-ANTIBODY)

Normal Values

- Titer <1:100.

Deviations from Normal

- A high antibody level may indicate such thyroid diseases as Hashimoto's thyroiditis and thyroid cancer.
- Increased antithyroglobulin antibodies are also seen with rheumatoid-collagen disease, pernicious anemia, thyrotoxicosis (Graves' disease), and lupus erythematosus.

Indications

- To aid in the differential diagnosis of thyroid diseases (e.g., Hashimoto's thyroiditis and cancer of the thyroid).

Contraindications

- None.

Procedure

1. Following standard venipuncture technique, approximately 3 to 5 ml of blood are collected in a red-top tube.
2. Pressure or a pressure dressing is applied to the venipuncture site.

Nursing implications

1. Assess the venipuncture site for bleeding.

ANTITHYROID MICROSOMAL ANTIBODIES (ANTIMICROSOMAL ANTIBODY TEST; MICROSOMAL ANTIBODY)

Normal Values

- Titer <1:100 (present in 5% to 10% of healthy people).

Deviations from Normal

- Elevated titers indicate Hashimoto's thyroiditis.
- Elevated titers also appear in patients with myxedema, thyroid carcinoma, granulomatous thyroiditis, lupus erythematosus, rheumatoid arthritis, autoimmune hemolytic anemia, and nontoxic nodular goiter.

Indications

- To aid in diagnosing Hashimoto's thyroiditis.

Contraindications

- None.

Procedure

1. Following standard venipuncture technique, 2 to 5 ml of blood are collected in a red-top tube.
2. Pressure or a pressure dressing is applied to the puncture site.

Nursing implications

1. Assess the venipuncture site for bleeding.

CORTISONE ADMINISTRATION TEST (DENT TEST)
Deviations from Normal

- Lowered serum levels indicate that hyperparathyroidism is not causing the client's hypercalcemia. Causes may be sarcoidosis, vitamin D intoxication, or bone metastasis.
- No change in the serum level indicates hyperparathyroidism.

Indications

- To differentiate the hyperparathyroid client from the client with hypercalcemia resulting from other causes.

Contraindications

- None.

Procedure
Client preparation

1. The client is assured that no complications result from the 10-day administration of cortisone. The importance of the client's maintaining his or her usual diet is stressed.
2. The cortisone acetate is administered orally with milk or with an antacid (if ordered) to protect the client from gastric irritation.

Procedure

1. A baseline calcium level determination is obtained before the test by following standard venipuncture technique.
2. A second calcium level determination is obtained after the 10-day cortisone course (see "Serum Calcium Test," p. 230).
3. Pressure or a pressure dressing is applied to the puncture sites.

Nursing implications

1. Assess the venipuncture sites for bleeding.

FREE THYROXINE INDEX (FTI)
Normal Values

- 0.9 to 2.3 ng/dl.

Deviations from Normal

- High FTI calculations suggest hyperthyroidism.
- Low FTI values suggest hypothyroidism.

Indications

- To diagnose hyperthyroidism and hypothyroidism, especially in clients with abnormalities in thyroxine binding protein levels.
- To evaluate the thyroid status of pregnant women and clients being treated with certain drugs (e.g., estrogen, phenytoin, salicylates) who have abnormal TBG levels.

Contraindications

■ None.

Procedure

1. See "T$_3$ Uptake and T$_4$ Tests," pp. 234 and 235.

GROWTH HORMONE STIMULATION TESTS

Growth hormone stimulation tests include the insulin tolerance test (ITT) and the growth hormone provocation test. These are two of several stimulation tests used to increase the pituitary's production of growth hormone, which is the primary growth hormone in the normal growth of children.

Normal Values (ITT)

■ Consistent rise in GH levels to over 20 ng/ml in conjunction with a decrease in blood glucose to less than 40 mg/dl, or less than 50% basal fasting level.
■ Pediatric: children may have no response, although the GH level is adequate. The combination of ITT and arginine as a stimulation test is the most definitive test for GH deficiency in children.
■ Normal response to use of arginine: GH level rises to 7 ng/ml.

Deviations from Normal

■ Increased GH response is found with hyperthyroidism and starvation (in arginine test).
■ Decreased GH response is found with cirrhosis, diabetes mellitus, hypothyroidism, obesity.

Indications

■ To assist with differential diagnosis of dwarfism and small stature.
■ To obtain information about the reserve capacity of GH. Although the GH level may be normal, the pituitary may not be capable of producing more GH when needed, such as with the stress of surgery.

Contraindications

- ITT is contraindicated in clients with ischemic heart disease, myocardial infarction, cerebrovascular disease, epilepsy, and low basal plasma cortisol levels.

Procedure
Client preparation

1. The procedure and purpose of the study are explained.
2. Fluids and food are withheld for 8 hours prior to the test.

Procedure

1. Following standard venipuncture procedure, a red-top tube of blood is drawn as a basal sample for glucose, cortisol, and GH.
2. Pressure is applied to the site.
3. An intravenous line is started if one is not already in place.
4. Insulin is given intravenously per physician's orders.
5. A red-top tube of blood is drawn every 15 minutes for the first hour, and every 30 minutes for the next 2 hours.

Nursing implications

1. Observe venipuncture sites for bleeding.
2. Closely monitor the client for signs and symptoms of hypoglycemia (e.g., dizziness, fainting, sweating, chest pain).

Nurse alert

1. Stop the test immediately if serious signs or symptoms of hypoglycemia occur.
2. Notify the physician.

GROWTH HORMONE SUPPRESSION TEST
See ''Glucose Tolerance Test,'' p. 268.

LONG-ACTING THYROID STIMULATION (LATS)
Normal Values

- Normally LATS does not appear in serum.

Deviations from Normal

- LATS appears in the serum of some hyperthyroid clients.
- LATS may appear in neonates whose mothers have Graves' disease.

Indications

- To evaluate clients with thyroid disease, especially clients with malignant exophthalmos and Graves' disease.

Contraindications

- None.

Procedure

Client preparation

1. The client is assessed to learn if he or she has had radio-active iodine within the past 2 days. Radioactive iodine in the blood may affect test results.

Procedure

1. Following standard venipuncture technique, approximately 5 ml of venous blood are collected in a red-top tube.
2. Pressure or a pressure dressing is applied to the venipuncture site.
3. The sample is sent to the lab for analysis. The lab is notified if the client has received ^{131}I within the past 2 days.

Nursing implications

1. Handle the blood sample gently. Hemolysis may interfere with test result interpretation.
2. Assess the venipuncture site for bleeding or hematoma.

SERUM CALCIUM TEST (TOTAL SERUM CALCIUM)

Normal Values

- 9.0 to 10.5 ng/dl (total).

Deviations from Normal

- Elevated serum calcium levels on three separate tests indicate hypercalcemia caused by metastatic tumor to the bone, hyperparathyroidism, nonparathyroid PTH-producing tumors (such as lung and renal carcinomas), vitamin D intoxication, sarcoidosis, and excessive ingestion of concentrated milk or calcium-containing antacids.

■ Thiazide diuretics may cause hypercalcemia by impairing the urinary excretion of calcium.

■ A serum parathormone blood level determination differentiates this condition from hyperparathyroidism (Fig. 7-1). Low levels indicate hypocalcemia, which occurs in clients who have hypoparathyroidism (usually following parathyroid surgery) and in clients with renal failure or rickets.

Indications

■ To evaluate parathyroid function and calcium metabolism.

Contraindications

■ None.

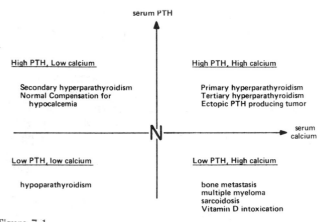

DIFFERENTIAL DIAGNOSIS USING CONCOMITANT SERUM PARATHORMONE
AND SERUM CALCIUM ASSAYS

serum PTH

High PTH, Low calcium

Secondary hyperparathyroidism
Normal Compensation for
   hypocalcemia

High PTH, High calcium

Primary hyperparathyroidism
Tertiary hyperparathyroidism
Ectopic PTH producing tumor

N — serum calcium

Low PTH, low calcium

hypoparathyroidism

Low PTH, High calcium

bone metastasis
multiple myeloma
sarcoidosis
Vitamin D intoxication

Figure 7-1
Graph showing various disease entities associated with concomitantly abnormal PTH and calcium levels. *N*, normality, which is marked by eucalcemia and a normal PTH level.

Procedure

Client preparation

1. The client is told if fasting is required for multichannel determinations.
2. The client is assessed for concurrent use of thiazide diuretics, which can cause hypercalcemia.

Procedure

1. Following standard venipuncture procedure, approximately 7 ml of blood are collected in a red-top tube.
2. Pressure or a pressure dressing is applied to the puncture site.

Nursing implications

1. Assess the puncture site for bleeding.

SERUM GROWTH HORMONE (GH); RIA

Normal Values

- Normal values of GH fluctuate throughout the day. A consistent secretion usually occurs during sleep.
- Adult: 0 to 8 ng/ml.
- Child: 0 to 10 ng/ml.

Deviations from Normal

- Increased secretion of GH is associated with adult acromegaly, bronchogenic cancer, gastric cancer, gigantism in children, infants with psychosocial deprivation syndrome, exercise, stress, sleep, ingestion of high levels of protein, L-dopa medication use, and increased levels of human placental lactogen in pregnant women.
- Decreased secretion of GH is associated with pituitary dwarfism in children, older children with psychosocial deprivation syndrome, ingestion of a glucose lead hyperglycemia, and doses of glucocorticoid.

Indications

- Serum GH measurement is used to assist in the diagnosis of disorders listed under ''Deviations from Normal'' as well as secreting pituitary tumors and idiopathic pituitary deficiencies.

Procedure

Client preparation

1. The procedure and purpose of the test are explained.
2. Fluids and food are withheld 8 hours before the test begins.
3. If ordered, the client is kept on bed rest for 30 minutes prior to drawing blood.
4. Following standard venipuncture procedure, a red-top tube of blood is drawn.
5. Pressure is applied to the site.

Nursing implications

1. Observe the venipuncture site for bleeding.

SERUM PARATHYROID HORMONE (PTH; PARATHORMONE TEST)

Normal Values

- <2,000 pg/ml.

Deviations from Normal

- Increased levels occur in clients with hyperparathyroidism or nonparathyroid, ectopic, PTH-producing tumors (as in lung and kidney carcinoma) or as a normal compensatory response to hypocalcemia in clients with renal failure or vitamin D deficiency (Fig. 7-1).
- Decreased levels appear in clients with hypoparathyroidism (mostly resulting from surgery) or as an appropriate response to hypercalcemia in clients with metastatic bone tumors, sarcoidosis, vitamin D intoxication, or milk-alkali syndrome (Fig. 7-1).

Indications

- To aid in the diagnosis of conditions listed under "Deviations from Normal" above.

Contraindications

- None.

Procedure
Client preparation

1. The client is kept on nothing by mouth (except water) after midnight the day of the study.

Procedure

1. Following standard venipuncture technique, the blood is drawn as required by the lab performing the PTH analysis.
2. If ordered, a serum calcium level determination is obtained at the same time. The serum PTH and serum calcium levels are important in differential diagnosis.
3. Pressure or a pressure dressing is applied to the venipuncture site.
4. Often the lab will then send the sample to a commercial lab for analysis by radioimmunoassay.

Nursing implications

1. Observe the venipuncture site for bleeding.
2. The client may eat after the specimen is drawn.

SERUM THYROXINE (T_4) TEST
Normal Values

- Murphy-Pattee: neonate, 10.1 to 20.0 µg/dl; 1 to 6 yrs, 5.6 to 12.6 µg/dl; 6 to 10 yrs, 4.9 to 11.7 µg/dl; 10 yrs, 4 to 11 µg/dl.
- Radioimmunoassay: 5 to 10 µg/dl.

Deviations from Normal

- Greater than normal levels indicate hyperthyroid states (e.g., Graves' disease, Plummer's disease, or toxic thyroid adenoma).
- Subnormal values appear in hypothyroid states (e.g., cretinism or myxedema).
- Elevated levels occur in pregnant clients and those taking oral contraceptives.

Indications

- To test thyroid function and diagnose conditions listed above.
- To detect hypothyroidism in infants.

Contraindications

- None.

Procedure
Client preparation

1. The client is evaluated to determine if she is pregnant or taking any oral contraceptives, since these conditions will alter serum thyroxine concentrations. The client also is assessed to learn if she is taking exogenous thyroxine medication, since this will affect the results. The physician is notified of any findings that may necessitate cancelling the study.

Procedure

1. Following standard peripheral venipuncture technique, one red-top tube of blood is collected.
2. For newborns, the standard procedure for a heel stick is followed to collect blood.
3. Pressure or a pressure dressing is applied to the puncture or stick site.
4. The sample is sent to the lab for analysis by either the Murphy-Pattee method or by radioimmunoassay.

Nursing implications

1. Observe the puncture site for bleeding.

SERUM TRIIODOTHYRONINE (T_3) TEST
Normal Values

- 110 to 230 ng/dl.

Deviations from Normal

- A T_3 level below normal indicates the client is in a hypothyroid state.

Indications

- To aid in diagnosing hypothyroidism.
- To aid in identifying hyperthyroidism, particularly in the client with a normal T_4 level (p. 234) but with the symptoms of hyperthyroidism.

Contraindications

- None.

Procedure

Client preparation

1. The client is assessed to learn if he or she is taking exogenous triiodothyronine medication, since this will affect the results.

Procedure

1. Following standard peripheral venipuncture technique, one red-top tube of blood is collected.
2. Pressure or a pressure dressing is applied to the puncture site.

Nursing implications

1. Observe the puncture site for bleeding.

T_3 RESIN UPTAKE (RT_3U) TEST

Normal Values

- 25% to 35%.

Deviations from Normal

- Increases or decreases in TBG and TBPA.

Indications

- To accurately assess the client's thyroid status.

Contraindications

- None.

Procedure

1. Following standard venipuncture technique, one red-top tube of blood is collected.
2. Pressure or a pressure dressing is applied to the venipuncture site.

Nursing implications

1. Assess the venipuncture site for bleeding.

THYROID-STIMULATING HORMONE (TSH) TEST (THYROID STIMULATION TEST)

Normal Values

- 1 to 4 μU/ml.
- Neonates <25 μIU/ml by 3 days of age.

Deviations from Normal

- TRH and TSH levels are elevated in primary hypothyroid states (e.g., surgical or radioactive thyroid ablation, burned-out thyroiditis, thyroid agenesis, congenital cretinism) or in taking antithyroid medications.
- Plasma levels of TRH and TSH are near zero in secondary hypothyroidism because the function of the hypothalamus or pituitary is faulty (because of tumor, trauma, or infarction) and TRH and TSH cannot be secreted.

Indications

- To detect primary hypothyroidism in newborns who have low screening T_4 levels.
- To differentiate pituitary from thyroid dysfunction.
- To distinguish primary from secondary hypothyroidism.
- A decreased T_4 and a normal or elevated TSH level can indicate a thyroid disorder. A decreased T_4 with a decreased TSH can indicate a pituitary disorder.

Contraindications

- None.

Procedure

1. Following standard venipuncture technique, one red-top tube of blood is collected.
2. A heel stick is performed for newborns.
3. Pressure or a pressure dressing is applied to the puncture site.

Nursing implications

1. Assess the venipuncture site for bleeding.

TSH STIMULATION TEST (THYROID STIMULATION TEST)

Normal Values

- Increased thyroid function with administration of exogenous TSH.

Deviations from Normal

- An increase of less than 10% in RAIU or less than 1.5 μg/dl rise in T_4 (or PBI) indicates a "primary" or thyroidal hypothyroid state.
- An RAIU increase of at least 1% or a T_4 level increase of 1.5 μg/dl or more indicates inadequate pituitary stimulation or an intrinsically normal thyroid (i.e., if the client's condition is secondary hypothyroidism).

Indications

- To differentiate "primary" or thyroidal hyperthyroidism from "secondary" or hypothalmic-pituitary hypothyroidism.

Procedure

Client preparation

1. The baseline levels of RAIU or T_4 are obtained as indicated.

Procedure

1. The TSH is administered intramuscularly for 3 days. Usually 5 to 10 units per day are ordered.

2. Using standard venipuncture technique, repeat blood samples are drawn to obtain RAIU and T_4 levels.
3. Pressure or pressure dressings are applied to the puncture sites.

Nursing implications

1. Assess venipuncture sites for bleeding.

TSH SUPPRESSION TEST (THYROID SUPPRESSION TEST)

Normal Values

- A 50% reduction in RAIU in response to T_3 administration.

Deviations from Normal

- Little or no decrease in TSH level indicates autonomous and overactive thyroid function (e.g., Graves' disease, Plummer's disease, or toxic adenomas).

Indications

- To assess whether normal homeostatic mechanisms control thyroid function.
- To aid in diagnosing overactive and autonomous thyroid function (see ''Deviations from Normal'' above).

Contraindications

- None.

Procedure

Client preparation

1. The client is assessed for iodine intake. A high iodine level will invalidate the test results.

Procedure

1. Following standard venipuncture technique, blood for the baseline RAIU or T_4 is drawn before the standard dose of T_3 is administered.
2. The T_3 dose is given orally as ordered for 7 days.

3. A new blood study is performed at the conclusion of this time by using standard venipuncture technique. Blood is collected in a red-top tube.
4. Pressure or a pressure dressing is applied to the puncture sites.

Nursing implications

1. Assess the venipuncture sites for bleeding.

THYROTROPIN-RELEASING HORMONE TEST (TRH TEST)

Normal Values

- Prompt rise in serum TSH to approximately twice the baseline level by 30 minutes after the dose of an IV bolus of TRH. (Response is normally greater in women than in men.)

Deviations from Normal

- Slight or no increase in TSH level occurs in hyperthyroidism.
- With secondary hypothyroidism (anterior pituitary failure) no TSH response occurs.
- A delayed rise in TSH indicates hypothyroidism (hypothalamic failure). Multiple injections of TRH may be needed to induce the appropriate TSH response in this case.
- Certain conditions (e.g., psychiatric primary depression, acute starvation) and medication therapy (aspirin, levodopa, or adrenocorticosteroids) depress TSH response to TRH.
- A blunted TSH response occurs in the majority of clients with primary depression.

Indications

- To aid in the detection of primary, secondary, and tertiary hypothyroidism.
- To differentiate primary from manic-depressive psychiatric illness and from secondary types of depression.

Contraindications

- None.

Procedure

Client preparation

1. The specific protocol for carrying out this test is obtained from the lab.
2. The client is assessed for medications that he or she is currently taking. Thyroxine, antithyroid drugs, estrogens, corticosteroids, or levodopa can modify the TSH response.

Procedure

1. The client needs a 500 μg IV bolus of TRH.
2. Blood samples are obtained at intervals by performing the standard venipuncture procedure. The maximum response usually occurs in 20 minutes, and the concentration returns to normal within 2 hours.
3. Pressure or pressure dressings are applied to venipuncture sites.

Nursing implications

1. Assess venipuncture sites for bleeding.
2. Indicate on the lab slip if the client is pregnant because TSH response is increased in pregnancy.

THYROXINE-BINDING GLOBULIN (TBG) TEST
Normal Values

- 12 to 28 μg/ml.

Deviations from Normal

- TBG levels are increased in clients with hypothyroidism.
- Levels are also increased in pregnancy and in clients taking estrogens, oral contraceptives, and long-term perphenazine medications.
- TBG levels may be decreased in clients with hyperthyroidism, nephrotic syndrome, malnutrition with hypoproteinemia, acromegaly, liver disease, uncompensated acidosis, acute stress, or surgical stress.

Indications

- To evaluate abnormal thyroid states not correlating with T_3 or T_4 values because an underlying TBG abnormality makes T_3 and T_4 test results inaccurate.
- To identify TBG abnormalities.

Contraindications

- None.

Procedure
Client preparation

1. The client is assessed for the use of such medications as estrogens, oral contraceptives, and long-term perphenazines, which can elevate TBG levels and skew the test results.

Procedure

1. Following standard venipuncture technique, 2 to 5 ml of blood are collected in a red-top tube.
2. Pressure or a pressure dressing is applied to the puncture site.
3. The sample is sent immediately to the lab for analysis.

Nursing implications

1. Handle the sample gently to prevent hemolysis.
2. Observe the venipuncture site for bleeding.

WATER DEPRIVATION TESTS

Several tests are used to assess antidiuretic hormone (ADH) secretion caused by water deprivation. These include the 24-hour Mosenthal test, the 12-hour Fishberg test, the 14- and 8-hour deprivation tests, and the renal concentration test. Each of these tests involve withholding all fluid intake over a set period of time while checking the client's urine and serum for changes in osmolarity, as well as checking the client for weight loss. Serum osmolarity is an indirect measurement of ADH. At present, serum measurement of ADH is in the research phase.

Normal Values

- Urine osmolarity greater than 800 mOsm/kg of water.
- Urine osmolarity greater than serum osmolarity.
- Serum osmolarity unchanged.

Deviations from Normal

- Nephrogenic diabetes insipidus.
- Neurohypophyseal diabetes insipidus.
- Primary polydipsia.

Indications

- Used to differentiate among possible causes of polyuria.
- Used to assess client's ability to produce ADH.

Contraindications

- None.

Procedure
Client preparation

1. The procedure and purpose of the test is explained, emphasizing that any fluid intake will invalidate the test.

Procedure

1. Following standard venipuncture procedure, one red-top tube of blood is drawn.
2. Pressure is applied to the site.
3. A clean-voided urine specimen is obtained and the amount recorded.
4. All fluids are withheld from the client for the duration of the test.
5. The client's weight is obtained and recorded at the beginning and end of the test and at other times during the test per physician's orders.
6. All urine is collected for the duration of the test.
7. Urine osmolarity is usually checked every hour or per physician's orders.

Nursing implications

1. Observe the venipuncture site for bleeding.
2. Post the hours of the urine collection on the client's door, above the bedpan hopper or in the bathroom, and in the utility room to prevent accidentally discarding the specimen.
3. Remove all fluids from the client's room.
4. Remind the client to void before defecating to avoid contaminating the urine.
5. Remind the client to not place toilet paper in the urine.

Nurse alert

1. Closely monitor the client for signs and symptoms of vascular collapse (e.g., orthostatic hypotension; dizziness; faintness; tachycardia; cold, clammy skin).

Urine Tests
URINE CALCIUM
Normal Values

- Ranges differ according to the client's diet.

Deviations from Normal

- Increased calcium excretion occurs in most clients with primary hyperparathyroidism.
- Hypercalciuria may also occur in clients with the following: idiopathic hypercalciuria, Cushing's syndrome, milk-alkali syndrome, osteoporosis, osteolytic bone disease, renal tubular acidosis, sarcoidosis, or vitamin D intoxication.
- Decreased values indicate hypoparathyroidism, malabsorption disorders, vitamin D deficiency, or dilute urine.

Indications

- To aid in diagnosing conditions listed under "Deviations from Normal" above.

Contraindications

- None.

Procedure
Client preparation

1. The procedure is explained to the client.
2. The nurse learns the specific diet regimen recommended by the performing lab. The client receives a written copy of any dietary restrictions.

Procedure

1. Collect a 24-hour urine specimen following the procedure outlined under ''Creatinine Clearance Test'' (p. 181), except for ''Client Preparation'' step 2 and ''Procedure'' step 3.

Nursing implications

1. See ''Creatinine Clearance Test,'' p. 181.
2. Disagreement exists as to whether the specimen should be collected with the client on a normal diet, a normal diet except for milk products, or a controlled 100 to 200 mg calcium diet. The reference values vary according to the type of diet.

Radiologic Laboratory Tests

Nuclear Scanning Tests
PROLACTIN RIA (PRL; LACTOGENIC HORMONE; LUTEOTROPHIN; MAMMOTROPIN)
Normal Values

- Prolactin increases during sleep and decreases during activity.
- Adult: female, 6 to 30 ng/ml; male, 5 to 18 ng/ml; child, neonate levels are elevated with progressive decrease to normal by 6 weeks of age.

Deviations from Normal

- The PRL is seldom decreased except in the instances of pituitary necrosis or infarction. An increase in PRL is found with amenorrhea, galactorrhea, hypothalmic tumors, and primary pituitary tumors.

Indications

- To assist in the diagnosis of those conditions listed under "Deviations from Normal."

Contraindications

- None.

Procedure

Client preparation

1. The procedure and purpose of the study are explained.

Procedure

1. All food and fluids, except for water, are withheld from the client after midnight the day of (or 8 hours before) the test.
2. The client is asked to stay on bed rest until the test is completed.
3. Following standard venipuncture, one red-top tube of blood is drawn.
4. Pressure is applied to the venipuncture site.

Nursing implications

1. Observe the venipuncture site for bleeding.

RADIOACTIVE IODINE UPTAKE (RAIU) TEST
Normal Values

- 2 hrs: 4% to 12% absorbed by thyroid.
- 6 hrs: 6% to 15% absorbed by thyroid.
- 24 hrs: 8% to 30% absorbed by thyroid.

Deviations from Normal

- Increased thyroid uptake of radioactive iodine occurs in hyperthyroid states. Decreased uptake occurs in hypothyroid conditions.

- If the client is iodine deficient, the uptake will be markedly and falsely increased.
- Rebound thyroid stimulation after discontinuation of suppressive doses of thyroid extract or antithyroid drugs will also falsely increase RAIU.
- The RAIU may be falsely elevated during the last trimester of pregnancy.
- Artificially decreased RAIU levels can occur in clients taking suppressive doses of thyroid extract or antithyroid drugs.
- Likewise previous intake of iodine (e.g., radiopaque dye) will increase the iodine pool and relatively decrease thyroid uptake of the radioactive iodine. Clients with diarrhea will have decreased absorption of tracer doses in the gastrointestinal (GI) tract, thereby decreasing RAIU test results.

Indications

- To assess thyroid function.

Contraindications

- A client who has taken thyroid or antithyroid drugs.
- A client who has had recent x-ray dye studies.
- A pregnant client.
- A client taking exogenous iodine preparations.
- A client who has recently had radioactive studies.

Procedure

Client preparation

1. The client must understand the exact time to return to the lab.
2. The client is assured that the dose of radioiodine used in this test is minute and therefore harmless. No isolation is necessary.
3. The client is questioned concerning the client's intake of iodine or thyroid hormones.
4. The client's intake of large amounts of iodine in food (fish, shellfish), drugs (saturated solution of potassium iodine, Lugol's solution, tolbutamide), antiseptics containing iodine, and iodinated contrast materials used in x-ray

studies is assessed. The client's use of thyroid or antithyroid drugs, TSH, estrogen, or barbiturates is noted. These iodine and thyroid preparations should be restricted for 1 week before testing. The physician is informed of any pertinent findings.

5. The client is advised of restrictions necessary before the study. Some hospitals prefer that the client be in the fasting state before taking the tracer dose. Others require that the client eat only a light breakfast before reporting for the study.

Procedure

1. A tasteless standard dose of radioactive iodine (usually ^{123}I) is given by mouth. If RAIU is to be determined at 2 hours, the iodine must be administered intravenously.
2. The client is then asked to return to the lab anywhere from 2 to 24 hours later (usually 24 hours).
3. When the client returns, a counter is placed over the client who is in the supine position.
4. The amount of radioactive iodine accumulated in the thyroid is calculated. The uptake of the iodine is expressed as a percentage of the thyroid uptake compared with the total of the administered dose.

$$RAIU = \frac{\text{Neck count of patient}}{\text{Standard dose given}} \times 100\%$$

5. A technician performs the study in the nuclear medicine department in approximately 30 minutes following the delay (between 2 and 24 hours) after the iodine ingestion or injection. A physician interprets the results.

Nursing implications

1. The client may eat 45 minutes after taking the tracer dose.

THYROID SCANNING (THYROID SCINTISCAN)
Normal Values

■ Normal size, shape, position, and function of the thyroid gland; no areas of decreased or increased uptake (Fig. 7-2).

Deviations from Normal

- A functioning nodule may represent benign adenoma or localized toxic goiter.
- A nonfunctioning nodule may represent a cyst, carcinoma, nonfunctioning adenoma or goiter, lymphoma, or a localized area of thyroiditis.

Indications

- To determine whether a neck or substernal mass arises from within or outside the thyroid.
- To indicate whether a thyroid nodule is functioning or nonfunctioning. Thyroid cancers are almost always nonfunctioning (cold) nodules.
- To assist in differentiating the two forms of hyperthyroidism: Graves' disease (diffusely enlarged hyperfunctioning thyroid gland) or Plummer's disease (nodular hyperfunctioning gland).
- To evaluate the success of medical treatment for hyperthyroidism.
- To demonstrate a primary thyroid tumor in a client with metastatic tumor without a known primary site.
- To determine areas of metastasis in a client with a well-differentiated form of thyroid cancer.

Contraindications

- See "RAIU," p. 247.

Procedure

1. See "RAIU" procedure.
2. A technician performs the study in the nuclear medicine department in approximately 30 minutes. A physician interprets the results.

Nursing implications

1. See "RAIU," p. 248.

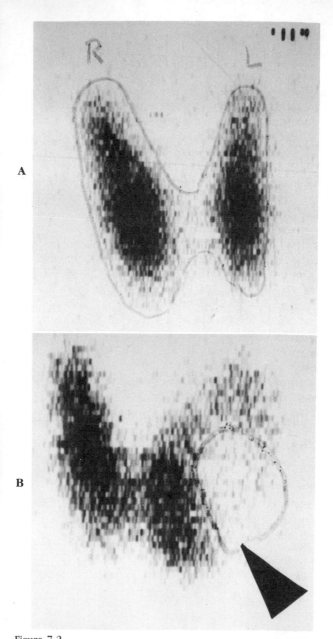

Figure 7-2

A, Normal thyroid scan. **B,** "Cold" area (arrow) on thyroid scan. **C,** "Hot" area (arrow) on thyroid scan.

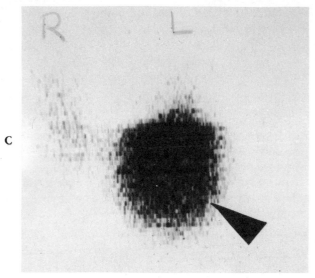

Figure 7-2, cont'd
For legend see opposite page.

Special Studies

Ultrasound Examination of the Thyroid (Thyroid Echogram)

Normal Values

- Normal size, shape, and position of the thyroid.

Deviations from Normal

- Abnormal size, shape, or position may indicate the presence of a cyst or solid nodule.

Indications

- To distinguish a cyst from a solid or mixed nodule, which will probably be cancerous. A cyst can simply be aspirated; carcinoma will probably require surgery.
- To determine the response of a thyroid mass to medical therapy when the test is repeated at intervals.

- To assess thyroid size, shape, and function in a pregnant client because radioactive iodine is harmful to the fetus.

Contraindications

- None.

Procedure
Client preparation

1. The client is assured that no discomfort is associated with this study. The client is told that the placement of the transducer will not affect breathing and swallowing.
2. The client is told that a liberal amount of lubricant will be applied to the neck to ensure effective transmission and reception of the sound waves.

Procedure

1. An ultrasonographer performs the study in the ultrasonography department in approximately 15 minutes.
2. The nonfasting, unsedated client is placed in the supine position.
3. Gel is applied to the client's neck.
4. An ultrasound technician passes a sound transducer over the nodule.
5. Photographs are taken of the image displayed, and these are evaluated by the ultrasound physician.

Nursing implications

1. After the study, help the client remove the lubricant from the neck.

Adrenal Glands

Clinical Laboratory Tests
Blood Tests
ADRENOCORTICOTROPIC HORMONE STIMULATION TEST (ACTH STIMULATION TEST)
Normal Values

- 40 μg/dl after 24-hour infusion.

Deviations from Normal

- An exaggerated response to ACTH stimulation occurs in cushingoid clients with bilateral adrenal hyperplasia.
- Little or no cortisol increase above baseline occurs in clients with hyperfunctioning adrenal tumors.
- In a client suspected of having Addison's disease, a plasma cortisol level between 10 and 40 μg/dl indicates that the adrenal gland is capable of function if stimulated. Thus the cause of adrenal insufficiency lies within the pituitary (hypopituitarism), and the client has secondary adrenal insufficiency.
- In a client suspected of having Addison's disease, little or no rise in the cortisol level indicates that the adrenal gland is capable of secreting cortisol (primary adrenal insufficiency) because of adrenal destruction from hemorrhage, infarction, autoimmunity, metastatic tumor, surgical removal of the adrenals, or congenital adrenal enzyme deficiency.

Indications

- To aid in diagnosing and determining the cause of Addison's disease or Cushing's syndrome.

Contraindications

- None.

Procedure
Client preparation

1. See "Client Preparation" for "Plasma Cortisol Test," p. 260.

Procedure

1. A baseline plasma cortisol level is obtained (see p. 260).
2. An IV infusion of synthetic alpha-ACTH (cosyntropin) in 1 L of normal saline is administered at the rate of 2 units per hour for 24 hours.
3. Peripheral venous blood for plasma cortisol level determination is again obtained 24 hours later and sent to the chemistry lab.

4. This test can also be performed by comparing the baseline urine hydroxysteroid excretion with stimulated hydroxycorticosteroid excretion. In normal clients stimulated hydroxysteroid excretion should exceed 25 mg/day.

5. The ACTH stimulation test can also be performed by administering 25 units of cosyntropin intravenously over an 8-hour period on 2 to 3 consecutive days. The response seen at the end of the second and third 8-hour period should approximate that seen after the continuous 24-hour infusion.

6. For the sake of convenience, a rapid ACTH stimulation test can be performed by giving an intramuscular (IM) injection of 25 units (0.25 mg) of cosyntropin and measuring plasma cortisol levels before and at 30- and 60-minute intervals after drug administration. Normal clients have an increase of cortisol of more than 7 μg/dl above baseline values.

Nursing implications

1. Accurately administer the cosyntropin as ordered. Perform the venipuncture for cortisol level determination or obtain a urine specimen at the exact time indicated.

DEXAMETHASONE SUPPRESSION TEST (PROLONGED/RAPID)

Normal Values

- Prolonged method: low dose, >50% reduction of plasma cortisol and 17-OCHS levels; high dose, >50% reduction of plasma cortisol and 17-OCHS levels.
- Cushing's syndrome: bilateral adrenal hyperplasia—low dose, no change; high dose, >50% reduction of plasma cortisol and 17-OCHS levels. Adrenal adenoma or carcinoma—low dose, no change; high dose, no change. Ectopic ACTH-producing tumor—low dose, no change; high dose, no change.
- Rapid method: nearly zero cortisol levels.

Deviations from Normal

- No reduction in plasma or urinary steroid levels on low-dose dexamethasone suppression indicates Cushing's disease caused by bilateral adrenal hyperplasia.
- In cushingoid clients who have autonomous adrenal tumors, pituitary ACTH will already be suppressed, and the tumor will secrete high levels of cortisol despite the dexamethasone. Therefore no reduction in plasma and urine steroid levels will occur with low-dose dexamethasone suppression. If, however, dexamethasone is administered in high enough doses to a client with adrenal hyperplasia, pituitary ACTH production can be suppressed, and plasma and urinary steroid levels can be expected to fall. In clients, however, with adrenal tumors or ectopic ACTH-producing tumors, still no plasma or urine steroid level reduction will occur even with high-dose suppression.

Contraindications

- None.

Procedure (Prolonged Method)
Client preparation

1. The procedure is explained to the client, who is given ample time to ask questions so that anxiety (stress) is diminished as much as possible. Stress can cause ACTH release and obscure the interpretation of test results.
2. See 24-hour urine collection for "OCHS," "Client Preparation," p. 262.

Procedure

1. The commonly performed classic dexamethasone suppression test is detailed below.

    Day 1: A baseline 24-hour urine test for corticosteroids (urinary 17-OCHS or urinary cortisol) is performed.

    Day 2: Same as day 1.

    Day 3: A low dose (0.5 mg) of dexamethasone is given by mouth every 6 hours, for a total of 2 mg/day. A 24-hour urine test for corticosteroids is performed (as on days 1 and 2).

Day 4: Same as day 3.

Day 5: A high dose (2.0 mg) of dexamethasone is given by mouth every 6 hours, for a total of 8 mg/day. A 24-hour urine test for corticosteroids is performed.

Day 6: Same as day 5.

2. The creatinine content is measured in all 24-hour urine collections to demonstrate the accuracy and adequacy of the collection period.

3. See 24-hour urine collection for ''OCHS,'' ''Procedure,'' p. 262.

4. Note that the urine sample for cortisol and 17-OCHS should not contain a preservative. The specimen is kept refrigerated or on ice during the collection period and is sent to the lab at the end of the 24-hour period.

Nursing implications

1. Administer the dexamethasone orally at the exact time it is ordered, with milk or an antacid (if ordered) to prevent gastric irritation. Administer a hypnotic, if ordered, to assure the client adequate sleep.

2. See pp. 262-263 for the nursing implications for a 24-hour urine collection for 17-OCHS. In studies such as the dexamethasone suppression test, when six continuous 24-hour urine collections are needed, no urine specimens are discarded except for the first one, after which the collection begins.

3. Assess the client for steroid-induced side effects by monitoring the client's weight daily, checking the urine for glucose and acetone, assessing serum potassium levels, and evaluating the client for evidence of gastric irritation.

Procedure (Rapid Method)

Client preparation

1. The study is explained to the client.

2. The client receives 1 mg of dexamethasone by mouth at 11 PM.

3. The client receives a barbiturate to ensure adequate sleep.

Procedure

1. At 8 AM the following morning, the client's cortisol level is determined (see "Plasma Cortisol Test," p. 260).

METYRAPONE TEST

Normal Values

- Baseline excretion of urinary 17-OCHS should be more than doubled.

Deviations from Normal

- Urinary levels of 17-OCHS are markedly increased in clients with adrenal hyperplasia.
- No response (no increase in urinary 17-OCHS levels) occurs to metyrapone in clients whose Cushing's syndrome results from adrenal adenoma or carcinoma.

Indications

- To differentiate adrenal hyperplasia from adrenal tumor by determining whether the pituitary-adrenal feedback mechanism is intact.

Contraindications

- None.

Procedure
Client preparation

1. The client is instructed in collecting the three 24-hour urine specimens needed for the study.
2. See "Client Preparation" for 24-hour urine collection for urinary 17-OCHS.
3. Before this study is performed, a baseline 24-hour urine specimen for 17-OCHS (p. 262) should be collected.

Procedure

1. A 24-hour urine collection for 17-OCHS (p. 262) is also obtained during and again 1 day after the oral administration of 500 to 750 mg of metyrapone, which is given every 4 hours for 24 hours.

Nursing implications

1. Chlorpromazine (Thorazine) interferes with the response to metyrapone and therefore should not be administered during this testing period.
2. See ''Nursing Implications'' for 24-hour collection for urinary 17-hydroxycorticosteroids.

Nurse alert

1. Because metyrapone inhibits cortisol production, assess the client for impending signs of addisonian crisis (muscle weakness, mental and emotional changes, anorexia, nausea, vomiting, hypotension, hyperkalemia, and vascular collapse). Addisonian crisis is a medical emergency that must be treated vigorously. Basically the immediate treatment includes replenishing steroids, reversing shock, and restoring blood circulation.

SERUM ADRENOCORTICOTROPIC HORMONE (ACTH) TEST
Normal Values

- 15 to 100 pg/ml.

Deviations from Normal

- In the client with *Cushing's syndrome,* a pituitary ACTH-producing tumor (rare), or a nonpituitary (ectopic) ACTH-producing tumor (usually in the lung, pancreas, thymus, or ovary) can cause bilateral hyperplasia. ACTH levels >200 pg/ml usually indicate ectopic ACTH production. If the ACTH level is below normal in a cushingoid client, an adrenal adenoma or carcinoma is the most probable cause of the hyperfunction.

- In clients with *Addison's disease,* an elevated ACTH level indicates primary adrenal gland failure (e.g., adrenal gland destruction caused by infarction, hemorrhage, or autoimmunity; surgical removal of the adrenals; congenital enzyme deficiency; or adrenal suppression after prolonged ingestion of exogenous steroids).
- An ACTH level below normal in a client with Addison's disease indicates that hypopituitarism is the most probable cause of the hypofunction.

Indications

- To help determine the cause of Cushing's syndrome or Addison's disease.

Contraindications

- None.

Procedure

Client preparation

1. Because stress of any kind can artificially increase the ACTH level, time should be given to answering the client's questions and providing emotional support.
2. The client is kept on nothing by mouth until the blood sample is drawn.

Procedure

1. Because ACTH levels are lowest at 8 AM and highest in the evening, the fasting blood is drawn between 8 and 10 AM.
2. Following standard venipuncture technique, a chilled, plastic, heparinized syringe is used to collect 20 ml of peripheral venous blood.
3. The blood is placed on ice and sent immediately to the chemistry lab for radioimmunoassay.

PLASMA CORTISOL TEST

Normal Values

- Morning specimen: 6 to 28 μg/dl.
- Afternoon specimen: 2 to 23 μg/dl.

Deviations from Normal

- Individuals with Cushing's syndrome often have top-normal plasma cortisol levels in the morning and do not exhibit a decline as the day proceeds.
- Low levels of plasma cortisol suggest Addison's disease (see "Urine Tests for 17-Hydroxycorticosteroids," p. 261).

Contraindications

- None.

Procedure

Client preparation

1. The procedure is explained to the client to minimize anxiety. Stress will cause elevated levels and complicate test interpretation. The client is observed for signs of physical stress (such as infection or acute illness) or emotional stress. If observed, these are reported to the physician.

Procedure

1. At 8 AM, after the client has adequate sleep, 7 to 10 ml of peripheral blood are obtained in a red-top tube.
2. Pressure or pressure dressing is applied to the puncture site.
3. The sample is usually sent to the chemistry lab for analysis.
4. Usually a second specimen is taken later in the day to identify the normal diurnal variation of the plasma cortisol levels. Although the level is at its nadir at midnight, this is an inconvenient time for the staff, client, and lab. Therefore the blood is obtained in a manner similar to the 8 AM collection at around 4 PM. One would expect the 4 PM value to be one third to two thirds of the 8 AM value.

Normal values may be transposed in individuals who have worked during the night and slept during the day for long periods of time.

Urine Tests
URINE TESTS FOR 17-HYDROXYCORTICOSTEROIDS AND 17-KETOSTEROIDS
Normal Values

- 17-Hydroxycorticosteroids (17-OCHS)
  Men: 5.5 to 15 mg/24 hr.
  Women: 5 to 13.5 mg/24 hr.
  Children: lower than adult values.
- 17-Ketosteroids (17-KS)
  Men: 8 to 15 mg/24 hr.
  Women: 6 to 12 mg/24 hr.
  Children: 12 to 15 yrs: 5 to 12 mg/24 hr.
  Under 12 yrs: <5 mg/24 hr.

Deviations from Normal

- Elevated levels of 17-OCHS appear in clients with hyperfunctioning of the adrenal gland (Cushing's syndrome), whether pituitary or adrenal tumor, bilateral adrenal hyperplasia, or ectopic ACTH-producing tumor causes the condition.
- Low values of 17-OCHS appear in clients with a hypofunctioning adrenal gland (Addison's disease) resulting from destruction of the adrenals (by hemorrhage, infarction, metastatic tumor, or autoimmunity), surgical removal of adrenals without appropriate steroid replacement, congenital enzyme deficiency, hypopituitarism, or adrenal suppression after prolonged exogenous steroid ingestion.
- Elevated 17-KS levels are frequently seen in clients with congenital adrenal hyperplasia and testosterone- or estrogen-secreting tumors of the adrenals, ovaries, or testes.
- Low levels of 17-KS occur in addisonian clients (see above) and in clients who have undergone removal of the ovaries or testes.

Indications

- To assess adrenal cortical function.

Contraindications

- None.

Procedure

Client preparation

1. The client must be told what is expected so that no urine is discarded. Valid interpretation of adrenal function depends on a complete 24 hour urine collection.
2. See pp. 181, "Client Preparation" for the "Creatinine Clearance Test" (except step 2) for 24-hour urine collection.
3. Many drugs can affect the results of these urine tests. Aspirin, acetaminophen, morphine, barbiturates, reserpine, furosemide, and thiazides artificially decrease measurements. Paraldehyde, monoamine oxidase inhibitors, spironolactone, cloxacillin, and licorice artificially raise them. Be certain the client receives none of these during the collection period.

Procedure

1. See "Creatinine Clearance Test," p. 181, except "Procedure" step 3.
2. Urine is collected over a 24-hour period in a 1-gallon urine container. A preservative is necessary for the 17-KS. The urine specimen is refrigerated or kept on ice during the entire collection period.
3. At the end of the collection period, the urine is sent to the chemistry lab, preferably during the 7 AM to 3 PM shift so that it can be evaluated immediately during routine lab working hours. The test is usually performed using a calorimetric technique.

Nursing implications

1. Be certain that none of the drugs mentioned in "Deviations from Normal" above is administered during the col-

lection period. On the lab slip, mention any medications the client is taking.

2. Emotional stress and physical stress (such as infection) may cause increased adrenal activity. These complications will alter the test results. Report any evidence of stress to the physician. In such a case the test should be rescheduled.

3. Encourage the client to take food and fluids during the 24-hour collection period, unless these are contraindicated for medical reasons.

Radiologic Laboratory Tests
X-Ray Tests
ADRENAL ANGIOGRAPHY
Normal Values

- Normal adrenal artery vasculature.

Deviations from Normal

- This technique easily detects both benign and malignant tumors of the adrenals (e.g., pheochromocytomas, adrenal adenomas, and carcinomas).
- Bilateral adrenal hyperplasia can also be seen.

Indications

- To diagnose benign and malignant adrenal tumors and belated adrenal hyperplasia.

Contraindications

- See "Renal Angiography."

Procedure

1. The procedure used in adrenal angiography is similar to that of renal angiography (see pp. 197-199). The only difference is that in adrenal angiography the inferior adrenal artery, a branch of the renal artery, must be cannulated for dye injection.

Nurse alert

1. The major complication of this test is anaphylaxis secondary to allergy to the iodinated dye. In clients with a pheochromocytoma, the dye reaction can precipitate a fatal episode of severe hypertension. Precautionary measures are
   necessary to prevent this complication. Propranolol (In-
   deral), a beta-blocker, and phenoxybenzamine (Dibenzy-
   line), an alpha-adrenergic blocker, are administered for
   several days before the study to avoid the precipitation of
   a malignant hypertensive episode.
2. Other complications include hemorrhage from the puncture
   site used for the arterial access and extremity eschemia or
   infarction from the dislodgement of an atherosclerotic
   plaque.
3. Occasionally arteriography (and venography) can induce
   serious hemorrhage within the adrenal that may cause necrosis of the glands, leading to Addison's disease. If an
   adrenal tumor is subsequently found and requires operative
   removal, the surgical procedure is technically more difficult after hemorrhage or infarction.

ADRENAL VENOGRAPHY

Normal Values

- Normal adrenal veins and normal adrenal vein hormone assay.

Deviations from Normal

- If the plasma cortisol level in blood obtained from one vein
  is markedly higher than that of the other, a unilateral adrenal tumor is causing the client's Cushing's syndrome. If
  plasma cortisol levels are bilaterally elevated, the cause of
  the Cushing's syndrome is bilateral adrenal hyperplasia.
- If the catecholamine level on one side is markedly higher
  than that of the other, a unilateral pheochromocytoma exists
  on the side of the elevated levels.
- If blood obtained from both sides is equally elevated, the
  client probably has bilateral adrenal pheochromocytomas

(this occurs more frequently in children and with the familial type of pheochromocytomas).

- If the adrenal venous blood samples are not elevated on either side in a client who has elevated peripheral blood catecholamine levels, the pheochromocytoma exists outside the adrenal (extraadrenal pheochromocytoma).

Indications

- To detect pathologic anatomy of the adrenal vein.

Contraindications

- An uncooperative client.
- A client allergic to iodinated dye who has not been desensitized (see ''Cardiac Catheterization,'' p. 13).

Procedure

Client preparation

1. The client is kept on nothing by mouth after midnight the day of the study.
2. The client is assessed for allergies to dye. If ordered, a steroid and antihistamine preparation is administered.
3. The client is usually given prednisone, 5 mg four times a day, and diphenhydramine (Benadryl), 25 mg four times a day, for 3 days before and 3 days after the test.

Procedure

1. The client is placed in the supine position on the x-ray table.
2. The client's groin is prepared in a sterile manner.
3. After the venipuncture site is locally anesthetized, the femoral vein is catheterized.
4. The catheter is passed into the adrenal vein.
5. Dye is injected to visualize the adrenal veins and to ensure that the catheter is indeed in the adrenal vein.
6. Blood is obtained and sent to the chemistry lab for assays.
7. In a client suspected of having a pheochromocytoma, appropriate pharmacologic beta- and alpha-adrenergic blocking agents are administered (propranolol [Inderal] and phenoxybenzamine [Dibenzyline], respectively) to prevent

the occurrence of a catecholamine-initiated malignant hypertensive episode when there is evidence of hypertensive crisis.

8. The radiologist performs this study in the angiography lab in approximately 1 hour.

Nursing implications

1. After the study, assess the client's vital signs frequently (normally every 15 minutes for four times, then every 30 minutes for four times, then every hour for four times, and then every 4 hours).

2. Assess the client suspected of having a pheochromocytoma for signs and symptoms of a hypertensive episode. If such an episode occurs, notify the physician immediately to obtain an order for appropriate alpha- and beta-adrenergic blocking agents.

3. After the study, assess the groin site for redness, pain, swelling, and bleeding with each vital sign check.

Nurse alert

1. A possible complication of this study is adrenal hemorrhage or necrosis caused by the pressure of the dye injection. This may cause Addison's disease. If adrenalectomy is subsequently indicated, the adrenal surgery would be technically more difficult to perform in the presence of adrenal hemorrhage or necrosis.

2. Another possible complication is allergic reaction to iodinated x-ray contrast material.

X-RAY STUDY OF THE SELLA TURCICA
Normal Values

- No abnormalities.

Deviations from Normal

- The presence of ACTH-producing tumors of the pituitary can cause Cushing's syndrome. Erosion and destruction of the normal sella turcica serves to diagnose these tumors.

Indications

▪ To diagnose ACTH-producing tumors of the pituitary.

Contraindications

▪ See "Contraindications" for "Skull X-Ray Study," p. 146.

Procedure

1. See "Skull X-Ray Study," p. 146.

Computerized Tomography Tests
COMPUTERIZED TOMOGRAPHY OF THE ADRENAL GLANDS (CT SCAN OF THE ADRENALS)

Normal Values

▪ No evidence of abnormality.

Deviations from Normal

▪ The presence of abnormalities suggesting one of the conditions listed under "Indications" below.

Indications

▪ To detect small tumors (adenomas, carcinomas, and pheochromocytomas) of the adrenal glands.
▪ To detect bilateral adrenal hyperplasia.
▪ To detect adrenal hemorrhage causing Addison's disease.

Contraindications

▪ See "CT of the Abdomen," p. 95.

Procedure
Client preparation

1. See "CT of the Abdomen," p. 95.

Procedure

1. See "CT of the Abdomen," p. 95.
2. A contrast agent may be administered orally to outline the

gut or intravenously to enhance visualization of the kidney.

Nursing implications

1. See "CT of the Abdomen," p. 95.

Endocrine Glands

Clinical Laboratory Tests
Blood Tests
GLUCOSE TOLERANCE TEST (GTT; ORAL GLUCOSE TOLERANCE TEST; OGTT)
Normal Values

	Serum	Whole Blood
Fasting: mg/dl	70-115	60-100 mg/dl
30 min: mg/dl	<200	<180
1 hr: mg/dl	<200	<180
2 hr: mg/dl	<140	<120
3 hr: mg/dl	70-115	60-100
4 hr: mg/dl	70-115	60-100

Deviations from Normal

- Markedly elevated serum glucose levels from 1 to 5 hours after glucose administration indicates diabetes mellitus. Glucose can also usually be detected in the diabetic client's urine.
- Persistent hyperglycemia after glucose loading can also be seen in nondiabetic clients with hyperthyroidism, acromegaly, infection, or ongoing chronic illness (e.g., cancer).
- Pregnant or obese clients may also show elevations. Drugs such as nicotine, aspirin, steroids, thiazides, and oral contraceptives may also cause glucose intolerance in nondiabetic clients.

Indications

- To diagnose diabetes mellitus.

Contraindications

- Clients with serious concurrent illness, endocrine disorders, or infection, because glucose intolerance will usually be observed even though the client may not be diabetic.

Procedure

Client preparation

1. Many clients are anxious about the procedure for this study, since approximately six venipunctures are required in a 4- to 5-hour period.
2. The client receives written instructions explaining the pretest dietary requirements. After at least 3 days of consuming a high-carbohydrate diet (at least 200 to 300 g), the client is kept on nothing by mouth (except water) after midnight the day of the test.
3. The client is encouraged to bring reading material or craft work to alleviate some of the boredom associated with this study.
4. The client is given the necessary urine containers with instructions regarding when specimens are needed.

Procedure

1. The nurse or technician draws the necessary serum glucose specimens. The client collects his or her own urine specimen. Nursing assistance is given as needed. The test requires about 5 hours and is performed in the outpatient department or in the client's hospital room.
2. Using standard venipuncture technique, a specimen for a fasting blood glucose test is obtained, and the client's urine is tested for glucose and acetone.
3. The client is then given a 100 g carbohydrate load, usually in the form of a carbonated sugar beverage (Glucola) or a cherry-flavored gelatin (Gel-a-dex). For children weighing less than 100 lb, 1 g of glucose per pound of body weight is given.
4. Serum and urine specimens for glucose level determination are obtained at 30 minutes, 1 hour, 2 hours, 3 hours, and 4 hours after the client's ingestion of the carbohydrate

load. Sometimes specimens are also obtained at 5 hours. The venipuncture sites are rotated.

5. Pressure or pressure dressings are applied to the venipuncture sites, which are then observed for bleeding.
6. All specimens must be clearly marked with the time at which they were obtained.
7. Occasionally a client is unable to absorb the oral glucose load (e.g., clients with prior gastrectomy, short bowel syndrome, or malabsorption).
8. The client should rest during the entire study because any exercise, even walking, can affect the glucose level.
9. In some instances an *intravenous glucose tolerance test* (IV-GTT) can be performed.
   a. A specimen of fasting blood glucose level determination is obtained.
   b. A 50% glucose solution (or glucose, 0.33 g/kg ideal body weight in adults; 0.5 g/kg body weight in children) is administered intravenously over a 3- to 4-minute period.
   c. Blood samples are obtained as indicated by the lab. Usually these are at 30-minute, 1-, 2-, and 3-hour intervals. The values for the IV-GTT differ slightly from the oral-GTT, since the IV glucose is absorbed more quickly.

Nursing implications

1. Encourage the client to drink water to help obtain the urine specimens.
2. Do not permit the client to have anything by mouth during the study (except water). Tobacco, coffee, and tea are not allowed.
3. Ensure that no drugs that alter GTT results (insulin or oral hypoglycemics) are given to the client during the test.
4. If the client has tremors, dizziness, euphoria, or other reactions during the study, obtain a blood specimen immediately. If the glucose level is too high, the test may need to be stopped and insulin administered.
5. Outpatients who feel faint during blood withdrawal should

be placed on a bed or stretcher in the supine position during venipuncture.

6. After the study, allow the client to eat and drink normally. Insulin or oral hypoglycemics may be administered, if ordered, after the study.

GLYCOSYLATED HEMOGLOBIN (HbA$_{1c}$; GLYCOHEMOGLOBIN)

Normal Values

- Vary with lab method employed.
- Adult: 2.2% to 4.8%.
- Child: 1.8% to 4.0%.
- Good diabetic control: 2.5% to 6%.

Deviations from Normal

- Fair diabetic control: 6.1% to 8%.
- Poor diabetic control: over 8%.

Indications

- To evaluate the success of diabetic treatment, which includes hypoglycemic agents, dietary therapy, insulin pumps, or client education programs.
- To compare and contrast the success of old and new forms of diabetic therapy.
- To aid in determining the duration of hyperglycemia in newly diagnosed diabetics.
- To provide a sensitive estimate of glucose imbalance in a client with a mild case of diabetes.
- To individualize diabetic control regimens.
- To provide a feeling of reward for many clients when the test shows that they have achieved good diabetic control.

Contraindications

- Falsely low values will occur in sickle cell anemia and in pregnancy.
- Falsely elevated values occur when the RBC lifespan is lengthened (as in thalassemia).

Procedure
Client preparation

1. The glycohemoglobin test and its potential to help monitor therapy are explained to the client. This test motivates most clients to follow their control regimen and to take a more active part in self-care.
2. The client is told that fasting is not indicated because short-term variations do not affect the level.

Procedure

1. Following standard venipuncture technique, 3 to 5 ml of blood are collected.
2. Pressure or a pressure dressing is applied to the puncture site.

Nursing implications

1. Observe the puncture sites for bleeding.

PLASMA INSULIN ASSAY
Normal Values

- 5 to 20 μU/ml.

Deviations from Normal

- Insulin/glucose ratio <0.3 occurs in clients with insulinoma.

Indications

- To diagnose insulinoma.
- To evaluate abnormal lipid and carbohydrate metabolism.
- At the present time, plasma insulin levels are not used in the diagnosis of diabetes mellitus.

Contraindications

- None.

Procedure
Client preparation

1. The client is kept on nothing by mouth (except water) for 8 hours before the study.

Procedure

1. Following standard venipuncture technique, a fasting blood sample is obtained.
2. Pressure or a pressure dressing is applied to the puncture site.

Nursing implications

1. If the serum insulin level will be measured during the GTT (p. 269), the blood samples should be drawn before the oral ingestion of the glucose load.
2. Observe the puncture sites for bleeding.

SERUM GLUCOSE TEST

Normal Values

- Adult: serum, 70 to 115 mg/dl; whole blood, 60 to 100 mg/dl.
- Child: 60 to 100 mg/dl; 30 to 80 mg/dl.

Deviations from Normal

- True glucose elevations generally indicate diabetes mellitus.
- Other possible causes of hyperglycemia include acute stress response (e.g., to surgery), Cushing's disease, hyperthyroidism, adenoma of the pancreas, pancreatitis, diuretics, and corticosteroid therapy.
- The most common cause of low serum glucose levels (hypoglycemia) is insulin overdose. Other causes of hypoglycemia include insulinoma, hypothyroidism, hypopituitarism, Addison's disease, and extensive liver disease.

Indications

- To diagnose metabolic diseases listed under ''Deviations from Normal'' above.
- To constantly monitor the insulin dosage administered to new diabetics.
- To diagnose an insulin reaction in a diabetic client.

Contraindications

- None.

Procedure
Client preparation

1. If fasting is required, the client is told that breakfast will be held until the blood is obtained.
2. The diabetic client is told that insulin or oral hypoglycemics will be withheld until after the blood is obtained.
3. If the client will have repeated blood glucose determinations (e.g., daily fasting and 3 PM blood glucose tests), the reason for this is explained.

Procedure

1. Following standard peripheral venipuncture technique, approximately 7 ml of venous blood are collected in a red- or gray-top tube. The blood should be obtained before insulin or hypoglycemic agents are administered.
2. Pressure or a pressure dressing is applied to the venipuncture site.
3. For diabetic clients being regulated on intermediate-acting insulins, fasting and 3 PM blood glucose tests are usually performed.

Nursing implications

1. Observe the puncture site for bleeding.
2. Ensure that the client receives a meal after the blood is obtained.

SERUM OSMOLALITY TEST
Normal Values

- 275 to 300 mOsm/kg.

Deviations from Normal

- In diabetic clients the number of glucose particles in the serum increases markedly, thus raising serum osmolality levels.
- Hypernatremia, ketosis, dehydration, and diabetes insipidus can also cause increased serum osmolality.

- Low serum osmolality usually results from fluid overload and inappropriate secretion of antidiuretic hormone (ADH).

Indications

- To aid in diagnosing conditions listed under "Deviations from Normal" above.

Contraindications

- None.

Procedure

1. Following standard venipuncture technique, peripheral venous blood is obtained in one red-top tube from a nonfasting client.
2. The sample is sent to the chemistry lab for serum osmolality measurement.
3. Pressure or a pressure dressing is applied to the puncture site.

Nursing implications

1. Observe the puncture site for bleeding.

TWO-HOUR POSTPRANDIAL GLUCOSE TEST (2-HOUR PPG; 2-HOUR POSTPRANDIAL BLOOD SUGAR; 2-HOUR PPBS)

Normal Values

- Serum: <140 mg/dl.
- Whole blood: <120 mg/dl.

Deviations from Normal

- An elevated glucose level 2 hours after the meal indicates diabetes mellitus.

Indications

- To screen clients for diabetes mellitus.

Contraindications

- None.

Procedure

Client preparation

1. The procedure is explained to the client, who is instructed to eat the entire meal consisting of at least 75 g of carbohydrates and then not to eat anything else or smoke until the blood is drawn. Smoking may increase the blood sugar.

Procedure

1. Following standard venipuncture procedure, 7 ml of peripheral venous blood are obtained in a gray- or red-top tube.
2. Pressure or a pressure dressing is applied to the puncture site.

Nursing implications

1. Observe the puncture sites for bleeding.

Urine Tests

URINE TEST FOR GLUCOSE AND ACETONE (URINE S & A; FRACTIONAL URINE)

Normal Values

- Negative for glucose and acetone.

Deviations from Normal

- Negative results for glucose and acetone are not necessarily indicative of a stabilized patient. Although these results would rule out hyperglycemia, the client could be hypoglycemic.

Indications

- To monitor insulin therapy in the diabetic client.

Procedure
Client preparation

1. The client should be able to test his or her urine confidently several times before being discharged from the hospital.
2. Fractional urine tests for glucose and acetone are performed at specified times during the day, generally before meals and at bedtime.

Procedure

1. A "double-voided" specimen is required.
2. The first specimen is discarded, and the client is given a glass of water (approximately 8 ounces) to drink.
3. A second specimen is then obtained and tested for glucose and acetone. The result obtained from this double-voided, or second, specimen accurately reflects the amount of glucose in urine that the kidney has recently filtered.

Nursing implications

1. Urine glucose and acetone are easily detected by using a Keto-Diastix or Multistix reagent strip.
   a. The reagent strip is completely immersed in a well-mixed urine specimen and removed immediately to avoid diluting out the reagents.
2. Urine testing for glucose can also be performed quickly and easily by the Clinitest method (a copper-reducing method).
3. Acetest tablets can detect acetone in urine.
4. Read the directions on the bottle or container of the reagent strips. Compare the color reaction with the manufacturer's color chart at the *exact* time specified. Check the expiration date on the bottle before use. Tightly close the bottle after removing the reagent strips.
5. If the client is receiving cephalothin (Keflin) intravenously or cephalexin (Keflex) orally, do not use Clinitest tablets, because false-positive results can be obtained. Vitamin C probenecid, chloramphenicol, levodopa, methyldopa, sulfonamides, tetracyclines, nalidixic acid, and high-dose salicylates also cause false-positive results with Clinitest tablets. Therefore use reagent strips for these clients.

SERUM PHOSPHATE (PHOSPHORUS) CONCENTRATION TEST

Normal Values

- Adults: 2.5 to 4.5 mg/dl.
- Children: 3.5 to 5.8 mg/dl.

Deviations from Normal

- Hypoparathyroidism, renal failure, or increased dietary or IV intake can cause hyperphosphatemia.
- Inadequate dietary ingestion of phosphorus, chronic antacid ingestion, hyperparathyroidism, and hypercalcemia resulting from other causes may result in hypophosphatemia. Symptoms include retarded skeletal growth in children, anorexia, dizziness, muscular weakness, waddling gait, skeletal and cardiac myopathies, decreased RBC oxygen transport, and RBC hemolysis.

Indications

- To aid in diagnosing hypophosphatemia or hyperphosphatemia.

Contraindications

- None.

Procedure

Client preparation

1. Some hospitals require the client be kept on nothing by mouth for 8 hours preceding the blood collection.

Procedure

1. Following standard venipuncture procedure, two red-top tubes are filled with peripheral venous blood.
2. Pressure or a pressure dressing is applied to the puncture site.

Nursing implications

1. Hemolysis must be avoided because it can release intracellular phosphate, which would artificially raise the phosphate level.
2. Observe the puncture site for bleeding.

Bibliography

Anthony, C.P., and Thibodeau, G.A.: Textbook of anatomy and physiology, ed. 11, St. Louis, 1983, The C.V. Mosby Co.

Cassmeyer, V.: Assessment of regulatory mechanisms. In Phipps, W.J., Long, B.C., and Woods, N.F., editors: Medical-surgical nursing: concepts and clinical practice, ed. 2, St. Louis, 1983, The C.V. Mosby Co.

Congdon, J.G.: Nursing assessment—the endocrine system. In Lewis, S.M., and Collier, I.C.: Medical-surgical nursing: assessment and management of clinical problems, New York, 1983, McGraw-Hill Book Co.

Estigarriba, J.A., and Lucus, C.P.: Elevated catecholamine levels in hypertension, Postgrad. Med. **73:**289, 1983.

Ganga, T.S.: Laboratory aids in thyroid problems, Van Nuys, Calif., 1981, Bioscience Laboratories.

Hammond, G.T.: Glycosylated hemoglobin and diabetes mellitus, Lab. Med. **12:**213, 1981.

Harris, E.: Dexamethasone suppression test, Am. J. Nurs. **82:**784-785, May 1982.

Harvey, A.M., Johns, R.J., Owens, A.H., and Ross, R.S., editors: The principles and practice of medicine, ed. 19, New York, 1976, Appleton-Century-Crofts.

Honigman, R.E.: Thyroid function tests, Nursing '82 **12**(4):68-71, April 1982.

Jones, S.G.: Adrenal patient: proceed with caution, RN **45**(1):67, Jan. 1982.

Joyce, M.A., Kuzich, C.M., and Murphy, D.M.: Those new blood glucose tests, RN **46**(4):46-52, April 1983.

Kee, J.L., and Tang, H.L.: Laboratory and diagnostic tests with nursing implications, Norwalk, Conn., 1983, Appleton-Century-Crofts.

Lafferty, F.N.: Primary hyperparathyroidism, Arch. Intern. Med. **141:**1761-1766, 1981.

McFarland, M.B., and Grant, M.M.: Nursing implications of laboratory tests, New York, 1982, John Wiley & Sons.

Metzger, M.J.: A new test for blood sugar, Am. J. Nurs. **83:**763-764, May 1983.

Morley, J.E., and Shafer, R.B.: Thyroid function screening in new psychiatric admissions, Arch. Intern. Med. **142:**591, 1982.

National Diabetes Data Group: Classification and diagnosis of diabetes mellitus and other categories of glucose intolerance, Diabetes **28:**1039, 1979.

Price, S., and Wilson, L.: Pathophysiology: clinical concepts of disease processes, ed. 2, New York, 1982, McGraw-Hill Book Co.

Rothfield, B.: Nuclear medicine endocrinology, Philadelphia, 1978, J.B. Lippincott Co.

Schottelius, B.A., and Schottelius, D.D.: Textbook of physiology, ed. 19, St. Louis, 1983, The C.V. Mosby Co.

Sherwood, M.J., et al.: A new reagent strip (Visidex) for determination of glucose in whole blood, Clin. Chem. **29:**438, 1983.

Smallridge, R.C., and Smith, C.E.: Hyperthyroidism due to thyrotropin-secreting pituitary tumors, Arch. Intern. Med. **143:**503, 1983.

Spiro, H.M.: Clinical gastroenterology, ed. 2, New York, 1977, MacMillan Publishing Co.

Treseler, K.M.: Clinical laboratory tests: significance and implications for nursing, Englewood Cliffs, N.J., 1982, Prentice-Hall, Inc.

Watts, N.B.: Diabetes mellitus: diagnostic and monitoring techniques, Lab. Mgmt. **20:**43, 1982.

Watts, N.B., and Keffer, J.H.: Practical endocrine diagnosis, ed. 3, Philadelphia, 1982, Lea & Febiger.

White, N.E., and Miller, B.K.: Glycohemoglobin: a new test to help the diabetic stay in control, Nursing '83 **13**(8):55-57, 1983.

Wright, B.T., et al.: Test for glucose in the urine: understanding test specificity and interferences, Pediatr. Nurs. **8**(1):44-45, 1982.

Reproductive System

8

Infertility
  Clinical laboratory tests
    Urine tests
      Hormone assay for urinary pregnanediol
  Radiologic laboratory tests
    X-ray tests
      Hysterosalpingography (uterotubography, uterosalpingography)
  Special studies
    Endoscopy
      Culdoscopy
      Laparoscopy (pelvic endoscopy)
    Cervical mucus test (Fern test)
    Endometrial biopsy
    Semen analysis
    Sims-Huhner test (postcoital test; postcoital cervical mucus test)
    Uterotubal insufflation (Rubin's test)
Pregnancy and the reproductive system
  Clinical laboratory tests
    Blood tests
      Fetal scalp blood pH
      Human placental lactogen (HPL)
      Pregnancy tests
      Rubella (German measles) antibody test (hemagglutination in-
        hibition [HAI] test)
      Serologic test for syphilis (VDRL, RPR, FTA)
      Serum alfa-fetoprotein (AFP) test
      TORCH test
      Toxoplasmosis antibody titer
    Urine tests
      Estriol excretion studies
      Human placental lactogen
      Pregnancy test

Radiologic laboratory tests
  X-ray tests
    X-ray pelvimetry (radiographic pelvimetry)
Special studies
  Endoscopy
    Amnioscopy
    Colposcopy
    Fetoscopy
  Amniocentesis
  Chlamydia smears
  Contraction stress test (CST, oxytocin challenge test)
  Gonorrhea culture
  Nonstress test
  Papanicolaou smear (Pap smear, Pap test, cytologic test for cancer)
  Ultrasonography
Newborn evaluation
  Clinical laboratory tests
    Blood tests
      Galactose-1-phosphate uridyl transferase (Gal-1-PUT)
      Phenylketonuria (PKU) test
  Special studies
    Barr body analysis (sex chromatin body, chromatin-positive body)
    Phenylketonuria (PKU) test

Infertility

Clinical Laboratory Tests

Urine Tests

HORMONE ASSAY FOR URINARY PREGNANEDIOL

Normal Values

- Increased excretion after ovulation to >1 mg/24 h for approximately 10 days.
- Preovulation level: 0.4 ± 0.1 mg/24 h.

Deviations from Normal

- A decrease in pregnanediol levels may precede a spontaneous abortion.
- Pregnanediol levels rise immediately after ovulation and normally during pregnancy because of placental progesterone production.

Indications

- To determine if and the exact time ovulation has occurred.
- To monitor the status of the placenta during pregnancy by performing repeated assays.
- To monitor progesterone supplementation in clients who have an inadequate luteal phase.

Contraindications

- None.

Procedure

Client preparation

1. See p. 181 for "Client Preparation" (except step 2) for the "Creatinine Clearance Test" for 24-hour urine collection. The specimen is refrigerated.
2. The client is told when and how she can get the results of this urinary assay.

Procedure

1. Progesterone determinations begin 4 to 6 days after a change in the biphasic curve (according to BBT measurements) when the client is being followed for an inadequate luteal phase.
2. A 24-hour urine specimen is collected in a standard specimen container and sent to the chemistry lab. See "Procedure" (except step 4) for 24-hour urine collection for "Creatinine Clearance Test."
3. During the entire collection, the specimen should be refrigerated.

Nursing implications

1. None.

Radiologic Laboratory Tests

X-Ray Tests

HYSTEROSALPINGOGRAPHY (UTEROTUBOGRAPHY; UTEROSALPINGOGRAPHY)

Normal Values

- Patent fallopian tube; no defects in uterine cavity.

Deviations from Normal

- Uterine tumors (e.g., leiomyomas), intrauterine adhesions, and developmental anomalies (e.g., uterus bicornis) can be recognized.
- Tubal obstruction caused by internal scarring, tumor, or kinking (resulting from pelvic adhesions) can also be seen.

Indications

- To aid in diagnosing fallopian tube obstruction.
- To document adequacy of surgical tubal ligation.

Contraindications

- A client with infections of the vagina, cervix, or fallopian tubes, for fear of extending the infection.
- A client with uterine bleeding, since contrast material might enter the open blood vessels.
- A client with suspected pregnancy, because the contrast material might induce abortion.

Procedure

Client preparation

1. Written instructions are helpful, since the procedure is usually scheduled on an outpatient basis at a later time.
2. Many clients fear that the results of this study may markedly affect their sexuality and fertility.
3. The woman is told what sensations she may feel during the test.
4. The client usually takes a laxative the night before the study, and an enema or suppository is given the morning of the study.

5. The test is best performed 4 to 5 days after completion of menstruation because debris may trap or transiently occlude the fallopian tubes. At this time one also avoids the risk of inducing abortion if an unknown pregnancy exists.
6. If ordered, mild sedatives or antispasmodics are administered before this study.
7. The client is assessed for allergy to iodinated dye.

Procedure

1. Immediately before the study a plain x-ray film of the abdomen is taken to ensure that the preparation adequately eliminated gastrointestinal (GI) gas and feces.
2. After voiding, the client is placed on the fluoroscopy table in the lithotomy position (as for pelvic examination).
3. A sterile cannula is inserted into the cervix and held in place by a tenaculum.
4. A 2-minute rest period is necessary to allow for relaxation of tubal spasm associated with cervical dilatation.
5. A few milliliters of dye are injected through the cannula during fluoroscopy, and x-ray films are taken.
6. More dye is then injected so that the entire upper genital tract (uterus and tubes) can be filled.
7. A gynecologist usually performs this test on an outpatient basis in the radiology department in approximately 15 minutes. A radiologist interprets x-ray films.

Nursing implications

1. During and after the study the client may feel transient menstrual cramping. Mild sedatives or antispasmodics are sometimes used. Dizziness, vaginal discharge (sometimes bloody) 1 to 2 days after the test, and shoulder pain from subphrenic irritation from the dye leaking into the peritoneal cavity may also occur.
2. After the study advise the client to wear a perineal pad because radiopaque material can stain her underclothing.
3. After the study observe the client for allergy to iodinated dye.

Nurse alert

1. A possible complication of the study is an allergic reaction to the iodinated contrast material.
2. Another possible complication is infection of the endometrium (endometritis) or fallopian tube (salpingitis) caused by using contaminated dye.

Special Studies
Endoscopy
CULDOSCOPY
Normal Values

- Normal-appearing reproductive organs.

Deviations from Normal

- The existence of tubal abnormalities.

Indications

- To use for tubal sterilization of obese women.
- To evaluate a client for infertility.
- To detect ectopic pregnancy.
- To assess unexpected pelvic pain or masses.
- Note that the indications for this study are reduced as a result of the introduction of laparoscopy.

Contraindications

- Clients unable to assume the knee-chest position.
- Clients with acute vulvar or vaginal infections.
- Clients with acute peritonitis.
- Clients with palpable masses in the cul-de-sac.
- Clients with previous pelvic surgery causing an adhesion of the bowel to the cul-de-sac.

Procedure
Client preparation

1. The preoperative and postoperative routines are explained. The stress associated with this study is minimized by factual information. A picture may be helpful.

2. The client is encouraged to verbalize her questions or fears regarding this study. Emotional support is provided.
3. Many clients fear the results of this study. A time is arranged for the client to call or to see her physician for the results.
4. The client is kept on nothing by mouth after midnight the day of the study.
5. The client receives preoperative preparation as for any minor vaginal surgery.

Procedure

1. The client is placed in the knee-chest position.
2. Spinal or local anesthesia is used.
3. A small incision is made in the posterior vaginal vault, and a culdoscope is passed into the cul-de-sac.
4. The pelvic and abdominal organs are then visualized and examined.
5. After the study the scope is removed.
6. No sutures are used to close the incision in the vaginal cuff.
7. The physician performs this study in the operating room in 1 hour.

Nursing implications

1. Inform the client that douching or intercourse is not permitted until the vaginal septum has healed. This healing takes approximately 1 to 2 weeks.
2. The client may take sitz baths 4 days after the procedure.
3. Mild oral analgesics may be ordered for discomfort.

LAPAROSCOPY (PELVIC ENDOSCOPY)
Normal Values

- Normal-appearing reproductive organs.

Deviations from Normal

- Abnormal-appearing organs suggest conditions listed under "Indications" below.

Indications

- To diagnose pelvic adhesions, ovarian tumors and cysts, and other tubal and uterine causes of infertility.
- To detect endometriosis, ectopic pregnancy, ruptured ovarian cyst, and salpingitis.
- To perform surgical procedures (e.g., biopsy specimen removal from abdominal organs, lysis of adhesions, removal of intraabdominal intrauterine devices [IUD], and tubal ligation) with the laparoscope.

Contraindications

- A client with localized peritonitis because laparoscopy may spread the infection throughout the abdominal cavity.
- A client who has had multiple operations because adhesions may have formed.
- A client with suspected intraabdominal hemorrhage, since blood will obscure visualization through the scope.

Procedure

Client preparation

1. The procedure is explained to the client as are the preoperative and postoperative routines.
2. If a biopsy is to be performed, the client's blood is typed and crossmatched before the study (if ordered).
3. The client is kept on nothing by mouth after midnight the day of the procedure. Food and fluid in the GI tract may result in pulmonary aspiration in the anesthetized client.
4. Some physicians will order a Fleet enema on the night before the study.
5. The abdomen is shaved and prepared, and the hospital's routine preoperative procedure is performed.
6. The client voids before going to the operating room.

Procedure

1. After induction of anesthesia (general or regional) the client is placed in a modified lithotomy of Trendelenburg (head-down) position so that the intestines move away from the pelvis, thus permitting better visualization of the pelvic organs.

2. After the abdominal skin is cleansed with povidone-iodine (Betadine), a blunt-tipped needle is inserted through a small incision in the subumbilical area into the peritoneal cavity.

3. The peritoneal cavity is filled with approximately 3 to 4 L carbon dioxide (pneumoperitoneum) to separate the abdominal wall from the intraabdominal viscera, thus enhancing visualization of pelvic and abdominal structures.

4. After pneumoperitoneum has been established, a trocar within a cannula is introduced into the peritoneal cavity.

5. The trocar is removed and the laparoscope (attached to a fiberoptic light source) is inserted (Fig. 8-1).

6. The pelvic organs and the upper abdomen are then examined.

7. After the desired procedure (e.g., inspection, tubal ligation, biopsy specimen removal) is completed the laparoscope is removed and the carbon dioxide is allowed to escape. The incision is closed with a few skin stitches and covered with an adhesive bandage.

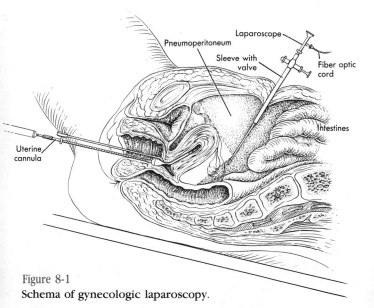

Figure 8-1
Schema of gynecologic laparoscopy.

8. A surgeon performs laparoscopy in the operating room in approximately 20 to 40 minutes.

Nursing implications

1. After the procedure, assess the client frequently for signs of bleeding (increased pulse, decreased blood pressure); perforated viscus (abdominal tenderness, guarding, and decreased bowel sounds); and acidosis (increased respiration rate). Normally, take vital signs every 15 minutes for four times, then every 30 minutes for four times, then every hour for four times, and then every 4 hours. Report any significant findings to the physician.
2. Keep the client on nothing by mouth after the study until she is fully alert and her "gag reflex" has returned.
3. If the client reports shoulder or subcostal discomfort (from pneumoperitoneum), assure her that this usually lasts only 24 hours. Minor analgesics usually relieve the discomfort.
4. The client may also have mild incisional pain.
5. If the results are not available immediately after the study, inform the client when she can obtain them.

Nurse alert

1. Because general anesthesia is used, all complications associated with it can occur (e.g., nausea, vomiting, respiratory abnormalities).
2. Because perforation of the gut and uncontrolled intraperitoneal bleeding may occur, some physicians prefer to perform this study on an inpatient basis. However, laparoscopy can be safely performed on an outpatient basis in most instances.
3. Acidosis may also result from carbon dioxide insufflation of the abdominal cavity during the procedure.

Cervical Mucus Test (Fern Test)
Normal Values

- Arborization, or ferning, of cervical mucus during midcycle.

Deviations from Normal

- Absence of ferning in premenopausal clients indicates an anovulatory state.
- Ferning of the cervical mucus is also absent in postmenopausal, castrated, or normally pregnant women (because of the presence of fern-inhibiting progesterone).

Indications

- To evaluate infertility by predicting the day of ovulation and determining whether ovulation occurs.

Contraindications

- None.

Procedure
Client preparation

1. This procedure is performed at midcycle to detect estrogen-induced ferning and is then repeated approximately 7 days later to detect the progesterone inhibition of ferning.

Procedure

1. The client is placed in the lithotomy position.
2. An unlubricated speculum is inserted into the vagina to expose the cervix.
3. A cotton-tipped applicator is gently inserted into the cervical canal and rotated.
4. The mucus that adheres to the cotton swab is spread on a clean glass slide and allowed to dry at room temperature. No staining is used.
5. The dried spread of mucus is then examined under the low-power lens of a microscope for the presence of ferning.
6. A physician performs this study, usually in the office or outpatient clinic, in approximately 15 minutes.

Nursing implications

1. The slides used for the mucus must be washed in distilled water because the electrolytes in tap water may produce false ferning.

2. Ferning may be inhibited if the cervix is traumatized during this procedure and blood mixes with the mucus.
3. Drape the client effectively to prevent unnecessary exposure.
4. Usually the client is given the results immediately after the test. If not, tell her when to call the physician for the results.

Endometrial Biopsy

Normal Values

- Presence of a "secretory-type" endometrium 3 to 5 days before normal menses; no abnormal cells.

Deviations from Normal

- The presence of a preovulatory "proliferative type" endometrium indicates that ovulation has not occurred.

Indications

- To determine if ovulation has occurred.
- To indicate estrogen effect in clients with suspected ovarian dysfunction or absence.
- To determine adequate circulating progesterone levels by identifying secretory endometrium.
- To diagnose endometrial cancer.
- To detect tuberculosis, polyps, or inflammatory conditions.

Contraindications

- A client in whom the cervix fails to visualize because of previous cervical position or previous surgery.
- A client with infections (such as trichomonal, monilial, or suspected gonococcal) of the cervix or vagina.

Procedure
Client preparation

1. The client is told that although momentary discomfort (menstrual-type cramping) is associated with this study, analgesics are not needed.

Procedure

1. The client is placed in the lithotomy position, and a bimanual pelvic examination is performed to determine the position of the uterus.
2. A suction tube-curet or an endometrial biopsy curet (Novak) is inserted into the uterus, and specimens are obtained from the anterior, posterior, and lateral walls. (Specimens are taken only from the lateral wall in infertility workups.)
3. The specimens are placed in a solution containing 10% formalin and are sent to the pathologist for histologic examination.
4. An obstetrician-gynecologist performs this study in the office in approximately 10 to 30 minutes.

Nursing implications

1. After the procedure, assess the client's vital signs at routine, regular intervals for the next 48 hours. Any temperature elevations (>100.4° F) should be reported to the physician, because this procedure may activate pelvic inflammatory disease (PID).
2. Advise the client to rest during the next 24 hours and to avoid heavy lifting to prevent uterine hemorrhage.
3. After the procedure, advise the client to wear a pad, because some vaginal bleeding is to be expected. Instruct the client to call her physician if excessive bleeding (requiring more than one pad per hour) occurs.
4. Inform the client that douching and intercourse are not permitted for 72 hours after the biopsy specimen removal.
5. Tell the client how to obtain her test results. Generally the report is available within 72 hours.

Nurse alert

1. Complications of this study include perforation of the uterus, uterine bleeding, and interference with early pregnancy. If lateral scrapings are used for hormone work-up, the chances of interfering with pregnancy are minimal, because most implantation occurs on the anterior or posterior surfaces.

Semen Analysis

Normal Values

- Volume: 2 to 6 ml.
- Sperm count (density): 20 to 200 million/ml.
- Sperm motility: 60% to 80% actively motile.
- Sperm morphology: 70% to 90% normally shaped.

Deviations from Normal

- Abnormal volume, density, motility, and morphology perhaps indicating infertility.

Indications

- To assess male fertility.
- To document adequate sterilization after a vasectomy.

Contraindications

- None.

Procedure
Client preparation

1. The client is told that a 3- to 5-day period of sexual abstinence is necessary before the semen collection. Prolonged abstinence before the collection should be discouraged, since the quality of the sperm cells, and especially their motility, may diminish.
2. The client is given the proper container for the sperm collection.
3. The explanation about collection and delivery should be matter of fact to avoid embarrassing the client.
4. If the specimen will be obtained at the client's home, he is told that the specimen must be brought to the lab for testing within 1 hour after collection and that it should be kept at room temperature. Exposure to heat during the transportation may alter sperm cell motility. The date of the previous semen emission and the collection time and date of the fresh specimen is recorded. The lab will refer to these dates.

5. The client is given time to discuss any questions or fears regarding the results of this study.
6. The client is told when and how to obtain the test results.

Procedure

1. After 3 to 5 days of sexual abstinence, the client ejaculates a semen specimen into a clean container.
2. For best results this specimen should be collected in the physician's office or lab by masturbation. Less satisfactory specimens can be obtained in the client's home by coitus interruptus or masturbation and delivered to the lab within 1 hour after collection.
3. If, for religious reasons, the client cannot obtain a specimen by masturbation or coitus interruptus, a plastic condom can be used. Rubber condoms should not be used.

Nursing implications

1. None.

Sims-Huhner Test (Postcoital Test; Postcoital Cervical Mucus Test)

Normal Values

- Cervical mucus adequate for sperm transmission, survival, and penetration; 6 to 20 active sperm per high-power field.

Deviations from Normal

- Present but inactive sperm cells indicate that the cervical environment is unsuitable (e.g., abnormal pH) for their survival.
- Lower than normal sperm count may indicate infertility.

Indications

- To aid in assessing causes for infertility.
- To document cases of suspected rape by testing vaginal and cervical secretions for sperm.

Contraindications

- None.

Procedure
Client preparation

1. No vaginal lubrication, douching, or bathing is permitted until after the vaginal cervical examination, because these factors will alter the cervical mucus.
2. This study is performed at the middle of the ovulatory cycle, because at this time the secretions should be optimal for sperm penetration and survival.
3. The study is performed after 3 days of sexual abstinence.

Procedure

1. The client is instructed to report to the physician for examination of her cervical mucus within 2 hours (some physicians suggest 4 to 8 hours) after coitus.
2. Precoital lubrication and postcoital douching, bathing, or voiding are not permitted.
3. After intercourse the client should rest in bed for 10 to 15 minutes to ensure cervical exposure to semen.
4. After resting, the client should wear a perineal pad until she is placed in the lithotomy position in the physician's office.
5. The cervix is then exposed by an unlubricated speculum.
6. The specimen is aspirated from the endocervix and delivered to the lab for analysis.
7. A physician performs this procedure in approximately 5 minutes. The specimen analysis is completed in 15 minutes.

Nursing implications

1. The client is told how and when she may obtain the results.

Uterotubal Insufflation (Rubin's Test)
Normal Values

- Patent fallopian tubes.

Deviations from Normal

- A pressure of 200 torr or more indicates tubal obstruction.
- A pressure rise to 160 to 200 torr with a rapid falling off when the tube opens indicates tubal spasm.

Indications

- To determine fallopian tube patency to aid in assessing fertility.
- To demonstrate spasm of the uterine end of the fallopian tube.

Contraindications

- A client with infections of the vagina, cervix, or fallopian tubes, because the procedure may spread such infections.
- A client with uterine bleeding, since gas may enter the open blood vessels and cause embolisms.
- A client with suspected pregnancy, because abortion may be induced.

Procedure

Client preparation

1. Written instructions are helpful, since the procedure is usually scheduled on an outpatient basis at a later date.
2. The client is told what sensations she may feel during the test. An apprehensive client will be more likely to show spastic obstruction of the fallopian tubes than a relaxed client.
3. Usually the client is instructed to take a laxative the night before the study and an enema or bisacodyl (Dulcolax) suppository the morning of the test.

Procedure

1. After voiding, the client is placed in the lithotomy position.
2. The pelvic area is cleansed and a vaginal speculum is introduced to expose the cervix.

3. After the vaginal lining and cervix are swabbed, a special sterile cannula with a rubber tip is inserted into the cervical canal.

4. The rubber tip of the catheter is pressed tightly against the external os to seal the opening and is held in place by a tenaculum.

5. A short rest period (2 minutes) is allowed to permit relaxation of any tubal spasm.

6. A controlled amount of carbon dioxide is administered at 60 cc per minute into the uterus. Air should never be used because it may cause air embolism.

7. A kymograph is used to record alterations in pressure and to demonstrate minor changes that peristaltic activity of the tubes can cause. To raise the intrauterine pressure to 100 torr takes approximately 1 minute.

8. A stethoscope is placed over the abdomen to detect gas flow into the abdomen.

9. If both fallopian tubes are blocked, the pressure will continue to rise until the flow of gas is stopped. Carbon dioxide flow should be stopped at 200 torr to prevent tubal rupture. The pressure will remain high until the cervical cannula is withdrawn.

10. After the study the client will feel pain caused by the irritation of the subdiaphragmatic areas. If no pain occurs, occlusion of the tubes may be suspected despite normal pressure curves.

11. Rubin's test is usually performed on an outpatient basis in the physician's office in approximately 30 minutes.

Nursing implications

1. After the study the client should rest for 2 to 3 hours. Pain, cramping, dizziness, nausea, and vomiting may be present and can be minimized by the client's reclining with the pelvis elevated so that gas will exit.

2. Clients whose results indicate tubal obstruction are usually upset after testing. Encourage them to verbalize their fears. Provide emotional support.

Pregnancy and the Reproductive System

Clinical Laboratory Tests
Blood Tests
FETAL SCALP BLOOD pH

Normal Values

- pH: 7.25 to 7.35.
- O_2 saturation: 30% to 50%.
- PO_2: 18 to 22 torr.
- PCO_2: 40 to 50 torr.
- Base excess: 0 to -10 mEq/L.

Deviations from Normal

- A decrease in pH occurs as a result of acidosis (increased hydrogen ion concentration). Fetal hypoxia is then indicated.

Indications

- To assess fetal acid-base status.
- To diagnose fetal distress.

Contraindications

- See "Amnioscopy," p. 311.

Procedure
Client preparation

1. See "Amnioscopy," p. 311.

Procedure

1. Amnioscopy (see p. 311) is performed with the mother in the lithotomy position.
2. Under sterile conditions the amnioscope is introduced into the vagina and the dilated cervix.
3. The fetal scalp is cleansed with an antiseptic and dried with a sterile cotton ball.
4. A small amount of petroleum jelly is applied to the fetal scalp to cause droplets of fetal blood to bead.
5. The skin on the scalp is pierced with a small metal blade.

6. Beaded droplets of blood are then collected in long, heparinized capillary tubes.
7. The tube is then sealed with wax and placed on ice to retard cellular respiration, which can alter the pH.
8. The physician performing the procedure then applies firm pressure to the puncture site to retard bleeding. Scalp blood sampling can be repeated as necessary.
9. A blood sample may be simultaneously obtained from the mother to aid in interpretation of the fetal pH and to reduce the frequency of false-positive results.
10. A physician performs this study in approximately 15 minutes.

Nursing implications

1. See ''Amnioscopy,'' p. 312.
2. After delivery of the infant, the nurse should assess the newborn and identify and document the puncture site(s).
3. The fetal scalp puncture site may be cleansed with an antiseptic solution and an antibiotic ointment applied.

Nurse alert

1. Complications of this procedure include continued bleeding from the puncture site, hematoma, ecchymosis, and infection.

HUMAN PLACENTAL LACTOGEN (HPL)
Normal Values

- Levels gradually rise until the 36th week of pregnancy and then tend to stabilize.

Deviations from Normal

- Values of <4 µg/dl are rarely found in the last 10 weeks of pregnancy. Low HPL levels may indicate fetal distress, threatened abortion, toxemia, intrauterine growth retardation, and postmaturity.
- High HPL levels may indicate maternal sickle cell disease, maternal liver disease, maternal diabetes mellitus, Rh sensitization, and multiple pregnancies.

Indications

- To diagnose conditions listed under "Deviations from Normal" above.

Contraindications

- None.

Procedure
Client preparation

1. If urine is collected, see "Client Preparation" for "Creatinine Clearance Test" (except step 2), p. 181.

Procedure

1. Urine collection: see "Procedure" for "Creatinine Clearance Test" (except step 4).
2. Blood collection.
   a. Following standard venipuncture technique, blood is collected.
   b. Pressure or a pressure dressing is applied.

Nursing implications

1. Assess the venipuncture site for bleeding.

PREGNANCY TESTS
Normal Values

- Negative unless client is pregnant.

Deviations from Normal

- A positive test may indicate pregnancy. Causes of false-negative results include (1) the test is performed too early in the pregnancy before a sufficient HCB level develops; (2) urine diluted by diuretic-induced excesses off excreted free water is used; and (3) the lab makes a technical error.
- False-positive results may occur (1) in some premenopausal or perimenopausal clients with gonadal hormone deficiencies caused by over production of pituitary gonadotropin, which can cause "HCG-like" positive reactions; and (2)

with the use of certain tranquilizers (especially promazine and its derivatives).

Indications

- To diagnose pregnancy; the tests do not necessarily indicate a normal pregnancy.
- To aid in diagnosing tumor activity because tumors also produce HCG.

Contraindications

- None.

Procedure
Client preparation

1. The client is told the time needed to obtain the test results and how to get the results from her physician.
2. If urine specimens are required, the client is given the urine container on the evening before the test so that she can provide a first-voided morning specimen. This specimen generally contains the greatest concentration of HCG.
3. If the client is using a home pregnancy testing kit, the need for her to still have antepartal health examinations should be emphasized.
4. If a blood sample is required, it is obtained as the lab indicates.

Procedure

1. *Urine:*
   a. Specimens should be collected in a standard container and taken to the lab.
   b. A first-voided morning specimen is preferred.
   c. Urine tests for pregnancy are usually recommended at least 2 weeks after the first missed menstrual period.
2. *Blood:*
   a. Blood samples are obtained according to the requirements of the specific test to be performed.
   b. Hemolysis of blood may interfere with test results.

Nursing implications

1. If peripheral venipuncture is used for obtaining the sample, check the puncture site for bleeding.

RUBELLA (GERMAN MEASLES) ANTIBODY TEST (HEMAGGLUTINATION INHIBITION [HAI] TEST)

Normal Values

- Lack of susceptibility to rubella if HAI titer is >1:10 to 1:20 or if complement-fixation test is positive.

Deviations from Normal

- A titer ≤1:8 indicates little or no rubella immunity. For a client with a rubella rash, taking an acute sample (taken about 3 days after the onset of the rash) and a convalescent sample (taken around 3 weeks later) confirms the rubella diagnosis.

·Indications

- To diagnose rubella.
- To assess a pregnant client's immunity to rubella at the first prenatal visit and later if she is exposed to rubella. A rise in antibody titer indicates that both the mother and the fetus have been infected by rubella. If the exposure occurred during the first trimester of pregnancy, the fetus is at risk for congenital heart defects, deafness, mental retardation, and cataracts.

Contraindications

- None.

Procedure

1. Following standard venipuncture technique, a blood sample is obtained.
2. Pressure or a pressure dressing is applied to the puncture site.
3. The sample is sent to the lab for analysis.

Nursing implications

1. Assess the puncture site for bleeding.
2. If the test shows a pregnant woman has little or no rubella immunity, she should be strongly advised to stay away from any small children, especially those with symptoms of an upper respiratory infection (prodromal symptoms of rubella) because infections may cause serious problems even as late as the fifth month of gestation. In addition, all hospital personnel associated with maternal and child care should be screened for rubella. Immunization is not done during pregnancy, but should be done after delivery for nonimmune mothers.

SEROLOGIC TEST FOR SYPHILIS (VDRL; RPR; FTA)

Normal Values

- Negative or nonreactive.

Deviations from Normal

- Positive results in any test may indicate syphilis but must be confirmed by the FTA-ABS test.
- With the VDRL and RPR, conditions such as mycoplasia, pneumonia, malaria, acute bacterial and viral infections, autoimmune diseases, and pregnancy can cause false-positive results.

Indications

- To diagnose syphilis.
- To screen for syphilis during a pregnant woman's first prenatal checkup.

Contraindications

- A client known to have a disease that can cause a false-positive result (see ''Deviations from Normal'' above).

Procedure
Client preparation

1. The clinical serology lab analyzing the sample may request that the specimen be drawn before meals. If so, the client

is instructed not to eat. The client is instructed to abstain from alcohol for 24 hours before the sample is drawn.

2. The client is assessed for other diseases that may cause a false-positive result.

Procedure

1. Following standard venipuncture technique a blood sample is collected.
2. Pressure or a pressure dressing is applied to the puncture site.
3. The sample is sent to the lab for analysis.

Nursing implications

1. Handle the sample gently because hemolysis can affect results.
2. If the test is positive, obtain a history of the client's recent sexual contacts so that these persons may be evaluated for syphilis.
3. If the test is positive, be sure that the client receives the appropriate antibiotic therapy.

SERUM ALFA-FETOPROTEIN (AFP) TEST
Normal Values

- <25 ng/ml.

Deviations from Normal

- Elevated serum AFP levels may indicate NTD (neural tube defects).
- Elevated levels may also indicate abortion, multiple pregnancy, and intrauterine fetal death.
- Because only *primary* liver tumors secrete AFP, levels >500 ng/ml indicate primary liver cancer in approximately 97% of cases.
- AFP levels may also be elevated in clients with Hodgkin's disease, lymphoma, and renal tumor.

Indications

- To aid in diagnosing NTD, abortion, multiple pregnancy, and intrauterine fetal death.
- To diagnose primary hepatocellular cancer.

Contraindications

- None.

Procedure

1. Following standard venipuncture technique, blood is collected.
2. Pressure or a pressure dressing is applied.
3. The sample is sent immediately to the lab for analysis.

Nursing implications

1. Assess the venipuncture site for bleeding.
2. If the AFP level is elevated, the client is referred for further testing.

TORCH TEST

The term TORCH (T = toxoplasmosis, O = other, R = rubella, C = cytomegalovirus, H = herpes) is applied to infections with recognized direct or indirect detrimental effects on the fetus.

Normal Values

- Negative.

Deviations from Normal

- Positive results.

Indications

- To diagnose the diseases listed above.

Contraindications

- None.

Procedure

Client preparation

1. See separate studies.

Procedure

1. Following standard venipuncture technique, blood is collected.
2. Pressure or a pressure dressing is applied.
3. The sample is sent immediately to the lab for analysis.
4. A cord blood sample may be obtained instead of a venous one.

Nursing Implications

1. Assess the venipuncture site for bleeding.

TOXOPLASMOSIS ANTIBODY TITER

Normal Values

- Titer <1:4 indicates no previous infection.
- Titer of 1:4 to 1:256 is generally prevalent in the general population.
- Titer >256 suggests a recent infection.

Deviations from Normal

- Persistently elevated or a rising titer on the Sabin-Feldman dye test or the indirect fluorescent antibody titer test in the infant 2 to 3 months of age indicates toxoplasmosis.
- A positive result on a complement-fixation test indicates active disease.

Indications

- To diagnose toxoplasmosis.

Contraindications

- None.

Procedure

1. Following standard venipuncture technique, 5 ml of blood is collected.
2. Pressure or a pressure dressing is applied.
3. The sample is sent to the lab for analysis. Some labs request that pregnancy be indicated on the lab slip.

Nursing implications

1. Assess the venipuncture site for bleeding.
2. Note that, if the infection is recognized in early pregnancy clinically or by seroconversion, abortion is usually recommended. If the infection occurs later in the pregnancy, treatment of the mother with triple sulfa may reduce the effect on the fetus.

Urine Tests
ESTRIOL EXCRETION STUDIES

Twenty-four-hour urine studies. Because urinary creatinine excretion is relatively constant (0.7 to 1.5 mg/dl), its determination can be used to assess the adequacy of the 24-hour urine collection. A serially increasing estriol-creatinine ratio is a favorable sign in pregnancy. If the estriol levels fall, early delivery of the fetus may be indicated.

Plasma estriol studies. (Urinary estriol excretion of 1 mg/24 h is approximately equivalent to 0.6 to 0.8 ng/ml of unconjugated plasma estriol.) The plasma estriol tests are more recent than the urinary studies, and their use is still limited and controversial.

Deviations from Normal

- Decreasing values suggest fetoplacental deterioration (failing pregnancy, dysmaturity, preeclampsia/eclampsia, complicated diabetes mellitus, anencephaly, fetal death).

Indications

- To assess fetal-maternal well-being.

Contraindications

- The client receiving barbiturates or steroids because these drugs may alter estriol levels.

Procedure
Client preparation

1. See p. 181 "Client Preparation" for the "Creatinine Clearance Test" (except step 2) for 24-hour urine collec-

tion. The client is told the importance of a complete collection. Every urine specimen must be included or the study must be started over. The specimen requires a preservative and must be kept on ice throughout the collection period.

2. If the woman is going to collect the 24-hour urine specimen at home, she is given the collection bottle (with the preservative) and instructed to keep the urine refrigerated.

Procedure

1. *Urine collection:* See "Procedure" for 24-hour urine collection for "Creatinine Clearance Test" (except step 4).
2. *Serum collection:*
   a. Following standard venipuncture technique, 5 ml of blood are collected in the manner specified by the lab. Some labs require a heparinized container.
   b. Pressure or a pressure dressing is applied.

Nursing implications

1. If blood was drawn, assess the puncture site for bleeding afterward.
2. Inform the client how and when to get the results of this study from her physician.

HUMAN PLACENTAL LACTOGEN

See p. 300.

PREGNANCY TEST

See p. 301.

Radiologic Laboratory Tests
X-Ray Tests
X-RAY PELVIMETRY (RADIOGRAPHIC PELVIMETRY)
Normal Values

- Transverse of midpelvis diameter >10.5 cm.

Deviations from Normal

- Transverse midpelvis diameter <10.5 cm indicates that delivery through the birth canal may be difficult.

Indications

- To assess the client suspected of carrying the fetus in an abnormal position (e.g., breech) when a vaginal delivery is anticipated.
- To assess the client who has had injury or disease of the bony pelvis or hips that may have caused pelvic distortion.
- To assess the client with clinically abnormal pelvic measurements.
- To assess the client who has a debilitating illness complicating the pregnancy and a clinically small or unfavorable pelvis.
- To assess the client who has a history of difficult delivery.
- To evaluate the primiparas client in early labor, with the fetus's head unengaged (to rule out cephalopelvic disproportion).
- To assess the client admitted for trial labor to rule out a contracted pelvis.
- To evaluate the client experiencing dysfunctional labor.
- To provide legal documentation in the rare cases in which vaginal delivery is attempted despite an anticipated difficult delivery.

Contraindications

- A client in early pregnancy because x-rays may damage the fetus.

Procedure
Client preparation

1. The client is told that she must remove all clothing and don a long x-ray gown. Having her put on the gown before she leaves the nursing unit is a good idea.

Procedure

1. A lateral x-ray film is taken with the client standing to detect the effect of gravity on engagement and to indicate

the position of the fetal head when it reaches the lower level of the birth canal.
2. The client may then be placed in the supine, lateral, and semirecumbent positions.
3. During the x-ray exposure the client, is asked to stop breathing.
4. A radiologic technician performs this study in the x-ray department in approximately 15 minutes.

Special Studies
Endoscopy
AMNIOSCOPY
Normal Values

- Normal color of amniotic fluid; no meconium staining.

Deviations from Normal

- The presence of meconium in the amniotic fluid possibly indicating fetal distress or death.

Indications

- To assess fetal well-being.
- To sample fetal blood.

Contraindications

- A client in labor.
- A client with premature membrane rupture.
- A client with active cervical infection (e.g., gonorrhea).

Procedure
Client preparation

1. The client is told that cervical dilation will be uncomfortable.

Procedure

1. The client is placed in the lithotomy position.
2. The cervix is dilated 2 cm.
3. An endoscope (amnioscope) is introduced into the cervical canal.

4. The color of the amniotic fluid is evaluated.
5. A physician performs the study in 10 to 15 minutes.

Nursing implications

1. After the study, assess the client for rupture of the membranes and for uterine contractions.
2. After the study the client may have vaginal discomfort and menstrual-type cramping.

COLPOSCOPY

Normal Values

- Normal vagina and cervix.

Deviations from Normal

- With this procedure, tiny areas of dysplasia, carcinoma in situ, and invasive cancer, which would be missed by the naked eye, can be visualized.

Indications

- To visualize abnormalities and remove biopsy specimens.
- To assess clients with abnormal vaginal epithelial patterns, cervical lesions, and suspicious Pap smears.
- To assess clients exposed to diethylstilbestrol in utero.
- To substitute, at times, for cone biopsy in evaluating the cause of abnormal cervical cytologic findings.

Contraindications

- An uncooperative client.
- A client with heavy menstrual flow.

Procedure

Client preparation

1. The very fact that this study is required will arouse anxiety in most women.
2. The sensations the client may feel during this study are explained: pressure pains from the speculum and minor discomfort when the biopsy specimen is removed.

Procedure

1. The client is placed in the lithotomy position.
2. A vaginal speculum is used to expose the vagina and the cervix.
3. After the cervix is sampled for cytologic findings, it is cleansed with a 3% acetic acid solution to remove excess mucus and cellular debris. The acetic acid also accentuates the difference between normal and abnormal epithelial tissues.
4. The colposcope is then focused on the cervix (especially the squamocolumnar junction), which is then carefully examined. Usually the entire lesion can be outlined and the most atypical areas selected for biopsy specimen removal.
5. A physician performs this procedure in approximately 5 to 10 minutes.
6. The client will need to be hospitalized for diagnostic conization if:
   a. Colposcopy and endocervical curettage do not explain the problem or match the cytologic findings of the Pap smear within one grade;
   b. The entire transformation zone is not seen;
   c. The lesion extends up the cervical canal beyond the vision of the colposcope.

Nursing implications

1. After the study the client may have some vaginal bleeding if biopsy specimens were taken. The client should wear a sanitary pad.
2. Inform the client when and how to obtain the results of this study (usually 2 to 3 days).

FETOSCOPY
Normal Values

- Normal fetus.

Deviations from Normal

- Abnormal fetus.

Indications

- To diagnose a severe malformation (e.g., neural tube defect [NTD]).
- To allow the drawing of blood samples for analysis for such conditions as sickle cell anemia, beta-thalassemia, and hemophilia.
- To allow the performing of fetal skin biopsies to detect primary skin disorders (e.g., ichthyosis).

Procedure
Client preparation

1. If ordered, meperidine (Demerol) is administered because it crosses the placenta and quiets the fetus, thus preventing excessive fetal activity that makes the procedure more difficult.

Procedure

1. The mother's abdominal wall is anesthetized with a local anesthetic.
2. Ultrasonography is used to locate the fetus and the placenta.
3. The endoscope is inserted.
4. A physician performs this study in a specialized room in approximately 30 minutes.

Nurse alert

1. A possible complication is amnionitis. Antibiotics may be given afterward to prevent this.

Amniocentesis
Normal Values

- Normal values depend on the reason for the study.

Deviations from Normal

- See indications.

Indications

- To assess fetal maturity status.
- To determine the sex of the fetus.
- To determine genetic and chromosomal aberrations (e.g., hemophilia, Down's syndrome, and galactosemia).
- To assess the status of the fetus affected by Rh isoimmunization.
- To determine the existence of hereditary metabolic disorders (e.g., cystic fibrosis).
- To assess anatomic abnormalities such as neural tube closure defects (myelomeningocele, anencephaly, and spina bifida).
- To detect fetal distress by meconium staining of the amniotic fluid resulting from relaxation of the anal sphincter.

Contraindications

- Clients with abruptio placentae, placenta previa, a history of premature labor (before 34 weeks) unless the client is receiving antilabor medication at this time, and incompetent cervix.

Procedure

Client preparation

1. The client is assured that precautions will be taken to minimize risk to both her and the fetus. Relaxation techniques such as focusing and slow breathing can help relieve some maternal anxiety.
2. The fetal heart rate is auscultated before and after the study to detect any ill effects related to the procedure.
3. The mother's blood pressure is taken.
4. The placenta should be localized before the study by ultrasound to permit selection of a site that will avoid placental puncture.

Procedure

1. The client is placed in a supine position, and the skin overlying the chosen site is prepared, draped, and locally anes-

thetized. Once the skin is pierced, the client will feel pressure, but not pain.
2. A 22-gauge, 5-inch spinal needle with a stylet is then inserted through the midabdominal wall and directed at an angle toward the middle of the uterine cavity.
3. The stylet is then removed and a sterile plastic syringe is attached.
4. Ten to fifteen milliliters of amniotic fluid are withdrawn, and the needle is removed.
5. The site is covered with an adhesive bandage.
6. The amniotic fluid is placed in a sterile siliconized glass container and transported to a special chemistry lab for analysis. Sometimes the specimen may be sent by air mail to another commercial lab. The results are usually not available for at least 3 weeks.
7. An obstetrician performs this study.

Nursing implications

1. If the woman felt dizzy or nauseated during the procedure, allow her to rest on her left side for several minutes before she leaves the examining room.
2. After the procedure the mother's blood pressure is checked and the fetal heart tone is then assessed.
3. Instruct the client to call her doctor if she has any fluid loss or temperature elevation.
4. Inform the client how she can obtain the results of this study from her physician. Be certain that the client knows the results are not available for at least 3 weeks.

Nurse alert

1. The potential risks of amniocentesis for the fetus include miscarriage, fetal injury, subsequent leak of amniotic fluid, infection (amnioitis), abortion, or premature labor.
2. Risks to the mother include hemorrhage, fetomaternal hemorrhage with possible maternal Rh isoimmunization, labor, amniotic fluid embolism, infection, abruptio placentae, and inadvertent damage to the bladder or intestines. Note: The probability of risk is less than 1%.

Chlamydia Smears

Normal Values

- Negative.

Deviations from Normal

- A gram stain of the smear showing polymorphonuclear leukocytes is diagnostic of *Chlamydia* infection.

Indications

- To diagnose *Chlamydia* infections.

Contraindications

- A client having a routine normal menses.

Procedure

1. See "Gonorrhea Culture," p. 320.
2. Note that no specific therapy exists for this infection. If the diagnosis is established early by viral culture or serology, abortion may be an option.

Contraction Stress Test (CST; Oxytocin Challenge Test)

Normal Values

- Negative.

Deviations from Normal

- The test is considered *positive* if consistent and persistent late deceleration of the fetal heart rate occurs with two or more uterine contractions.
- The test is considered *equivocal* if inconsistent late decelerations occur, therefore the test should be repeated 24 hours later.
- The test is considered *unsatisfactory* if the results cannot be interpreted (e.g., because of hyperstimulation of the uterus or excessive maternal movement), and again it should be repeated.

Indications

- To assess fetoplacental adequacy in any high-risk pregnancy in which fetal well-being is threatened, including pregnancies marked by diabetes, hypertensive disease of pregnancy (toxemia), intrauterine growth retardation, Rh-factor sensitization, history of stillbirth, postmaturity, or low estriol levels.

Contraindications

- A client with multiple pregnancy.
- A client with premature ruptured membrane.
- A client with placenta previa.
- A client with abruptio placentae.
- A client with previous hysterotomy.
- A client with previous vertical or classic cesarean section; however, if necessary, the CST may be performed if carefully monitored and controlled.
- A client with a pregnancy of less than 33 weeks.

Procedure

Client preparation

1. The necessity of the test usually raises realistic fears in the mother. Verbalization and providing factual information is encouraged.
2. Breathing exercises and relaxation are practiced with the client before the study.
3. If the procedure is electively performed, the client is kept on nothing by mouth in case labor occurs as a result of testing.

Procedure

1. After emptying her bladder, the client is placed in the semi-Fowler's position and tilted slightly to one side to avoid venal caval compression by the enlarged uterus.
2. The client's blood pressure is checked every 10 minutes to avoid hypotension, which may cause diminished placental blood flow and a false-positive test result.

3. Blood pressure is then checked routinely every 15 minutes throughout the test.

4. An external fetal monitor is placed over the abdomen to record the fetal heart tones, and an external tocodynamometer is attached to the abdomen at the fundal region to monitor uterine contractions.

5. The output of the fetal heart tones and the uterine contractions is recorded on a two-channel strip recorder.

6. Baseline fetal heart rate and uterine activity are monitored for 15 to 20 minutes.

7. If uterine contractions are detected during this pretest period, oxytocin is withheld and the response of the fetal heart tone to spontaneous uterine contractions is monitored.

8. If no spontaneous uterine contractions occur, oxytocin (Pitocin) is administered by IV infusion using a pump (IVAC pump) at 0.5 to 1.0 mU/minute.

9. The rate of oxytocin infusion is increased every 20 minutes until the client is having three ''moderate-quality'' contractions per 10-minute period. The fetal heart rate pattern is recorded.

10. The oxytocin infusion is then discontinued, while fetal heart rate monitoring is continued for another 30 minutes until the uterine activity has returned to its preoxytocin state.

11. The body metabolizes oxytocin in approximately 20 to 25 minutes.

12. Analgesics are administered during the study, if ordered. The need for narcotics must be carefully assessed, because these drugs may affect the fetal heart rate tracing.

13. For the *breast stimulation* or *nipple stimulation* technique the nipples are stimulated for about 15 minutes by gentle twisting. If sufficient contractions do not result from nipple stimulation, the standard CST procedure is performed.

14. A nurse performs this test in the labor and delivery unit on an outpatient basis in approximately 2 hours. A physician is available.

Nursing implications

1. Monitor the client's blood pressure and the fetal heart rate before, during, and after the study, as indicated. Record these signs and the oxytocin infusion rate every 15 minutes on the monitor strip.
2. Administer the oxytocin by means of an infusion pump, because the infusion pump can be more precisely controlled than manual methods.
3. Discontinue the IV line after the study and apply an adhesive bandage to the site.
4. Continue the fetal monitoring for 30 minutes.
5. Assess the IV site for bleeding.
6. Many clients will have this study repeated at weekly intervals until delivery. This regimen is tiring and anxiety-producing for the clients, and they and their partners require much support.

Gonorrhea Culture
Normal Values

- No evidence of *Neisseria gonorrhoeae*.

Deviations from Normal

- Evidence of *Neisseria gonorrhoeae* indicating gonorrhea.

Indications

- To diagnose gonorrhea.

Contraindications

- The female client having a routine, normal menses.

Procedure
Client preparation

1. The female client is instructed to refrain from douching and bathing prior to a *cervical* culture.
2. The client is draped appropriately to avoid unnecessary exposure.

Procedure

1. Cervical culture:
   a. The female client is placed in the lithotomy position.
   b. A nonlubricated vaginal speculum is inserted to expose the cervix.
   c. Cervical mucus is removed with a cotton ball held in ring forceps.
   d. A sterile cotton-tipped swab is inserted into the endo-cervical canal and moved from side to side.
2. Anal canal culture:
   a. An anal culture of the female or male is taken by inserting a sterile, cotton-tipped swab about 1 inch into the anal canal.
   b. If stool contaminates the swab, a repeat swab is taken.
3. Urethral culture:
   a. The urethral specimen should be obtained from the male prior to voiding.
   b. The culture material is obtained by inserting a sterile swab gently into the anterior urethra.
4. Oropharyngeal culture:
   a. One can best obtain a throat culture by depressing the tongue with a wooden blade (tongue blade) and touching the posterior wall of the throat with a sterile cotton swab.
5. The specimens are obtained in a sterile manner. Sterile disposable gloves should be worn.
6. All specimens are handled as though they were capable of transmitting disease.
7. After the cultures are obtained, the swabs are placed in the Thayer-Martin medium and rolled from side to side. The swabs are then discarded.
8. The culture bottle is labeled and sent to the microbiology lab as soon as possible after specimen collection (at least within 30 minutes).

Nursing implications

1. Obtain the specimens before initiating any antibiotic therapy.

2. If culture results were positive, sexual partners should be evaluated and treated. If the results are positive in a pregnant client, treatment during pregnancy can prevent possible fetal complications (e.g., ophthalmia neonatorium) and maternal complications.

Nonstress Test
Normal Values

- "Reactive" fetus (heart rate acceleration associated with fetal movement).

Deviations from Normal

- If the test detects a nonreactive fetus (i.e., no fetal heart rate acceleration with fetal movement) within 40 minutes, the client is a candidate for the CST.

Indications

- To screen high-risk pregnancies.
- To select clients who may require CST. A nonstress test is now routinely performed before the CST to avoid the complications associated with oxytocin administration.

Procedure
Client preparation

1. The client is assured that no discomfort or adverse effects are associated with this study.
2. Verbalization of the client's fears is encouraged. The necessity for this study usually raises realistic fears in the expectant mother.
3. If the client is hungry, sending her to the cafeteria before initiating the nonstress test may be helpful because a high maternal serum glucose level enhances fetal activity.
4. The client empties her bladder before the study begins.

Procedure

1. The client is placed in the Sim's position.
2. An external fetal monitor is placed on the abdomen to record the fetal heart rate. The mother can indicate the occur-

rence of fetal movement by pressing a button on the fetal monitor whenever she feels the fetus move.

3. Fetal heart rate and fetal movement are concomitantly recorded on a two-channel strip graph.

4. The fetal monitor is then observed for fetal heart rate accelerations associated with fetal movement.

5. If the baby is quiet for 20 minutes, fetal activity is stimulated by external methods, such as rubbing the mother's abdomen, compressing the abdomen, ringing a bell near the abdomen, or placing a pan on the abdomen and banging on the pan.

6. A nurse performs this study in 20 to 40 minutes. A physician is available.

Papanicolaou Smear (Pap Smear; Pap Test; Cytologic Test for Cancer)

Normal Values

- No abnormal or atypical cells found.

Indications

- To detect neoplastic cells in cervical and vaginal secretions.
- To follow certain abnormalities (e.g., infertility).

Contraindications

- A woman who is currently having a routine, normal menses.

Procedure

Client preparation

1. The procedure is explained to the client, who is assured that she will be appropriately draped to prevent unnecessary exposure.

2. Determine if the client has douched or tub bathed during the 24 hours before the Pap smear. Douching and tub baths may wash away cellular deposits, which are desired in the specimen.

3. Determine if the client is menstruating.

Procedure

1. The client is placed in the lithotomy position.
2. An examining light is positioned for good visualization of the pelvic area.
3. A nonlubricated vaginal speculum is inserted to expose the cervix.
4. Material is collected from the cervical canal by rotating a moist, saline cotton swab or spatula within the cervical canal and also in the squamocolumnar junction.
5. The cells are immediately wiped across a clean glass slide and fixed either by immersing the slide in equal parts of 95% alcohol and ether or by using a commercial spray. The secretions must be fixed before drying occurs, because drying will distort the cells and make interpretation difficult.
6. The slide is labeled with the client's name. The client's name, age, and parity, the date of her last menstrual period, and the reason for the cytologic examination should be written on the request form.
7. A physician or a nurse obtains the smear in approximately 10 minutes.

Nursing implications

1. After the study, inform the client how to obtain the test results. Usually the office will notify the client only if further evaluation is necessary. If the smear was abnormal, assure the client that this does not necessarily mean that she has a malignancy. Many clients associate a suspicious test with malignancy and become frightened. Provide emotional support.

Ultrasonography
Normal Values

- Normal fetal and placental size and position.

Deviations from Normal

- The detection of an abnormal pregnancy.

Indications

- To make an early diagnosis of normal and abnormal pregnancy (e.g., ectopic or abdominal pregnancy).
- To identify multiple pregnancies.
- To differentiate a tumor (e.g., a hydatidiform mole) from a normal pregnancy.
- To determine the age of the fetus by the diameter of its head.
- To measure the rate of fetal growth. Sequential cephalometry can detect intrauterine growth retardation of the fetus. A disparity in BPDs in the second trimester can detect problems with twins. Sequential scans showing lack of growth, loss of fetal outline, and an increased number of echoes coming from within the fetal body can determine fetal death.
- To identify placental abnormalities such as abruptio placentae and placenta previa.
- To determine the position of the placenta.
- To make differential diagnoses of various uterine and ovarian enlargements (e.g., polyhydramnios, benign and malignant neoplasms, cysts, and abscesses).
- To determine fetal position.

Contraindications

- A client who has recently had a GI contrast study because the barium causes severe distortion of the sound waves.
- A client with air-filled bowels because gas does not transmit the sound waves well.

Procedure
Client preparation

1. The procedure is explained to the client, who is assured that this study has no known deleterious effect on maternal or fetal tissues even when repeated several times.
2. The client is given three or four glasses (200 to 350 ml) of water or other liquids 1 hour before the examination and is instructed *not* to void until after ultrasonography is completed. The fluid will permit better transmission of the sound waves and enhance visualization of the uterus.

3. The client is told that no pain is associated with this study. The client may have some discomfort because she will have a full bladder and the urge to void. Some clients may be uncomfortable lying on a hard x-ray table.

4. The client is told that a liberal amount of gel or lubricant will be applied to her skin to enhance the transmission and reception of the sound waves. The gel will feel cold.

Procedure

1. The client is placed in the supine position on the examining table.

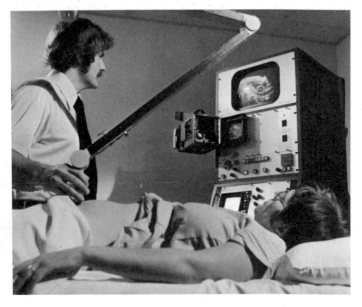

Figure 8-2
Ultrasonography is a safe, painless method of scanning a client's abdomen with high-frequency sound waves to follow fetal growth and development.
(Courtesy March of Dimes.)

2. The ultrasonographer (usually a radiologist) applies a greasy, conductive paste to the abdomen.
3. A transducer is then passed vertically and horizontally over the skin, and pictures are taken of the reflections (Fig. 8-2).
4. During the ultrasound examination, the fetal structures should be pointed out to the mother. Seeing the fetus during ultrasound may promote prenatal attachment.
5. The ultrasonographer performs the study in the ultrasound room in approximately 20 minutes.

Nursing implications

1. After the study, remove the lubricant from the client's skin and allow the client an opportunity to void.

Newborn Evaluation

Clinical Laboratory Tests

Blood Tests

GALACTOSE-1-PHOSPHATE URIDYL TRANSFERASE (GAL-1-PUT)

Normal Values

- 18.5 to 28.5 U/g hemoglobin.

Deviations from Normal

- Increased levels indicate galactosemia.

Indications

- To diagnose galactosemia.

Contraindications

- None.

Procedure

1. Following standard heel-stick procedure, 1 ml of blood is collected.

2. One of the screening tests is performed. Popular ones include:
   a. *Paigen assay* (a bacterial inhibition test), which depends on the presence of elevated blood galactose level, and so milk feeding is necessary.
   b. *Beutler assay,* which measures Gal-1-PUT and does not depend on milk feeding.
3. Both tests can be performed on filter-paper blood spots.

Nursing implications

1. If the test results for galactosemia are positive, dietary therapy should begin at once. Galactose-containing foods, especially milk, are removed from the diet.

PHENYLKETONURIA (PKU) TEST
Normal Values

- Blood: negative (<4 mg/dl). Level >8 to 12 mg/dl indicates PKU.
- Urine: no green coloration.

Deviations from Normal

- Elevated levels are diagnostic of phenylketonuria.

Indications

- To diagnose phenylketonuria.

Contraindications

- None.

Procedure
Client preparation

1. The purpose of the test and the method of performing this test are explained to the parent(s).
2. The infant's feeding patterns are assessed before the PKU test is performed. An inadequate amount of protein prior to performing the test can cause false-negative results.

3. Urine tests for PKU are commonly performed on the infant's first well-baby examination. This schedule is vitally important if the infant was not checked for PKU while in the hospital. The infant must be at least 6 weeks of age for appropriate screening with the urine test.

4. If the infant is discharged early or if a feeding problem (such as vomiting) has existed, the test may be falsely negative. To prevent this the test should be performed several days after discharge.

Procedure

1. Blood is collected by heel stick.
   a. The blood is placed on a filter paper for the Guthrie test.
2. *Urine* tests can also be used to detect PKU in infants who are at least 6 weeks of age, and are usually performed at the baby's first checkup.
   a. For the *diaper test,* 10% ferric chloride is dropped on a freshly wet diaper. A green spot indicates probable PKU.
   b. The *Phenistix test* is performed by pressing a test stick against a wet diaper or dipping it in urine. A green color reaction indicates probable PKU.
3. A nurse performs this study in less than 2 minutes. Blood is usually collected on the infant's discharge day from the hospital.

Nursing implications

1. If the results of the test are positive, dietary control must begin immediately to prevent brain damage. For this control, Lofenalac is substituted for milk. Later, strained foods low in protein are added to the diet. Dietary treatment is monitored by blood and urine testing.

2. Women with PKU, who wish to have children, should be instructed to begin a low phenylalanine diet prior to conception and continue it throughout the pregnancy. The risk of producing a mentally retarded infant is high if the mother remains on a general diet.

Special Studies

Barr Body Analysis (Sex Chromatin Body; Chromatin-Positive Body)

Normal Values

- Depends on the sex of the child.

Deviations from Normal

- A lack of Barr body in a female indicates Turner's syndrome (XO).
- Normal males (XY) have no Barr bodies. A male with Klinefelter's syndrome (XXY) would have one Barr body.
- An XXX female has two Barr bodies.
- A false lowering of sex chromatin Barr bodies may occur if specimens are taken during the first week of life.

Indications

- To aid in assigning a sex to an infant when ambiguity of the newborn's genitalia makes assigning sex to the infant difficult.
- To detect sex chromosome abnormalities (e.g., Turner's syndrome and Klinefelter's syndrome).

Contraindications

- None.

Procedure

Client preparation

1. Ample time for verbalization of feelings is allowed.
2. Clients and families with potential or confirmed chromosomal abnormalities often have much anxiety.

Procedure

1. Buccal cells are obtained by scraping the oral mucosa and smearing the cells onto a glass slide.
2. After chemical fixation and staining, the cells are studied. Assessment of the results, together with the secondary sexual characteristics and genitalia of the client, permit pre-

sumptive diagnosis of certain sex chromosome abnormalities. If necessary, chromosome *karyotyping* (systematic arrangement of photographed chromosomes to demonstrate structure and number) can confirm the results.
3. A technician performs the buccal smear in less than 5 minutes. A pathologist studies the smears.

Phenylketonuria (PKU) Test

See p. 328.

Bibliography

Anthony, C.P., and Thibodeau, G.A.: Textbook of anatomy and physiology, ed. 11, St. Louis, 1983, The C.V. Mosby Co.

Atkinson, L., Schearer, S., Harkairy, O., and Lincoln, R.: Prospects for improved contraception, Family planning perspectives **12:**173, 1980.

Austin, J.M., Cain, M.G., Hicks, J., and Wolf, F.S.: The Gravlee method—an alternative to the Pap smear? Am. J. Nurs. **83**(7):1057-1058, July 1983.

Becker, C.: Comprehensive assessment of the healthy gravida, JOGN Nurs. **11**(6):375-378, 1982.

Benson, R.C., editor: Current obstetric and gynecologic diagnosis and treatment, Los Altos, Calif., 1982, Lange Medical Publications.

Bernstein, J., and Mattox, J.H.: An overview of infertility, JOGN Nurs. **11**(5):309, 1982.

Bobak, I.M., and Jensen, M.D.: Essentials of maternity nursing, St. Louis, 1984, The C.V. Mosby Co.

Bolognese, R.L., Schwartz, R.H., and Schneider, J., editors: Perinatal medicine management of the fetus and neonate, ed. 2, Baltimore, 1982, Williams & Wilkins.

Brodish, M.S.: Perinatal assessment, JOGN Nurs. **10**(1):42-46, Jan./Feb. 1981.

Emerson, E.A.: Assessment and classification of the high-risk maternal–fetal unit, In Vestal, K.W., and McKenzie, C.A., editors: High-risk perinatal nursing, Philadelphia, 1983, W.B. Saunders Co.

Friedman, B.M.: Infertility workup, Am. J. Nurs. **81**(11):2040-2046, Nov. 1981.

Garcia, C., et al.: Current therapy of infertility, 1982-1983, St. Louis, 1983, The C.V. Mosby Co.

Jensen, M.D., Benson, R.C., and Bobak, I.M.: Maternity care—the nurse and the family, St. Louis, 1981, The C.V. Mosby Co.

Josten, L.: Prenatal assessment guide for illuminating possible problems with parenting, MCN 6(2):113-117, 1981.

Lieber, M.T.: "Nonstress" antepartal monitoring, MCN 5(5):335-339, 1980.

Lum, S.B., Lartz, R., and Barnett, E.: Reappraising newborn eye care, Am. J. Nurs. 80(9):1602-1603, Sept. 1980.

Maternal serum alpha-fetoprotein measurement in antenatal screening for anencephaly and spina bifida, Report of a V.K. Collaborative Study on Alpha-fetoprotein in Relation to Neural Tube Defects, Lancet 2:1323, 1977.

McCusker, M.P.: The subfertile couple, JOGN Nurs. 11(3):157, 1982.

McDonough, M., Sheriff, D., and Zimmel, P.: Parent's responses to fetal monitoring, MCN 6:32-34, 1981.

Moore, M.L.: Realities on childbearing, ed. 2, Philadelphia, 1983, W.B. Saunders Co.

Neilson, J.P., and Hood, V.D.: Ultrasound in obstetrics and gynecology, Br. Med. Bull. 36(3):249-255, 1980.

Patrick, J., et al.: Patterns of gross fetal body movements over 24-hour observation intervals during the last 10 weeks of pregnancy, Am. J. Obstet. Gynecol. 142:363-371, 1982.

Rayburn, W.F.: Clinical implications from monitoring fetal activity, Am. J. Obstet. Gynecol. 144(8):967-979, 1982.

Reeder, S.J., Mastroianni, L., and Martin, L.L.: Maternity nursing, ed. 15, Philadelphia, 1983, J.B. Lippincott Co.

Schottelius, B.A., and Schottelius, D.D.: Textbook of physiology, ed. 19, St. Louis, 1983, The C.V. Mosby Co.

Seeds, A.E.: Maternal–fetal acid-base relationships and fetal scalp blood analysis. In Makowski, E.L., editor: Clinical Obstetrics and Gynecology, High Risk Obstetrics, vol. 21, no. 2, pp. 579-591, New York, 1978, Harper & Row.

Vestal, K.W., and McKenzie, C.A., editors: High-risk perinatal nursing, Philadelphia, 1983, W.B. Saunders Co.

Willis, S.E., and Sharp, E.S.: Hypertension in pregnancy: prenatal detection and management, Am. J. Nurs. 82(5):798-808, May 1982.

Ziegel, E.E., and Cranley, M.S.: Obstetric nursing, ed. 8, New York, 1984, Macmillan Publishing Co.

Hematologic System

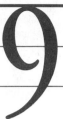

Clinical laboratory tests
  Blood tests
    Bleeding time test (Ivy bleeding time)
    Blood typing
    Coagulating factors concentration
    Complete blood count and differential count (CBC and diff, hemogram)
    Delta-aminolevulinic acid test (ΔALA, aminolevulinic acid, ALA)
    Direct Coombs' test
    Disseminated intravascular coagulation (DIC) screening
    Euglobulin lysis time test
    Fibrin degradation products test (fibrin split products, FSP, fibrinogen degradation products)
    Folic acid (folate)
    Glucose-6-phosphate-dehydrogenase (G6PD)
    Hemoglobin electrophoresis
    Indirect Coombs' test (blood antibody screening)
    Iron level and total iron-binding capacity test (Fe and TIBC)
    Partial thromboplastin time (activated) test (PTT test)
    Peripheral blood smear
    Platelet count
    Prothrombin time test (Pro-time, PT test)
    Reticulocyte count test
    Serum ferritin
    Serum haptoglobin test
    Sickle cell test (sickle cell preparation, sickledex, Hgb S test)
    Whole blood clot retraction test
  Urine tests
    Schilling test (vitamin B_{12} absorption test)
    Urinary porphyrins and porphobilinogens

Special studies
Bone marrow examination (bone marrow biopsy, bone marrow aspiration)

Clinical Laboratory Tests

Blood Tests
BLEEDING TIME TEST (IVY BLEEDING TIME)
Normal Values

- 1 to 9 minutes.

Deviations from Normal

- Prolonged bleeding times occur in decreased platelet counts, infiltration of marrow by primary or metastic tumor, consumption of platelets during disseminated intravascular coagulation (DIC), increased platelet destruction (e.g., in primary and secondary thrombocytopenia and hypersplenism), inadequate platelet function, increased capillary fragility, and ingestion of antiinflammatory drugs (e.g., aspirin or indomethacin).

Indications

- To evaluate vascular and platelet factors associated with hemostasis.

Contraindications

- None.

Procedure
Client preparation

1. The client is assessed for aspirin ingestion during the week preceding the test.

Procedure

1. The skin of the inner part of the forearm is cleansed with alcohol or povidone-iodine (Betadine).

2. A blood pressure cuff (tourniquet) is placed on the arm above the elbow, inflated to 40 torr, and maintained at this pressure during the study.
3. A small laceration is then made 3 mm deep into the skin, and the time is recorded.
4. Bleeding ensues and the blood is blotted clean at 30-second intervals.
5. When no new bleeding occurs, the time is recorded. The time interval (from the beginning to the end of bleeding) is calculated and called the bleeding time.
6. The blood pressure cuff is removed, and an adhesive bandage is applied to the client's arm.
7. If the bleeding persists for more than 10 minutes, the test is stopped and a pressure dressing is applied.
8. A physician performs this test at the client's bedside.

Nursing implications

1. Assist the physician in performing the test.
2. Apply a dressing to the client's forearm after the study. Assess the arm for subsequent bleeding. Apply a pressure dressing if oozing of blood is noted.
3. If the client is on anticoagulants, include this information with the test results.
4. The client with a factor deficiency may have a normal bleeding time but subsequently ooze blood from the test site 20 minutes after the original bleeding has stopped. Pressure should be applied to the wound.

Nurse alert

1. A rare complication is laceration of a muscle, tendon, artery, or vein.
2. Infections usually do not occur if appropriate skin preparation and aftercare are given.

BLOOD TYPING
Deviations from Normal

- Mismatch of antigens.

Indications

- To detect antibodies to the recipient's blood in the donor's blood.
- To screen all pregnant women for incompatibility with the fetus' blood.
- To advise the mother whether she is a candidate for Rhogam (Rh immunoglobulin) after the delivery.

Contraindications

- None.

Procedure
Client preparation

1. The client is assessed for a previous allergic reaction to transfused blood products.

Procedure

1. Following standard venipuncture technique, 14 ml of blood are collected.
2. Pressure or a pressure dressing is applied.

Nursing implications

1. Assess the venipuncture site for bleeding.

COAGULATING FACTORS CONCENTRATION
Normal Values

- 50% to 200% of "normal."

Deviations from Normal

- See Table 9-1.

Indications

- To identify the factor(s) involved in the coagulating defect so that appropriate blood component replacement can be administered (see Table 9-2).

Contraindications

- None.

Procedure

Client preparation

1. The procedure is explained to the client.

Procedure

1. Following standard venipuncture technique, blood is collected.
2. Pressure or a pressure dressing is applied.

Table 9-1   Conditions that may result in coagulation factor deficiency

Condition	Factor Diminished
Liver disease	I, II, V, VII, IX, X, XI
Disseminated intravascular coagulation (DIC)	I, V, VIII
Fibrinolysis	I, V, VII
Congenital deficiency	I, II, V, VII, VIII, IX, X, XI
Heparin administration	II
Warfarin ingestion	II, VII, IX, X, XI
Autoimmune disease	VIII

Table 9-2   Minimum concentration of coagulation factors required for adequate fibrin production

Factor	Minimum Hemostatic Level (mg/dl)	Blood Components*
I	60-100	C, FFP, FWB
II	10-15	P, WB, FFP, FWB
V	5-10	FFP, FWB
VII	5-20	P, WB, FFP, FWB
VIII	30	C, FFP, VIII CONC
IX	30	FFP, FWB
X	8-10	P, WB, FFP, FWB
XI	25	P, WB, FFP, FWB

*Blood components capable of providing specific factor: *C*, cryoprecipitate; *FFP*, fresh frozen plasma; *FWB*, fresh whole blood (<24 hours old); *P*, unfrozen banked plasma; *WB*, banked whole blood; *VIII CONC*, factor VIII concentrate.

Nursing implications

1. Assess the venipuncture site for bleeding.
2. Test results usually require 1 to 7 days, depending on whether the specimen must be sent to a commercial lab or whether the hospital lab can perform the test.

COMPLETE BLOOD COUNT AND DIFFERENTIAL COUNT (CBC AND DIFF; HEMOGRAM)

Red Blood Cell (RBC) Count

Normal values

- Vary according to sex and age.
- Men: 4.7 to 6.1 million/mm^3.
- Women: 4.2 to 5.4 million/mm^3.
- Infants and children: 3.8 to 5.5 million/mm^3.
- Newborns: 4.8 to 7.1 million/mm^3.

Deviations from normal

- A client with an RBC count below 10% of the expected norm is anemic.
- Causes for low RBC values include hemorrhage (e.g., gastrointestinal bleeding or trauma), hemolysis (e.g., glucose 6-phosphate dehydrogenase deficiency, spherocytosis, secondary splenomegaly), dietary deficiency (e.g., iron or vitamin B_{12}), genetic aberrations (e.g., sickle cell anemia or thalassemia), drug ingestion (e.g., chloramphenicol, hydantoins, quinine), marrow failure (e.g., fibrosis, leukemia, antineoplastic chemotherapy), chronic illness (e.g., tumor or sepsis), and other organ failure (e.g., renal disease).
- The body's requirement for greater oxygen-carrying capacity (e.g., at high altitudes) may physiologically induce an RBC level greater than normal.
- Diseases that produce chronic anoxia (e.g., congenital heart disease) also provoke physiologic increase in RBCs.
- Polycythemia vera, a neoplastic condition, involves uncontrolled production of RBCs.

Hemoglobin (Hgb) Concentration
Normal values

- Vary with age and sex.
- Men: 14 to 18 g/dl.
- Women: 12 to 16 g/dl (pregnancy <11 g/dl).
- Children: 11 to 16 g/dl.
- Newborns: 14 to 24 g/dl.

Deviations from normal

- Deviations from normal closely parallel those for the RBC count above.
- In addition, hemoglobin concentration more accurately reflects changes in plasma volume.
- Dilutional overhydration decreases the concentration.
- Dehydration tends to cause an artificially high value.
- Values are decreased during pregnancy.

Hematocrit (Hct)
Normal values

- Vary with age and sex.
- Men: 42% to 52%.
- Women: 37% to 47% (pregnancy >33%).
- Children: 31% to 43%.
- Infants: 30% to 40%.
- Newborns: 44% to 64%.

Deviations from normal

- Abnormal values indicate the same pathologic states as do abnormal RBC counts and hemoglobin concentrations (see above).

Mean Corpuscular Volume (MCV)
Normal values

- Vary with sex and age.
- Adults and children: 80 to 95 μm^3.
- Newborns: 96 to 108 μm^3.

Deviations from normal

- A macrocytic (abnormally large) RBC count occurs when the MCV value is increased, most commonly in megaloblastic anemias (e.g., vitamin B_{12} or folic-acid deficiency).
- A microcytic (abnormally small) RBC count occurs when the MCV value is decreased (e.g., iron-deficiency anemia or thalassemia).

Mean Corpuscular Hemoglobin (MCH)
Normal values

- Adults and children: 27 to 31 pg.
- Newborns: 32 to 34 pg.

Deviations from normal

- Because macrocytic cells usually have more hemoglobin and microcytic cells generally have less hemoglobin, the causes for these values closely resemble those for the MCV value (see above).

Mean Corpuscular Hemoglobin Concentration (MCHC)
Normal values

- Adults and children: 32 to 36 g/dl (or 32% to 36%).
- Newborns: 32 to 33 g/dl (or 32% to 33%).

Deviations from normal

- Hypochromic cells have a hemoglobin deficiency and occur when values are decreased (e.g., iron-deficiency anemia and thalassemia). See boxed material on p. 341.

White Blood Cell Count (WBC)
Normal values

- Total WBCs: adults and children over 2 years old, 5000 to 10,000/mm³; children 2 years old and younger, 6200 to 17,000/mm³; newborns: 9000 to 30,000/mm³.
- Differential count: neutrophils, 55% to 70%; lymphocytes, 20% to 40%; monocytes, 2% to 8%; eosinophils, 1% to 4%; basophils, 0.5% to 1%.

Categories of Anemia According to the RBC Indexes (MCV, MCH, MCHC)

Normocytic, normochromic anemia
 Chronic illness (such as sepsis or tumor)
 Acute blood loss
 Aplastic anemia (such as chloramphenicol toxicosis)
 Acquired hemolytic anemias (such as from a prosthetic cardiac valve)
Microcytic, hypochromic anemia
 Iron deficiency
 Thalassemia
 Lead poisoning
Microcytic, normochromic anemia
 Renal disease (because of the loss of erythropoietin)
Macrocytic, normochromic anemia
 Vitamin B_{12} or folic-acid deficiency
 Hydantoin ingestion

Deviations from normal

- An increased total WBC count (leukocytosis) usually indicates infection or leukemic neoplasia.
- Trauma or stress, either emotional or physical, can increase the WBC count.
- Leukopenia (a decreased WBC count) occurs in many forms of bone marrow failure (e.g., after antineoplastic therapy or in agranulocytosis), overwhelming infections, dietary deficiency, and autoimmune diseases.
- Elevation of any one type of leukocyte (e.g., neutrophil, which is important in fighting microbial invasion) may indicate a specific disease. See boxed material on p. 342.

Indications

- To screen clients upon admission to the hospital.
- To aid in diagnosing conditions listed under "Deviations from Normal" above.

Contraindications

■ None.

Procedure

1. Following standard venipuncture technique, 5 to 7 ml of blood are collected in a lavender-top (oxalate-containing)

Differential Categories for Diagnosis of Disease Processes Based on Leukocyte Elevation

Elevated neutrophil count (neutrophilia)
  Physical or emotional stress
  Acute suppurative infection
  Myelocytic leukemia
  Trauma
  Ketoacidosis
Decreased neutrophil count (neutropenia)
  Aplastic anemia
  Myelotoxic drugs (as in chemotherapy)
  Dietary deficiency
  Overwhelming bacterial infection (especially in the aged)
Elevated lymphocyte count (lymphocytosis)
  Chronic bacterial infection
  Viral infection
  Lymphocytic leukemia
  Multiple myeloma
  Infectious mononucleosis
Decreased lymphocyte count (lymphocytopenia)
  Leukemia
  Antineoplastic drugs
  Sepsis
  Immune deficiency diseases
Elevated eosinophil count (eosinophilia)
  Parasitic infestation
  Allergic reactions
  Eczema
  Leukemia
  Autoimmune diseases
Decreased eosinophil count (eosinopenia)
  Increased adrenal steroid production

vacutainer. The blood specimen is tilted up and down to mix the oxalate with the blood. A 20-gauge needle is used.
2. Capillary blood sticks of the finger may be performed for some individual tests.
3. Pressure or a pressure dressing is applied.

Nursing implications

1. Assess the venipuncture site for bleeding.

DELTA-AMINOLEVULINIC ACID TEST (ΔALA; AMINOLEVULINIC ACID, ALA)

Normal Values

- 1 to 7 mg/24 h.

Deviations from Normal

- Elevated levels occur in lead poisoning, porphyrias, hepatitis, and hepatic carcinoma.
- Certain medications (e.g., penicillin, barbiturates, griseofulvin) may cause elevated levels.

Indications

- To screen for lead poisoning.
- To aid in the diagnosis of certain genetic deficiencies of porphyrin metabolism (the porphyrias).

Contraindications

- None.

Procedure

Client preparation

1. The test and the method for collecting the 24-hour urine specimen are explained to the client.
2. If the client has a Foley catheter in place, the drainage bag should be protected during the collection period by a dark plastic bag to prevent light exposure.
3. See "Client Preparation" for 24-hour urine collection for "Creatinine Clearance Test" (except step 2), p. 181.

Procedure

1. The client, with assistance as needed, collects a 24-hour urine specimen in a light-resistant container.
2. A preservative is used.
3. The specimen is kept on ice or refrigerated during the entire collection period.
4. See "Procedure" for 24-hour urine collection for "Creatinine Clearance Test" (except step 4), p. 181.

Nursing implications

1. Indicate on the lab slip any medications the client is currently taking. Some medications (e.g., penicillin, barbiturates, and griseofulvin) may cause false-positive results.
2. Because the chronic ingestion of lead leads to anemia and eventually to vomiting, stupor, or convulsions, the source of lead (e.g., paint) should be found and removed. The child and his or her family should be referred to a community health nurse for follow-up in the community setting.

DIRECT COOMBS' TEST

Normal Values

- Negative; no agglutination.

Deviations from Normal

- Many diseases (e.g., erythroblastosis fetalis, lymphomas, lupus erythematosus, mycoplasmal infection, and infectious mononucleosis) and some drugs (e.g., alpha-methyldopa, levodopa, penicillin, and quinidine) are associated with the production of autoantibodies against RBCs. These antibodies result in hemolytic anemia.
- Frequently the production of these autoantibodies against RBCs is not associated with any disease, and the resulting hemolytic anemia is called idiopathic.

Indications

■ To evaluate suspected transfusion reaction.

Procedure

1. Following standard venipuncture technique, blood is collected in a red-top container.
2. Pressure or a pressure dressing is applied.
3. In newborns, venous blood from the umbilical cord is used.

Nursing implications

1. Assess the venipuncture site for bleeding.

DISSEMINATED INTRAVASCULAR COAGULATION (DIC) SCREENING

Fig. 9-1 provides a summary of DIC pathophysiology and effects. When a client with a bleeding tendency is suspected of having DIC, a series of readily performed lab tests should be performed (Table 9-3). The tests are all presented elsewhere in this chapter.

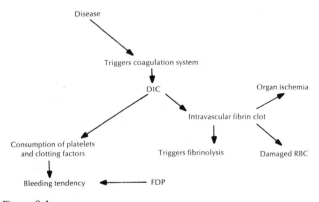

Figure 9-1
Pathophysiology of disseminated intravascular coagulation, which may result in bleeding tendency, organ ischemia, and hemolytic anemia.

Table 9-3   DIC screening tests

Test	Positive Result
Bleeding time	Prolonged
Platelet count	Decreased
Prothrombin time	Prolonged
Activated partial thromboplastin time	Prolonged
Fibrinogen (factor I concentration)	Decreased
Fibrin degradation products	Present
RBC smear	Damaged RBCs and decreased number of platelets
Euglobulin lysis time	Normal or prolonged

EUGLOBULIN LYSIS TIME TEST
Normal Values

- 90 minutes to 6 hours.

Deviations from Normal

- Rapid (short) euglobulin time may indicate primary fibrinolysis resulting from streptokinase administration, cancer of the prostate, shock, and other conditions.

Indications

- To differentiate fibrinolysis from DIC, which usually presents a normal euglobulin time.
- To monitor streptokinase or urokinase therapy used to dissolve clots in deep-vein thrombophlebitis.

Contraindications

- None.

Procedure

1. Following standard procedure, a peripheral venipuncture is performed, and 4.5 ml of blood are collected in a chilled oxalate-containing tube.
2. Pressure or a pressure dressing is applied.

Nursing implications

1. See "PT Test," p. 358, and "PTT Test," p. 353.

FIBRIN DEGRADATION PRODUCTS TEST (FIBRIN SPLIT PRODUCTS; FSP; FIBRINOGEN DEGRADATION PRODUCTS)

Normal Values

- < 10 µg/ml.

Deviations from Normal

- A high level of fibrin degradation products indicates increased fibrinolysis as in DIC and primary fibrinolytic disorders.

Indications

- To aid in diagnosing DIC and primary fibrinolytic disorders.

Contraindications

- None.

Procedure

1. Following standard venipuncture technique, blood is collected in a blue-top tube.
2. Pressure or a pressure dressing is applied.

Nursing implications

1. Assess the venipuncture site for bleeding.
2. See "PTT Test," p. 353.

FOLIC ACID (FOLATE)

Normal Values

- 5 to 20 μg/ml.

Deviations from Normal

- Decreased levels may occur in pregnancy.
- Decreased levels occur in clients with folic-acid anemia (megaloblastic anemia), hemolytic anemia, malnutrition, malabsorption syndrome, malignancy, liver disease, sprue, and celiac disease.
- Some drugs (e.g., anticonvulsants, antimalarials, alcohol, aminopterin, and methotrexate) are folic-acid antagonists and therefore interfere with nucleic acid synthesis.
- Elevated levels of folic acid occur with pernicious anemia.

Indications

- To evaluate hemolytic disorders.
- To detect folic-acid anemia (where the red blood cells are abnormally large, causing a megaloblastic anemia).

Contraindications

- None.

Procedure

Client preparation

1. The client should avoid alcoholic beverages prior to the test.

Procedure

1. Following standard venipuncture technique, 7 to 9 ml of blood are collected in a red-top tube.
2. Pressure or a pressure dressing is applied.

Nursing implications

1. Assess the venipuncture site for bleeding.
2. Prevent hemolysis of blood by gently handling specimen.

GLUCOSE-6-PHOSPHATE-DEHYDROGENASE (G6PD)

Normal Values

- 8 to 18.6 U/g hemoglobin.

Deviations from Normal

- Levels of G6PD may be increased in clients with pernicious anemia, myocardial infarction, hepatic coma, hyperthyroidism, chronic blood loss, and other megaloblastic anemias.

Indications

- To aid in detecting conditions listed above in "Deviations from Normal."
- To determine if the hemolytic anemia results from lack of G6PD.

Contraindications

- None.

Procedure

1. Following standard venipuncture technique, blood is collected.
2. Pressure or a pressure dressing is applied.
3. The sample is sent immediately to the lab for analysis.

Nursing implications

1. Assess the venipuncture site for bleeding.
2. If the test indicates that a lack of G6PD exists, the client should receive the list of drugs that can precipitate hemolysis (see above).
3. Clients with the Mediterranean variation of this disease should not eat fava beans.
4. Teaching the client to read the labels on any over-the-counter drugs for the presence of products (e.g., aspirin and phenacetin) that can cause hemolytic anemia is important.

HEMOGLOBIN ELECTROPHORESIS

Normal Values

- Hgb A_1: 95% to 98%.
- Hgb A_2: 2% to 3%.
- Hgb F: 0.8% to 2%.
- Hgb S: 0%.
- Hgb C: 0%.

Deviations from Normal

- Increased levels of Hgb F may indicate prolonged chronic hypoxia (e.g., congenital cardiac abnormalities) or hemoglobinopathies, which hinder the transportation of adequate amounts of oxygen (e.g., thalassemia).
- Hgb S is associated with sickle cell anemia.
- The presence of Hgb C may result in mild hemolytic anemia.

Indications

- To aid in diagnosing conditions listed under "Deviations from Normal" above.

Contraindications

- A client who has received a blood transfusion within the previous 12 weeks because the donor's blood may, if normal, mask and dilute abnormal hemoglobin variation that may exist in the recipient.

Procedure
Client preparation

1. The client is assessed to be certain that he or she has not had any blood transfusions within 12 weeks.

Procedure

1. Following standard venipuncture technique, 7 ml of blood are collected in a lavender-top or a EDTA-containing tube.
2. Pressure or a pressure dressing is applied.

Nursing implications

1. Assess the venipuncture site for bleeding.

INDIRECT COOMBS' TEST (BLOOD ANTIBODY SCREENING)
Normal Values
- Negative.

Deviations from Normal
- Clumping indicates the presence of antibodies against the recipient's RBCs.
- Circulating antibodies against RBCs may also occur in a pregnant woman who is Rh negative and is carrying an Rh-positive fetus.

Indications
- To screen transfusion recipients for compatibility with donor blood.

Contraindications
- None.

Procedure
1. Following standard venipuncture technique, 7 ml of blood are collected from the proposed recipient in a red-top vacutainer (without an anticoagulant).
2. Pressure or a pressure dressing is applied.

Nursing implications

1. Assess the venipuncture site for bleeding.

IRON LEVEL AND TOTAL IRON-BINDING CAPACITY TEST (Fe AND TIBC)
Normal Values
- Iron: 60 to 190 μg/dl.
- TIBC: 250 to 420 μg/dl.
- Dividing the serum iron level by the TIBC gives the percentage of saturation:

$$\text{Transferrin saturation (\%)} = \frac{\text{Serum iron level}}{\text{TIBC}} \times 100\%$$

Deviations from Normal

- A low iron level may indicate anemia resulting from many causes, including insufficient iron intake, inadequate gut absorption, increased requirements (e.g., growing children), and loss of blood (e.g., menstruation, bleeding peptic ulcer, colon neoplasm).
- A decreased serum iron level, an elevated TIBC, and a low transferrin saturation value are characteristic of iron-deficiency anemia.
- A decrease in the MCV and MCHC indexes is also found.
- A low serum iron level, a decreased iron-binding capacity, and a normal transferrin saturation characterize chronic illness (e.g., infections, neoplasia, cirrhosis).
- Pregnancy is marked by high levels of protein, including transferrin. Because of high iron requirements, finding low serum iron levels, high TIBC, and a low percentage of transferrin saturation is not unusual in late pregnancy.
- Increased intake or absorption of iron (e.g., hemochromatosis) leads to elevated iron levels. Because in such cases the TIBC is unchanged, the percentage of transferrin saturation is high. Excess iron is usually deposited in the brain, liver, and heart, causing severe dysfunction of these organs.

Indications

- To aid in diagnosing conditions discussed above.

Contraindications

- A client who recently received transfusions.
- A client who recently ingested a meal with a high iron content.
- A client with a hemolytic disease that may be associated with an artificially high iron content.

Procedure
Client preparation

1. The client is kept on nothing by mouth (except water) for 12 hours before the test.
2. The client is assessed for a history of blood transfusions and recent meals high in iron content.

Procedure

1. A 20-gauge needle is used because a smaller needle may traumatize the RBC, resulting in hemolysis. Some labs require the use of an iron-free needle and container.
2. Following standard venipuncture technique, 7 ml of blood are obtained and placed in a red-top tube.
3. Pressure or a pressure dressing is applied.

Nursing implications

1. Assess the puncture site for bleeding.

PARTIAL THROMBOPLASTIN TIME (ACTIVATED) TEST (PTT TEST)

Normal Values

- 30 to 40 seconds.

Deviations from Normal

- Because factors II, IX, and X are vitamin K–dependent factors produced in the liver, hepatocellular disease or biliary obstruction can reduce their concentration and thus prolong the PTT.

Indications

- To assess the intrinsic system and the common pathway of clot formation.
- To determine the appropriate dose of heparin by monitoring the dosage by the PTT. Heparin provides therapeutic anticoagulation.

Contraindications

- None.

Procedure

Client preparation

1. The client is told that the blood is being drawn to assess how quickly it clots.
2. Usually the PTT specimen is drawn daily, 30 minutes to 1

hour before heparin administration. The heparin dosage may be altered, depending on the results.

Procedure

1. Following standard venipuncture technique, blood is collected in a blue-top tube. The tube must be completely full to prevent an incorrect PTT value resulting from the extra citrate within the tube.
2. Pressure or a pressure dressing is applied.

Nursing implications

1. Assess the venipuncture site for bleeding.
2. If the client is receiving anticoagulants or has coagulopathies, bleeding time will be increased.
3. Assess the client to detect possible bleeding (i.e., check for blood in the urine and all excretia and assess the client for bruises, petechiae, and low back pain).
4. If severe bleeding occurs, the anticoagulant effect of heparin can be reversed by parenteral administration of protamine sulfate.

PERIPHERAL BLOOD SMEAR

Normal Values

- Normal quantity of RBCs, WBCs, and platelets; normal size, shape, and color of RBCs; normal white cell differential count.

Deviations from Normal

- See the boxed material on pp. 356 and 357 for a list of RBC variables, possible deviations, and causes of anemia.
- An increased number of immature WBCs may indicate leukemia.
- A decreased WBC count indicates marrow failure caused by drugs, chronic disease, neoplasia, or fibrosis.

Contraindications

- To aid in diagnosing conditions listed under ''Deviations from Normal'' above.

Procedure

1. A finger stick is performed in the hematology lab by a technician who also prepares the slide. A physician examines the slide.
2. The finger is cleaned with alcohol.
3. A finger stick is performed, and a drop of blood is spread on a slide.

PLATELET COUNT

Normal Values

- 150,000 to 400,000/mm^3.

Deviations from Normal

- Counts below 100,000/mm^3 constitute *thrombocytopenia* (decreased number of platelets). Causes include reduced production (secondary to bone marrow failure or infiltration), sequestration (secondary to hypersplenism), accelerated destruction of platelets (secondary to antibodies, infections, prosthetic heart valves), consumption (secondary to disseminated intravascular coagulation), and platelet loss from hemorrhage.
- *Thrombocytosis* exists when counts are greater than 400,000/mm^3. Conditions associated with thrombocytosis include severe hemorrhage, polycythemia vera, leukemia, postsplenectomy syndromes, and various malignant disorders.

Indications

- To detect thrombocytosis and thrombocytopenia.
- To signal the possibility for spontaneous bleeding when the count falls below 15,000/mm^3.

Contraindications

- None.

Procedure

1. Following standard venipuncture technique, 5 to 7 ml of blood are collected in a lavender-top tube.
2. Pressure or a pressure dressing is applied.

RBC Variables, Possible Deviations, and Causes of Anemia

RBC size
  Microcytes (small RBC)
    Iron deficiency
    Hereditary spherocytosis
    Thalassemia
  Macrocytes (larger size)
    Vitamin B_{12} or folic acid deficiency
    Reticulocytosis secondary to increased erythropoiesis
      (RBC production)
    Occasional liver disorder
    Postsplenectomy anemia
RBC shape
  Spherocytes (small and round)
    Hereditary spherocytosis
    Acquired immunohemolytic anemia
  Elliptocytes (crescent or sickled)
    Hereditary elliptocytosis
    Sickle cell anemia
  Leptocytes, or "target cells" (thin and less hemoglobin)
    Hemoglobinopathies
    Thalassemia
  Spicule cell
    Uremia
    Liver disease
    Bleeding ulcer
RBC color
  Hypochromic (pale)
    Iron deficiency
    Thalassemia
    Cardiac disease
  Hyperchromasia (more colored)
    Concentrated hemoglobin usually caused by dehydration

RBC Variables, Possible Deviations, and Causes of Anemia—cont'd

RBC intracellular structure

Nucleus (because the maturation process of the RBC results in the loss of the nucleus, nucleated RBCs [normoblasts] seen in the peripheral smear indicate increased RBC production)

"Normal" for infant's blood

Physiologic response to RBC deficiency (as in hemolytic anemias, sickle cell crisis, transfusion reaction, and erythroblastosis fetalis)

Physiologic response to hypoxemia (as in congenital heart disease and congestive heart failure)

Marrow-occupying neoplasm or fibrotic tissue (as in myeloma and leukemia)

Basophilic stippling (refers to bodies enclosed or included in the cells)

Lead poisoning

Reticulocytosis (see p. 359)

Howell-Jolly bodies (small, round remnants of nuclear material)

Postsplenectomy

Hemolytic anemia

Megaloblastic anemia

Heinz bodies (small, irregular particles of hemoglobin)

Drug-induced RBC injury

Hemoglobinopathies

Hemolytic anemia

Nursing implications

1. Assess the venipuncture site for bleeding.

PROTHROMBIN TIME TEST (PRO-TIME; PT TEST)
Normal Values

- 11 to 12.5 seconds; 85% to 100%.

Deviations from Normal

- Many diseases and drugs are associated with decreased levels of these factors, including hepatocellular liver disease (e.g., cirrhosis, hepatitis, and neoplastic invasive processes), obstructive biliary disease (e.g., bile duct obstruction secondary to tumor or stones or intrahepatic cholestasis secondary to sepsis or drugs), and coumarin ingestion (used to prevent coagulation in clients with thromboembolic disease, e.g., pulmonary embolism, thrombophlebitis, and arterial embolism).

Indications

- To evaluate clotting adequacy.
- To monitor the adequacy of coumarin therapy. Appropriate coumarin therapy should prolong PT by one and a half to two times the control value (or 20% to 30% of the normal value if percentages are used).
- To differentiate parenchymal liver disease from obstructive biliary disease by using the PT to determine the client's response to parenteral vitamin K administration (10 mg, IM, twice daily).

Contraindications

- None.

Procedure
Client preparation

1. If the client is receiving warfarin (a coumarin derivative), the PT specimen should be drawn before the client receives the daily dose. The daily dose may be increased,

decreased, or kept the same, depending on the PT test results for the day.

Procedure

1. Following standard venipuncture technique, collect one or two blue-top tubes (containing sodium citrate). The tubes *must* be filled to capacity to prevent artificially prolonging PT test results because of extra citrate in the tube.
2. Pressure or a pressure dressing is applied.

Nursing implications

1. Assess the venipuncture site for bleeding.
2. The bleeding time will be prolonged if the client is taking warfarin or if the client has any coagulopathies.
3. If the PT is markedly prolonged, evaluate the client for bleeding tendencies (i.e., check for blood in the urine and all excretia and assess the client for bruises, petechiae, and low back pain).
4. If severe bleeding occurs, the anticoagulant effect of warfarin can be reversed by the slow parenteral administration of vitamin K (phytonadione).
5. Because of drug interactions, the client is instructed not to take any medication unless the physician specifically ordered it.

RETICULOCYTE COUNT TEST
Normal Values

- Adults and children: 0.5% to 2% of total erythrocytes.
- Infants: 0.5% to 3.1% of total erythrocytes.
- Newborns: 2.5% to 6.5% of total erythrocytes.
- Reticulocyte index: 1.

Deviations from Normal

- A normal or low reticulocyte count in an anemic client indicates that the marrow production of RBC is inadequate and is perhaps the cause of the anemia (e.g., aplastic anemia, iron deficiency, and B_{12} deficiency).

- An elevated reticulocyte count found in clients with a normal hemogram indicates RBC overproduction (polycythemia vera).
- A reticulocyte index below 1 in an anemic client indicates that the bone marrow response is inadequate in its ability to compensate (e.g., iron deficiency or vitamin B_{12} deficiency):

$$\text{Reticulocyte index} = \text{Reticulocyte count (\%)} \times \frac{\text{Patient's hematocrit}}{\text{Normal hematocrit}}$$

Indications

- To determine the adequacy of bone marrow function.

Contraindications

- None.

Procedure

1. See "Complete Blood Count," p. 338.

SERUM FERRITIN
Normal Values

- 12 to 300 mg/L (RIA).
- Male: mean = 123 ng/ml.
- Female: mean = 56 ng/ml radiometric assay.

Deviations from Normal

- Ferritin is decreased in iron-deficiency anemia and normal or increased in other forms of anemia and diseases affecting the liver such as cirrhosis, cancer, hepatitis, leukemia, and Hodgkin's disease.
- Inflammatory diseases can also elevate ferritin as an acute phase reactant.

Indications

- Serum ferritin is used primarily to differentiate iron-deficiency anemia from other anemias. It is also used to monitor therapy for clients with chronic renal failure on hemodialysis and with clients being treated for iron deficiency or excess.

Contraindications

- None.

Procedure

Client preparation

1. The purpose and procedure are explained.

Procedure

1. Following standard venipuncture procedure, one red-top tube of blood is drawn.
2. Pressure is applied to the site.

Nursing implications

1. Observe the site for bleeding.
2. Continue to monitor the venipuncture site for bleeding with clients with liver disease.

SERUM HAPTOGLOBIN TEST

Normal Values

- 100 to 150 mg/dl.

Deviations from Normal

- Hemolytic anemia associated with intravascular destruction of RBCs produces a transient reduced serum haptaglobin level.
- Haptoglobins are also decreased with primary liver disease unassociated with hemolytic anemias because the diseased liver is unable to produce these glycoproteins.
- Elevated haptoglobin concentrations are found in many inflammatory diseases and can therefore be used as a nonspecific test of disease in a way similar to that of a sedimentation rate test (see p. 421).

Indications

- To detect intravascular destruction of RBCs and thus aid in diagnosing conditions listed above in ''Deviations from Normal.''

Contraindications

■ None.

Procedure
Client preparation

1. The client is assessed for signs of ongoing infection that could falsely elevate the results.

Procedure

1. Following standard venipuncture technique, blood is collected.
2. Pressure or a pressure dressing is applied.

Nursing implications

1. Assess the venipuncture site for bleeding.

SICKLE CELL TEST (SICKLE CELL PREPARATION; SICKLEDEX; Hgb S TEST)

Normal Values

■ No sickle cells. A negative test indicates that the client has no or very little Hgb S.

Deviations from Normal

■ The presence of sickle cells indicates sickle cell anemia.

Indications

■ To screen for sickle cell anemia and sickle cell trait.

Contraindications

■ The client who received a blood transfusion within 3 months before the time of the test.

Procedure

1. Following standard venipuncture technique, 7 ml of blood are collected in a lavender-top vacutainer.
2. Pressure or a pressure dressing is applied.
3. The sample is sent immediately to the lab for analysis.

Nursing implications

1. Assess the venipuncture site for bleeding.
2. If the test is positive, the family should be offered genetic counseling. A client with one recessive gene (heterozygous) is said to have sickle cell *trait*. A client with two recessive genes (homozygous) has sickle cell *anemia*.
3. Clients with sickle cell anemia should avoid situations in which hypoxia may occur (e.g., strenuous exercise, air travel in unpressurized aircraft, and travel to high-altitude regions).

WHOLE BLOOD CLOT RETRACTION TEST

Normal Values

- 50% to 100% clot retraction in 1 to 2 hours.
- Complete retraction within 24 hours.
- This test is only reliable if the hematocrit and fibrinogen (factor I) concentration (see Table 9-2) are within normal limits.

Deviations from Normal

- With a platelet deficiency (thrombocytopenia), the clot retraction will be slower and the clot formation will stay soft and watery.
- If fibrinolysins are present, no clot retraction will occur. Poor white blood retraction occurs with thrombasthenia (abnormal platelets), anemia, and Waldenstrom's macroglobulinemia.

Indications

- To determine if bleeding disorders may be caused by thrombocytopenia (decreased platelet count). Platelets play a vital role in hemostasis and blood clotting.

Contraindications

- None.

Procedure

1. Following standard peripheral venipuncture technique, 5 to 7 ml of venous blood are collected in a red-top tube.
2. Clot retraction is then timed and evaluated.
3. Pressure or a pressure dressing is applied.

Nursing implications

1. Assess the venipuncture site for bleeding.
2. Avoid excessive probing during the venipuncture if a co-agulation disorder is suspected.
3. Handle the specimen carefully to avoid hemolysis.
4. If the clot retraction is to be evaluated on the floor, it should be accurately timed and carefully evaluated for contraction.

Urine Tests
SCHILLING TEST (VITAMIN B_{12} ABSORPTION TEST)

Normal Values

- Excretion of 8% to 40% of radioactive vitamin B_{12} within 24 hours.

Deviations from Normal

- Decreased levels of vitamin B_{12} occur in clients with pernicious anemia, malabsorption syndrome, liver diseases, hypothyroidism, and sprue.

Indications

- To detect the occurrence of vitamin B_{12} absorption to aid in diagnosing conditions listed above under ''Deviations from Normal.''

Contraindications

- A client who has had a radionuclide scan within 10 days because the previous test could alter the current test results.

Procedure
Client preparation

1. Written and verbal instructions should be given to the client.
2. The client should not take laxatives in the evening prior to the test because they could decrease the rate of vitamin B_{12} absorption.
3. The client is kept on nothing by mouth for 8 to 12 hours prior to the test. Food should not be given until after the client receives the IM injection.
4. The client must receive the injection of the nonradioactive vitamin B_{12} at the exact time specified. Otherwise the liver will absorb the radioactive vitamin B_{12}, which will then not be excreted in the urine.
5. The procedure for collection of the 24-hour urine specimen is explained. (See "Client Preparation" for "Creatinine Clearance Test," except step 2, p. 181.)
6. The lab guidelines regarding refrigeration are followed.
7. Clients with elevated BUN levels (p. 177) may be required to collect the urine specimens for longer periods of time, since impaired renal function may slow excretion of vitamin B_{12}.
8. The client is assured that the tracer dose of radioactive vitamin B_{12} will not be harmful to himself or herself or others. The dose is extremely small.

Procedure

The test can be performed in one or two stages. Clients excreting a normal amount of radioactive vitamin B_{12} in the first stage require no further testing. The second stage is performed if the first stage showed a decreased percentage of radioactive vitamin B_{12} to confirm the diagnosis of pernicious anemia.

First stage (without intrinsic factor)

1. After being kept on nothing by mouth for 8 to 12 hours before the test, the client collects and discards a urine specimen.

2. The client then receives an oral dose of radioactive vitamin B_{12} and begins a 24- to 48-hour urine collection.
3. After 1 to 2 hours the client receives an IM injection of nonradioactive vitamin B_{12} to saturate tissue binding sites and to permit some excretion of radioactive vitamin B_{12} in the urine. The client can resume eating after the IM injection of vitamin B_{12}.

Second stage (with intrinsic factor)

1. After taking nothing by mouth for 8 to 12 hours prior to the test, the client voids and discards the urine specimen.
2. The client receives an oral dose of radioactive vitamin B_{12} and human intrinsic factor.
3. A 24-hour urine collection is begun.
4. After 2 hours the client receives an IM dose of nonradioactive vitamin B_{12}. The client can resume eating after the IM injection.
5. After administration of intrinsic factor and vitamin B_{12} in the second stage, most clients excrete normal amounts of radioactive B_{12}. The second stage is usually performed within 1 week after the first stage.

Nursing implications

1. If the client had a decreased excretion of vitamin B_{12} in the first stage of the test, explain that the second stage of the test is usually performed within 1 week.

URINARY PORPHYRINS AND PORPHOBILINOGENS
Normal Values

- Porphyrins: 50 to 300 mg/24 h.
- Porphobilinogens: 1.5 to 2 mg/24 h or negative.

Deviations from Normal

- An increased porphyrins level may result in certain disease states (e.g., abnormal porphyrin metabolism, liver disease, lead poisoning, and pellagra).
- Disorders in porphyrin metabolism also cause porphobilinogen.
- Abnormalities may also be drug (usually lead) induced.

Indications

■ To aid in diagnosing conditions listed under "Deviations from Normal" above.

Contraindications

■ None.

Procedure
Client preparation

1. The procedure for the 24-hour urine collection is explained to the client.
2. See "Client Preparation" for 24-hour urine collection for "Creatinine Clearance Test" (except step 2), p. 181.

Procedure

1. See "Procedure" for 24-hour urine collection for "Creatinine Clearance Test" (except step 4).
2. The urine is collected in a dark specimen bottle with a preservative to prevent degradation of the light-sensitive porphyrin.
3. Porphobilinogens are usually evaluated with the porphyrin test or by a single, fresh-voided random urine specimen.
4. The specimen should be protected from light and taken immediately to the lab for analysis.

Special Studies

Bone Marrow Examination (Bone Marrow Biopsy; Bone Marrow Aspiration)
Normal Values

■ Active erythroid cell, myeloid cell, and megakaryocyte (platelet) production.

Deviations from Normal

Findings	Possible Causes
Increased marrow leukocyte precursors	Leukemias or leukemoid reactions Physiologic marrow compensation for infection
Decreased marrow leukocyte precursors	Myelofibrosis Old age Metastatic neoplasia Agranulocytis following radiation therapy or chemotherapy
Increased marrow RBC precursors	Polycythemia vera Physiologic compensation to hemorrhage or hemolytic anemias
Decreased marrow RBC precursors	Erythroid hypoplasia following radiation therapy or chemotherapy Receiving of toxic drugs or marrow replacement by fibrotic tissues Neoplasms
Increased marrow platelet precursors (megakaryocytes)	Acute hemorrhage Chronic myeloid leukemia Physiologic compensation in clients with secondary hypersplenism
Decreased marrow platelet precursors	Radiation therapy or chemotherapy Neoplastic or fibrotic marrow infiltrative disease Aplastic anemia
Increased marrow lymphocyte precursors	Infections (e.g., mononucleosis) Lymphocytic leukemia Lymphoma
Increased marrow plasma cells (plasmocytes)	Multiple myelomas Hodgkin's disease Hypersensitivity state Rheumatic fever and other chronic inflammatory diseases

Indications

- To evaluate hematopoiesis.
- To detect drug-induced or idiopathic myelofibrosis (usually via biopsy).
- To detect leukemias, multiple myelomas, and diffusely metastatic tumors and polycythemia vera (usually via biopsy).
- To aid in diagnosing conditions listed under "Deviations from Normal" above.

Contraindications

- An uncooperative client.
- A client with a coagulopathy (e.g., hemophilia) because severe hemorrhage can occur.

Procedure

Client preparation

1. The client is encouraged to verbalize fears because many clients are anxious concerning this study.
2. The coagulation studies performed on the client before the study are assessed. Any evidence of coagulopathy is reported to the physician.
3. An order for sedatives is obtained if the client appears extremely apprehensive before the study.

Procedure

1. Bone marrow aspiration:
   a. Bone marrow aspiration is performed on the sternum, iliac crest, anterior or posterior iliac spines, and proximal tibia (in children).
   b. The client is positioned on his or her back or side, according to the site selected.
   c. The area overlying the bone is prepared and draped in a sterile manner.
   d. The overlying skin, soft tissue, and the periosteum of the bone are infiltrated with lidocaine (Xylocaine).
   e. A large-bore needle (14-gauge) containing a stylus is slowly advanced through the soft tissues and into the outer table of the bone.

    f. Once inside the marrow, the stylus is removed and a syringe is attached.

    g. One half to two milliliters of bone marrow are aspirated, smeared on slides, and allowed to dry.

    h. The slides are then sprayed with a preservative and taken to the pathology lab.

2. Bone marrow biopsy:

    a. A physician performs bone marrow biopsy in 10 to 20 minutes.

    b. The procedure may require general anesthesia.

    c. The iliac spines or the site of suspected tumor provides the biopsy specimen.

    d. See steps 1c and 1d above under ''Bone Marrow Aspiration.''

    e. The skin and soft tissues overlying the bone are incised.

    f. A core biopsy instrument is screwed into the bone.

    g. The biopsy specimen is obtained and sent to the pathology lab for analysis.

3. A trained nurse or physician performs the procedure, usually in the client's room, in 10 to 20 minutes.

Nursing implications

1. Assist the physician or nurse in obtaining the specimen.

2. During the study, remind the client to remain still. If the client moves, the needle could accidentally puncture a vital organ.

3. Label the slides appropriately with the client's name, date, and room number.

4. After the needle is removed, apply pressure to arrest the scant amount of bleeding from the puncture site. Pressure will usually stop any bleeding from the biopsy or aspiration site.

5. Apply an adhesive bandage.

6. Ice packs may be used to help control bleeding. Uncontrolled hemorrhage can lead to hematoma formation, which can be uncomfortable.

7. Observe the puncture site for bleeding. Tenderness and erythema may indicate infection.

8. After the study, assess the client for signs of shock (increased pulse, decreased blood pressure) and pain. Normally, keep the client on bed rest for 30 to 60 minutes after the study. After that time, allow the client to resume normal activity.

9. Some clients complain of tenderness at the puncture site for several days after the study. Administer mild analgesics as ordered.

Nurse alert

1. Complications include severe bleeding (especially if the client has a coagulopathy), infection (especially if the client is leukopenic), and puncture of the heart or great vessels when the test is performed on the sternum.

Bibliography

Anthony, C.P., and Thibodeau, G.A.: Textbook of anatomy and physiology, ed. 11, St. Louis, 1983, The C.V. Mosby Co.

Block, M.H.: Text—atlas of hematology, Philadelphia, 1976, Lea & Febiger.

Boggs, D.R., and Winkelstein, A.: White cell manual, ed. 4, Philadelphia, 1983, F.A. Davis.

Corbett, J.V.: Laboratory tests in nursing practice, Norwalk, Conn., 1982, Appleton-Century-Crofts.

Crosby, W.: Red cell mass: its precursors and its perturbations, Hosp. Pract. **16:**71-81, 1980.

Fischbach, F.: A manual of laboratory diagnostic tests, ed. 2, Philadelphia, 1984, J.B. Lippincott Co.

Franklin, F.I., and others: The many facets of hemophilia, JAMA **228:**85, 1974.

Godwin, M., and Baysinger, M.: Understanding antisickling agents and the sickling process, Nurs. Clin. North Am. **18**(1):207, 1983.

Jennings, B.M.: Nursing assessment—hematologic system. In Lewis, S.M., and Collier, I.C., editors: Medical-surgical nursing: assessment and management of clinical problems, New York, 1983, McGraw-Hill Book Co.

Kenny, M.W.: Sickle cell disease, Nurs. Times **76:**1582-1584, 1980.

Kozak, A.: Blood therapy: processing blood for transfusion, Am. J. Nurs. **79:**931-934, 1979.

Markus, S.: Taking the fear out of bone marrow examinations, Nursing '81 **11**(4):64-67, 1981.

McGann, M.A., and Triplett, D.A.: Laboratory evaluation of the fibrinolytic system, Lab. Med. **14**:18, 1983.

Petersdorf, R.G., editor: Harrison's principles of internal medicine, ed. 10, New York, 1983, McGraw-Hill Book Co.

Schottelius, B.A., and Schottelius, D.D.: Textbook of physiology, ed. 19, St. Louis, 1982, The C.V. Mosby Co.

Walsh, P.N.: Oral anticoagulant therapy, Hosp. Pract. **18**:101, 1983.

Williams, W.J., and others: Hematology, ed. 2, New York, 1977, McGraw-Hill Book Co.

Xistris, D.M.: Problems of the blood and blood-forming organs. In Phipps, W.J., Long, B.C., and Woods, N.F., editors: Medical-surgical nursing: concepts and clinical practice, ed. 2, St. Louis, 1983, The C.V. Mosby Co.

Autoimmune System

10

Clinical laboratory tests
  Blood tests
    Anti-DNA binding antibody
    Antimitochondrial and antismooth muscle antibodies
    Antinuclear antibody (ANA) test
    Anti-RNP
    C-reactive protein
    Complement assay
    HLA-B27 antigen
    Cryoglobulin test
    Estimated sedimentation rate
    Immunoglobulin electrophoresis
    LE cell prep
    Mono spot test (mononuclear heterophile test or heterophile antibody test)
    Rheumatoid factor
    Serum aldolase
    Serum protein electrophoresis
    Warm/cold agglutinins
Radiologic laboratory tests
  X-ray tests
    X-ray of the knee joint
Special studies
  Synovial fluid analysis

Clinical Laboratory Tests

Blood Tests

ANTI-DNA BINDING ANTIBODY

Normal Values

- 0% to 15% binding by Farr assay or absent by Crithidia assay.

Deviations from Normal

- Systemic lupus erythematosus (SLE).
- Sjögren's syndrome.
- Rheumatoid arthritis.
- Lupus nephritis.

Indications

- To assist in making the diagnosis of SLE.

Contraindications

- None.

Procedure

Client preparation

1. The procedure and purpose of the study are explained.

Procedure

1. Following standard venipuncture procedure, one red-top tube of blood is drawn.
2. Pressure is applied to the site.

Nursing implications

1. Observe the venipuncture site for bleeding.

ANTIMITOCHONDRIAL AND ANTISMOOTH MUSCLE ANTIBODIES

Normal Values

- No antimitochondrial antibodies at titers >1:5.
- No antismooth muscle antibodies at titers >1:30.

Deviations from Normal

- Antismooth muscle antibodies are present in only about 30% of the clients with primary biliary cirrhosis. The majority of clients with chronic hepatitis, however, have antismooth muscle antibodies.
- Antimitochondrial antibodies appear in most clients with primary biliary cirrhosis.
- Infectious mononucleosis, acute hepatitis, and hepatomas can cause false-positive readings.

Indications

- To diagnose chronic hepatitis via the antismooth muscle antibodies titer.
- To aid in diagnosing biliary cirrhosis via the antimitochondrial antibodies titer.

Contraindications

- None.

Procedure

1. Following standard venipuncture technique, 7 ml of blood are collected in a red-top tube.
2. Pressure or a pressure dressing is applied to the puncture site.

Nursing implications

1. Assess the puncture site for bleeding.
2. Be sure to check the site also for ongoing bleeding. Jaundiced clients often may have coagulopathies associated with vitamin K deficiency.

Nurse alert

1. Avoid contact with the needles used to withdraw the blood, since the client may have chronic hepatitis.

ANTINUCLEAR ANTIBODY (ANA) TEST

Normal Values

- No antinuclear antibodies detected in a titer of greater than 1:32.

Deviations from Normal

- Elevated titers occur in 95% of clients with systemic lupus erythematosus (SLE).
- Although other diseases may also cause an elevated titer, if the ANA test is negative, the client probably does not have SLE.

Indications

- To screen for SLE.

Contraindications

- None.

Procedure

1. Following standard venipuncture technique, 7 ml of blood are collected in a red-top tube.
2. Pressure or a pressure dressing is applied to the puncture site.

Nursing implications

1. Observe the puncture site for bleeding.
2. See "LE Cell Prep," p. 382.

ANTI-RNP

Normal Values

- Absent.

Deviations from Normal

- Mixed connective tissue disease.
- Systemic lupus erythematosus (SLE).
- Sjögren's syndrome.
- Scleroderma.

Indications

- To assist in the diagnosis of the diseases listed under "Deviations from Normal."

Contraindications

■ None.

Procedure
Client preparation

1. The procedure and purpose of the test are explained.

Procedure

1. Following standard venipuncture procedure, one red-top tube of blood is drawn.

Nursing implications

1. Observe the site for bleeding.

C-REACTIVE PROTEIN
Normal Values

■ <6 μg/ml.

Deviations from Normal

■ See "SED Rate," p. 421.

Indications

■ See "SED Rate," p. 421.

Contraindications

■ None.

Procedure

1. Following standard venipuncture technique, 7 ml of blood are collected in a red-top tube.
2. Pressure or a pressure dressing is applied to the site.

Nursing implications

1. Observe the puncture site for bleeding.
2. See "SED Rate," p. 421.

COMPLEMENT ASSAY

Normal Values

- Total complement: 41 to 90 hemolytic units.
- C_3 = 70 to 176 mg/dl.
- C_4 = 16 to 45 mg/dl.

Deviations from Normal

- The complement assays are decreased in autoimmune diseases (e.g., lupus erythematosus and serum sickness).

Indications

- To detect autoimmune diseases.
- To follow the course of autoimmune disease.
- C_3 and C_4 components are particularly helpful in detecting autoimmune disease and following its course.

Contraindications

- None.

Procedure

Client preparation

1. See "LE Cell Prep," p. 382.

Procedure

1. Following standard venipuncture procedure, 7 ml of blood are collected in a red-top tube.
2. Pressure or a pressure dressing is applied to the puncture site.

Nursing implications

1. Observe the puncture site for bleeding.
2. See "LE Cell Prep," p. 382.

HLA-B27 ANTIGEN

Normal Values

- No antigen present.

Deviations from Normal

- The antigen occurs in 80% to 90% of clients with ankylosing spondylitis and Reiter's syndrome.

Indications

- To confirm the diagnosis of the above disease.

Contraindications

- None.

Procedure

1. The technician is instructed to be especially gentle with the venipuncture. These clients usually have painful joints, and for them extending an arm completely for venipuncture is difficult.
2. Following standard venipuncture, 10 ml of blood are drawn and collected in a heparinized solution.
3. Pressure or a pressure dressing is applied.

Nursing implications

1. Observe the puncture site for bleeding.

CRYOGLOBULIN TEST

Normal Values

- No cryoglobulins detected.

Deviations from Normal

- Serum levels greater than 5 mm are associated with myeloma, macroglobulinemia, and leukemia.
- Globulin levels less than 1mm/cc can be associated with systemic lupus erythematosus, rheumatoid arthritis, infectious mononucleosis, viral hepatitis, cirrhosis, endocarditis, and glomerulonephritis.
- Globulin levels between 1 and 5 mm are associated with rheumatoid arthritis.

Indications

- To detect levels of cryoglobulin that may be associated with one of the specific disease entities mentioned above.

Contraindications

- None.

Procedure

Client preparation

1. The client is kept on nothing by mouth for 8 hours prior to obtaining the specimen if the lab requires this preparation.

Procedure

1. Following standard venipuncture technique, 10 ml of blood are drawn and collected in a red-top tube *prewarmed* to body temperature.
2. Pressure or a pressure dressing is applied to the puncture site.

Nursing implications

1. If cryoglobulins are found, warn the client to avoid cold temperatures to minimize Raynaud's symptoms.
2. Note that clients with cryoglobulins may have diseases associated with coagulation defects. Observe the puncture site for possible bleeding or hematoma.

ESTIMATED SEDIMENTATION RATE

See p. 421.

IMMUNOGLOBULIN ELECTROPHORESIS

Normal Values

- IgG: 565 to 1,765 mg/dl.
- IgA: 85 to 385 mg/dl.
- IgM: 55 to 375 mg/dl.

Deviations from Normal

- Increased levels occur with autoimmune disorders.
- Abnormal levels also occur with multiple myeloma, macro-globulinemia, hypergammaglobulinemias or hypogammag-lobulinemias, hepatitis, and cirrhosis.

Indications

- To diagnose conditions listed above.

Contraindications

- None.

Procedure

Client preparation

1. See "LE Cell Prep," p. 382.
2. Some labs require that the client fast for 12 hours prior to the drawing of the sample.

Procedure

1. Following standard venipuncture technique, 7 ml of blood are collected and placed in a red-top tube.
2. Pressure or a pressure dressing is applied to the site.

Nursing implications

1. Observe the puncture site for bleeding.
2. See "LE Cell Prep," p. 382.

LE CELL PREP

Normal Values

- No LE cells seen.

Deviations from Normal

- Seventy to eighty percent of the clients with active SLE have a positive LE prep. Clients with SLE have antibodies against the constituents of nuclei within their own cells.
- Drugs (e.g., dilantin, isoniazid, procainamide, and hydral-azine) can cause false-positive LE cell preps.
- Steroids may tend to suppress LE cell production.

Indications

- To aid in diagnosing SLE.
- To monitor SLE treatment.

Contraindications

- None.

Procedure
Client preparation

1. The client is assessed for the use of drugs known to alter the test results (see above).

Procedure

1. Following standard venipuncture technique, one red-top tube of blood is collected.
2. Pressure or a pressure dressing is applied.

Nursing implications

1. Assess the puncture site for bleeding.
2. Because clients with SLE have immunologic disorders, they are at risk for infection. Be sure the clients understand the signs of infection that may occur at the venipuncture site. Instruct clients to notify their physician if they recognize these signs.

MONO SPOT TEST (MONONUCLEAR HETEROPHILE TEST OR HETEROPHILE ANTIBODY TEST)
Normal Values

- No infectious mononucleosis antibody in titers >1:56.

Deviations from Normal

- When IgM antibodies are present in serial dilutions of greater than 1:56, infectious mononucleosis can be strongly considered. False-positives, however, occasionally occur in clients with lymphoma or systemic lupus erythematosus.
- Clients with Burkitt's lymphoma, leukemia, and some GI cancers also have a false-positive test.

- Narcotic addicts may also have high titers of infectious mononucleosis heterophile antibodies.

Indications

- To diagnose infectious mononucleosis.

Contraindications

- None.

Procedure

1. Following standard venipuncture technique, 7 ml of blood are collected in a red-top tube.
2. Pressure or a pressure dressing is applied to the puncture site.

Nursing implications

1. Assess the puncture site for bleeding.
2. The results are available in approximately 1 hour.

RHEUMATOID FACTOR

Normal Values

- No rheumatoid factor present.
- <60 units/ml by nephelometric testing.

Deviations from Normal

- Positive rheumatoid factor titers (those found in a dilution >1:80) occur in 80% of clients with rheumatoid arthritis.
- Rheumatoid factor occurring in titer <1:80 may indicate diseases such as lupus erythematosus, scleroderma, and other autoimmune diseases.
- Rheumatoid factor is also occasionally seen in tuberculosis, chronic hepatitis, infectious mononucleosis, and subacute bacterial endocarditis.

Indications

- To aid in diagnosing rheumatoid arthritis and, secondarily, autoimmune disease.

Contraindications

■ None.

Procedure

Client preparation

1. See "LE Cell Prep," p. 382.

Procedure

1. Following standard venipuncture technique, 7 ml of blood are collected in a red-top tube.
2. Pressure or a pressure dressing is applied.

Nursing implications

1. Observe the puncture site for bleeding.
2. See "LE Cell Prep," p. 382.

SERUM ALDOLASE

Normal Values

■ 3.0 to 8.2 Sibley-Lehninger units/dl.

Deviations from Normal

■ The serum aldolase level is high in muscular dystrophies, dermatomyositis, and polymyositis.
■ The level is also increased with gangrenous processes, muscular trauma, and muscular infectious diseases (e.g., trichinosis).
■ Elevated levels are also noted in chronic hepatitis, obstructive jaundice, and cirrhosis.

Indications

■ To differentiate neurologic diseases (e.g., poliomyelitis, myasthenia gravis, and multiple sclerosis) that cause weakness from muscular diseases. Elevated aldolase levels occur in primary muscular disorders.

Contraindications

■ None.

Procedure
Client preparation

1. The client is kept on nothing by mouth after midnight the day of the study until the sample is drawn.

Procedure

1. Following standard venipuncture technique, 7 ml of blood are collected in a red-top tube.
2. Pressure dressing or pressure is applied to the puncture site.

Nursing implications

1. Assess the puncture site for bleeding.
2. See "SGOT," pp. 3 or 70.

SERUM PROTEIN ELECTROPHORESIS
Normal Values

- Total protein: 6.6 to 7.9 g/dl.
- Albumin: 3.3 to 4.5 g/dl.
- Alpha$_1$-globulin: 0.1 to 0.4 g/dl.
- Alpha$_2$-globulin: 0.5 to 1.0 g/dl.
- Beta-globulin: 0.7 to 1.2 g/dl.
- Gamma globulin: 0.5 to 1.6 g/dl.

Deviations from Normal

- Several electrophoretic patterns (variations of concentrations of the protein components) are associated with specific disease entities (e.g., malnutrition, chronic liver disease, nephrotic syndrome, acute/chronic inflammation, rheumatoid-connective tissue diseases, multiple myeloma, gammopathies, and immune deficiencies.
- Many diseases are associated with an increase or decrease in just one protein component. The protein electrophoresis identifies that specific component.
- Many drugs (e.g., aspirin, bicarbonates, chlorpromazine, corticosteroids, isoniazid, phenacemide, salicylates, neomycin, sulfonamides, and tolbutamide) can affect protein

component concentrations. The medication history must be considered in interpreting any specific pattern.

Indications

■ To aid in diagnosing conditions listed above under "Deviations from Normal."

Contraindications

■ None.

Procedure
Client preparation

1. A medication history is obtained to determine if the client is taking any drug that may affect the results (see above).

Procedure

1. Following standard venipuncture technique, 7 ml of blood are collected in a red-top tube.
2. Pressure or a pressure dressing is applied to the puncture site.

Nursing implications

1. Assess the venipuncture site for bleeding.
2. If the client is suspected of having an immune globulin abnormality, take extra precautions to prevent infection.

WARM/COLD AGGLUTININS
Normal Values

■ Cold agglutinins: no agglutination in titers <1:16.
■ Febrile (warm) agglutinins: no agglutination in titers ≤1:80.

Deviations from Normal

■ Titers >1:80 for warm agglutinins are considered positive and result from such infectious diseases as salmonellosis, rickettsial diseases, brucellosis, and tularemia.
■ For cold agglutinins titers >1:16 indicate infections by other agents, particularly *Mycoplasma pneumoniae*.

Indications

- To diagnose conditions listed above.

Contraindications

- None.

Procedure

Client preparation

1. The client is assessed to be sure that he or she has not been exposed to marked abnormalities in temperature that may affect the respective agglutination testing.

Procedure

1. For cold agglutinins the red-top tube is prewarmed to above 37° C. For warm agglutinins the red-top tube is cooled.
2. Following standard venipuncture technique, 7 ml of blood are collected in a red-top tube.
3. Pressure or a pressure dressing is applied to the puncture site.
4. The sample is taken immediately to the lab so that no hemolysis will occur.

Nursing implications

1. Observe the puncture site for bleeding.

Nurse alert

1. Under no circumstances should the cold agglutinin specimen be refrigerated or the febral agglutinin specimen heated.

Radiologic Laboratory Tests

X-Ray Tests
X-RAY OF THE KNEE JOINT
See p. 392.

Special Studies

Synovial Fluid Analysis

See "Arthrocentesis," p. 399.

Bibliography

Beyers, M., and Dudas, S.: The clinical practice of medical-surgical nursing, ed. 2, Boston, 1984, Little, Brown & Co.

Brunner, L.S., and Suddarth, D.S.: Textbook of medical-surgical nursing, ed. 5, Philadelphia, 1984, J.B. Lippincott Co.

Buergin, P.: Assessment of the musculoskeletal system. In Phipps, W.J., Long, B.C., and Woods, N.F., editors: Medical-surgical nursing: concepts and clinical practice, ed. 2, St. Louis, 1983, The C.V. Mosby Co.

Cohen, S., and Viellion, G.: Patient assessment: examining joints of the upper and lower extremities, Am. J. Nurs. **81:**763-786, 1981.

Convery, F.R., and Convery, M.M.: Examination of the joints. In Kelly, W.N., and others, editors: Textbook of rheumatology, Philadelphia, 1981, W.B. Saunders Co.

Fries, J.F.: General approach to the rheumatic disease patient. In Kelly, W.N., and others, editors: Textbook of rheumatology, Philadelphia, 1981, W.B. Saunders Co.

Fudenberg, H.H., editor: Basic and clinical immunology, ed. 3, Los Altos, Calif., 1980, Lange Medical Publications.

Gilliland, B.C., and Mannik, M.: Approaches to disorders of the joints. In Petersdorf, R.G., and others, editors: Harrison's principles of internal medicine, ed. 10, New York, 1983, McGraw-Hill Book Co.

Gilliland, B.C., and Mannik, M.: Rheumatoid arthritis. In Petersdorf, R.G., and others, editors: Harrison's principles of internal medicine, ed. 10, New York, 1983, McGraw-Hill Book Co.

Groenwald, S.L.: Physiology of the immune system, Heart Lung **9:**645-650, 1980.

Kunkel, H.G.: The immunopathology of SLE, Hosp. Pract. **15:**47, 1980.

Lind, M.: The immunologic assessment: a nursing focus, Heart Lung **9:**658-661, 1980.

Lloyd, W., and Schur, P.H.: Immune complexes, complement, and anti-DNA in exacerbations of systemic lupus erythematosus (SLE), Medicine **60:**208, 1981.

Long, B.C.: Assessment of the integument and immune status. In Phipps, W.J., Long, B.C., and Woods, N.F., editors: Medical-surgical nursing: concepts and clinical practice, ed. 2, St. Louis, 1983, The C.V. Mosby Co.

Long, B.C., Wright, E.R., and Phipps, W.J.: Problems associated with impaired immune response. In Phipps, W.J., Long, B.C., and Woods, N.F., editors: Medical-surgical nursing: concepts and clinical practice, ed. 2, St. Louis, 1983, The C.V. Mosby Co.

Mannik, M., and Gilliland, B.C.: Systematic lupus erythematosus. In Petersdorf, R.C., and others, editors: Harrison's principles of internal medicine, ed. 10, New York, 1983, McGraw-Hill Book Co.

Notman, D.D., and others: Profiles of antinuclear antibodies in systemic rheumatic diseases, Ann. Intern. Med. 83:464, 1975.

Rana, A.N., and Luskin, A.: Immunosuppression, autoimmunity, and hypersensitivity, Heart Lung 9:651-657, 1980.

Ravel, R.: Clinical laboratory medicine: clinical application of laboratory data, ed. 4, Chicago, 1984, Year Book Medical Publishers, Inc.

Zvaifler, N.J.: Etiology and pathogenesis of rheumatoid arthritis. In McCarty, D.J., editor: Arthritis and allied conditions, Philadelphia, 1979, Lea & Febiger.

Skeletal System

11

Clinical Laboratory Tests

Urine Tests

URIC ACID TEST

Normal Values

- Serum: males, 2.1 to 8.5 ml/dl; females, 2.0 to 6.6 ml/dl; children, 2.5 to 5.5 ml/dl.
- Urine: 250 to 750 mg/24 h.

Deviations from Normal

- Elevated uric acid levels (hyperuricemia) may occur in clients with gout.
- A catabolic enzyme deficiency stimulating purine metabolism may cause elevated levels.
- Cancer in which purine and DNA turnover is great may lead to hyperuricemia.
- Other causes of hyperuricemia may include alcoholism, leukemias, metastatic cancer, multiple myeloma, hyperlipoproteinemia, diabetes mellitus, renal failure, stress, lead poisoning, and dehydration from diuretic therapy.
- Ketoacids (as occur in diabetic or alcoholic ketoacidosis) may compete with uric acid for tubular excretion and can cause decreased uric acid excretion.
- Many causes of hyperuricemia production go undefined and are therefore labeled as *idiopathic*.
- Increased serum levels may also be clinically associated with arthritis, soft-tissue deposits of uric acid (tophi), and uric acid kidney stones.
- Decreased uric acid levels are not associated with any clinical symptoms and are usually the result of poor liver function.

Indications

- To diagnose conditions listed under "Deviations from Normal" above.
- To allow the treatment of increased levels of uric acid in clients who have no symptoms of gout.

Contraindications

- None.

Procedure
Client preparation

1. See "Client Preparation" for 24-hour urine specimen for "Creatinine Clearance Test" (except step 2), p. 181.

Procedure
Blood

1. Following standard venipuncture procedure, two red-top tubes of blood are collected from a vein in the arm.
2. Pressure or a pressure dressing is applied.

Urine

1. See "Procedure" for 24-hour urine specimen for "Creatinine Clearance Test" (except step 4), p. 181.

Nursing implications

1. Observe the venipuncture site for bleeding.
2. See "Nursing Implications" for 24-hour urine specimen for "Creatinine Clearance Test," p. 181.
3. If the uric acid levels are high, instruct the client to avoid foods high in purine (e.g., liver, kidney, heart, brain, sweet breads, sardines, anchovies, and mince meat). Foods with a moderate amount of purine nitrogens include poultry, fish, asparagus, mushrooms, peas, and spinach.
4. Instruct clients with elevated levels to decrease alcoholic intake because alcohol causes a renal retention of urate.

Radiologic Laboratory Tests

X-Ray Tests
ARTHROGRAPHY
Normal Values

- Normal bursae, menisci, ligaments, and articular cartilage of the joint.

Deviations from Normal

■ Bones with the meniscus, cartilage, and ligaments are clearly visualized. Joint derangement and synovial cysts are also made visible.

Indications

■ To diagnose the cause for persistent, unexplained knee and shoulder pain (see "Deviations from Normal" above).

Contraindications

■ A pregnant client.
■ A client with active arthritis, joint infection, or allergy to radiopaque material.

Procedure
Client preparation

1. The physician obtains written and informed consent before the procedure begins.
2. Prior to the study the client is assessed for allergies to iodine dye. If allergies exist, the physician is notified.

Procedure

1. The procedure is performed under local anesthetic using sterile technique.
2. The client is placed in the supine position on an examining table.
3. The skin overlying the desired joint is aseptically cleansed and anesthetized.
4. The needle is inserted into the joint space, and fluid is aspirated to prevent dilution of the contrast agent and thus diminish the quality of the x-ray films.
5. With the needle still in place, the aspirating syringe is removed and a syringe containing dye is replaced.
6. The contrast agent(s) is injected.
7. The needle is removed and the joint manipulated to afford distribution of the contrast material. The client may be asked to walk a few steps or to pass the joint through range-of-motion exercises.

8. X-ray films are then taken with the joint held in various positions.
9. A physician performs the procedure in approximately 30 minutes.

Nursing implications

1. After the study the client usually rests the joint for at least 12 hours.
2. An elastic bandage is usually applied to the knee joint and left in place for several days.
3. After the test, ice may be applied to the joint if swelling occurs.
4. Some clients may require a mild analgesic (e.g., aspirin or acetaminophen [Tylenol]) for minor discomfort. Report any increase in pain or swelling to the physician.
5. After the test, tell the client that he or she may hear crepitant noises in the joint. These symptoms are normal and usually disappear in 1 to 2 days. The noise is a result of air injected into the joint during the procedure.

BONE SCAN
See p. 415. See p. 415.

LUMBOSACRAL SPINAL X-RAY STUDY
See p. 140.

X-RAY OF THE LONG BONES
Normal Values

▪ No evidence of fracture, tumor, infection, or congenital abnormalities.

Deviations from Normal

▪ Abnormalities suggesting conditions listed under ''Indications.''

Indications

- To detect an infection involving a bone (osteomyelitis) when the client has a severe or chronic infection overlying a bone.
- To follow growth patterns by serial x-rays of a long bone (usually the wrist).
- To detect a fracture.
- To document and follow the healing of a fracture.
- To detect joint destruction and bone spurring as a result of persistent arthritis.
- To reveal the presence of fluid.

Contraindications

- None.

Procedure

Client preparation

1. Any injured locations of the body should be carefully handled.
2. The client is told that holding the extremity still while the x-ray picture is taken is important. Holding still can sometimes be a difficult task, especially when the client has severe pain associated with a recent injury.
3. To avoid exposure from scattered radiation, the testes, ovaries, or pregnant abdomen should be appropriately shielded during the procedure.
4. The large equipment and the fear of being taken away from their parents usually frightens young children requiring x-ray films. Many x-ray departments allow the parent(s) to accompany the child and provide the parent(s) with lead shielding.

Procedure

1. The client is asked to place the involved extremity in several positions, and an x-ray film is taken of each one.
2. An x-ray technician usually performs this test in several minutes in the x-ray department.

Nursing implications

1. Although no pain is associated with these x-ray films, many clients (especially those with arthritis) are extremely uncomfortable lying on a hard x-ray table. After the x-ray films are taken, these clients may receive an analgesic or local heat applications for relief of joint pain.

Special Studies

Endoscopy
ARTHROSCOPY
Normal Values

- Normal ligaments, menisci, and articular surfaces of the joint.

Deviations from Normal

- Abnormal anatomical findings (see ''Indications'' below).

Indications

- To evaluate the knee for meniscus cartilage or ligament.
- To aid in providing differential diagnosis of acute and chronic knee disorders.
- To provide a safe and convenient alternative to open surgery (arthrotomy) because the surgical instruments can be passed directly through the arthroscope for performing the surgery.
- To monitor the progression of disease.
- To monitor the effectiveness of a particular therapy.
- To record visual findings by attaching a camera to the arthroscope.

Contraindications

- A client with ankylosis, because maneuvering the instrument into a joint stiffened by adhesives is almost impossible.
- A client with local skin or wound infections because of the risk of sepsis.

Procedure

Client preparation

1. Routine preoperative procedure is followed.
2. The client must be kept on nothing by mouth after midnight the day of the study.
3. Prior to the procedure, many orthopedic surgeons recommend that clients learn crutch walking. Crutches must be used after arthroscopy until the client can walk without limping.
4. Prior to the procedure, hair in the area of 6 in. above or below the joint is removed by shaving or by a depilatory cream.

Procedure

1. This procedure is commonly performed with a local anesthetic. It may, however, also be performed with the client under spinal or general anesthesia, especially when knee surgery is anticipated.
2. The client is placed on his or her back on an operating table.
3. The client's leg is carefully surgically scrubbed, elevated, and wrapped with an elastic bandage from the toes to the lower thigh to drain as much blood from the leg as possible.
4. A tourniquet is placed on the client's leg. If a tourniquet is not used, a fluid solution may be instilled into the client's knee immediately before insertion of the arthroscope to distend the knee and to help reduce bleeding.
5. The foot of the table is lowered so the client's knee is at about a 45-degree angle.
6. The stocking is opened, and a local anesthetic is administered.
7. A small incision is made in the skin of the knee.
8. The arthroscope (a lighted instrument) is inserted in and out of the joint space to visualize the inside of the knee joint.
9. Although the entire joint can be viewed from one puncture site, additional punctures often are necessary for better visualization.

10. After the area is examined, biopsy or appropriate surgery can be performed and the arthroscope removed.
11. The joint is irrigated clean.
12. Pressure is applied to the knee to remove the irrigating solution.
13. After a few stitches are placed in the skin, a pressure dressing is applied over the incision site.
14. An orthopedic surgeon performs the procedure in the operating room in 15 to 30 minutes.

Nursing implications

1. After the procedure, take the vital signs frequently according to the hospital routine. Assess the neurovascular status of the affected leg by checking pulses, color, temperature, and sensation.
2. Observe the client for signs of infection, including fever, swelling, increased pain and redness, or drainage at the incision site.
3. After the procedure, any discomfort the client has can usually be relieved by a mild analgesic (e.g., aspirin or acetaminophen [Tylenol]).
4. After the study, instruct the client to elevate the knee when sitting and to avoid twisting the knee.
5. After the procedure the client can usually walk on the knee with crutches as soon as the test is complete. However, this action depends on the extent of the procedure and the physician's protocol. The client should be taught isometric quadriceps exercises and instructed to perform them as per the physician's protocol.
6. After the study, examine the incision site for bleeding and apply ice to reduce pain and swelling.
7. The client can resume the normal diet after the study.

Nurse alert

1. The rare complications of this procedure may include infection, hemarthrosis, swelling, thrombophlebitis, joint injury, and synovial rupture.

Arthrocentesis with Synovial Fluid Analysis (Synovial Fluid Analysis; Joint Aspiration)

Normal Values

- Synovial fluid is clear straw-colored, and viscous, with few white blood cells, no crystals, and a good mucin clot.
- Chemical test values (such as glucose determination) should approximate those found in the blood stream.

Deviations from Normal

- Viscosity can be grossly evaluated by forcing synovial fluid from a syringe. Fluid of high viscosity forms a string several inches long, while fluid of low viscosity drips like water.
- Viscosity is reduced in clients with inflammatory arthritis.
- The *mucin clot test*, which correlates with the viscosity, is performed by adding acetic acid to joint fluid. The formation of a tight, ropy clot indicates qualitatively good mucin and the presence of adequate molecules of intact hyaluronic acid. Mucin clot is of poor quality and quantity in inflammatory joint diseased (e.g., rheumatoid arthritis).
- Synovial fluid should not form a fibrin clot because normal joint fluid does not contain fibrinogen. The fluid will clot only if blood entered the joint during the aspiration or in the presence of an inflammatory effusion.
- The *synovial fluid glucose* value is usually within 10 ml/dl of the serum glucose value. For proper interpretation, the synovial fluid glucose and the serum glucose should be drawn simultaneously after the client has fasted for 6 hours. Because synovial fluid glucose level falls with increasing inflammation, in septic arthritis the synovial fluid glucose may be less than 50% of the serum glucose. A low synovial glucose level may also occur with rheumatoid arthritis.
- *Cell counts* normally reveal that joint fluid contains fewer than 200 white blood cells/mm^3. A high percentage of neutrophils (over 75%) occurs in most cases of untreated acute bacterial infectious arthritis.

- *Gram stains* are performed for tubercle bacilli. Bacterial, fungal, and viral cultures are obtained when these diseases are suspected.
- *Crystals* may appear when the fluid is examined under polarized light. The presence of crystals indicates gout.
- *Complement levels* may also be assessed. The complement level may be decreased in clients with systemic lupus erythematosus and in those with rheumatoid arthritis, perhaps because of consumption of complement by the antigen-antibody complexes within the joint cavity.

Indications

- To aid in diagnosing the conditions listed above.
- To aid in the differential diagnosis of gout and pseudogout.
- To detect the presence of gonococci, a major cause of joint infection.
- To establish the diagnosis of infection, crystal-induced arthritis, synovitis, or neoplasms involving the joint.
- To identify the cause of joint effusion.
- To follow the progression of joint disease.
- To inject antiinflammatory medications (mostly common corticosteroids) into a joint area.

Contraindications

- A client with skin or wound infections because of the risk of sepsis.

Procedure
Client preparation

1. Prior to the study the client is usually kept on nothing by mouth after midnight the day of the test to prevent alterations of the chemical determinations (e.g., glucose) that will be performed with the study. If glucose testing of the synovial fluid is not to be performed, the client need not restrict food before the test.

Procedure

1. The client lies on his or her back with the knee fully extended.

2. The knee to be examined is locally anesthetized to minimize pain.
3. The area is meticulously cleansed because this procedure is performed under strict sterile technique.
4. A needle is then inserted through the skin and into the joint space.
5. A small amount of fluid is obtained for analysis.
6. Sometimes the joint area may be wrapped with an elastic bandage to compress free fluid into a certain area to enhance maximal collection of fluid.
7. If a corticosteroid is to be injected, a syringe containing the steroid preparations is attached to the needle and injected.
   a. The needle is then removed.
   b. Pressure is applied to the site, and a bandage is applied.
8. Sometimes blood is drawn from the vein in the arm after the study to compare chemical tests on the blood with chemical studies on the synovial fluid.
9. A physician performs the procedure in the office or at the client's bedside.

Nursing implications

1. After the study, assess the joint for any pain, fever, or swelling, which may indicate infection. Ice may be applied to decrease pain and swelling.
2. After the study the client will usually resume his or her usual activity. The client should, however, avoid strenuous use of the joint for the next several days.
3. After the study the client may resume a normal diet.
4. The specimen should be sent to the lab immediately after the procedure is completed. All specimens should be collected in the appropriate containers. Anticoagulants should be added as the lab indicates.

Nurse alert

1. Complications of arthrocentesis include joint infection and hemorrhage into the joint areas.

Bibliography

Anthony, C.P., and Thibodeau, G.A.: Textbook of anatomy and physiology, ed. 11, St. Louis, 1983, The C.V. Mosby Co.

Brunner, L.S., and Suddarth, D.S.: Textbook of medical-surgical nursing, ed. 5, Philadelphia, 1984, J.B. Lippincott Co.

Buergin, P.: Assessment of the musculoskeletal system. In Phipps, W.J., Long, B.C., and Woods, N.F., editors: Medical-surgical nursing: concepts and clinical practice, ed. 2, St. Louis, 1983, The C.V. Mosby Co.

Cohen, S., and Viellion, G.: Programmed instruction: patient assessment: examining joints of the upper and lower extremities, Am. J. Nurs. 81(4):763-786, April 1981.

Farrell, J.: Arthroscopy, Nursing '82 12(5):73-75, May 1982.

Gilliland, B.C., and Mannik, M.: Approaches to disorders of the joints. In Petersdorf, R.G., and others, editors: Harrison's principles of internal medicine, ed. 10, New York, 1983, McGraw-Hill Book Co.

Krane, S.M., and Holick, M.F.: Metabolic bone disease. In Petersdorf, R.G., and others, editors: Harrison's principles of internal medicine, ed. 10, New York, 1983, McGraw-Hill Book Co.

Krane, S.M., and Potts, J.T.: Disorders of bone and bone mineral metabolism. In Petersdorf, R.G., and others, editors: Harrison's principles of internal medicine, ed. 10, New York, 1983, McGraw-Hill Book Co.

Lee, Y.T.: Bone scanning in patients with early breast carcinoma: should it be a routine staging procedure? Cancer 47:486, 1981.

Ravel, R.: Clinical laboratory medicine, ed. 4, Chicago, 1984, Year Book Medical Publishers, Inc.

Schreck, I.R.: Musculoskeletal physiology and assessment. In Beyers, M., and Dudas, S., editors: The clinical practice of medical-surgical nursing, ed. 2, Boston, 1984, Little, Brown & Co.

Tucker, S.M., and others, editors: Patient care standards, ed. 3, St. Louis, 1984, The C.V. Mosby Co.

Wassel, A.: Nursing assessment of injuries to the lower extremities, Nurs. Clin. North Am. 16(4):739-748, Dec. 1981.

Cancer Tests

12

Clinical Laboratory Tests

Blood Tests

ALPHA-FETOPROTEIN (AFP)

Normal Values

- <25 ng/ml.

Deviations from Normal

- Elevated levels may indicate the presence of liver neoplasms and germ cell tumors of the testicle or ovaries.
- In newborns, elevated levels may indicate hepatitis or biliary atresia.

Indications

- To detect and follow the clinical course of clients with tumors (hepatomas, hepatoblastomas, teratoblastomas, and other embryonic tumors of the gonads).
- To differentiate neonatal hepatitis from biliary atresia in the newborn.

Contraindications

- See "AFP," p. 305.

Procedure

1. See "AFP," p. 305.

CEA
See p. 34.

5-HYDROXY INDOLE ACETIC ACID (5-HIAA)

Normal Values

- 2 to 9 mg/24 h (women lower than men).

Deviations from Normal

- In clients known to have carcinoid tumor, rising levels of 5-HIAA indicate worsening of tumor; falling levels indicate a response to antineoplastic tumor.

- Elevated levels in the undiagnosed client may indicate carcinoid tumor.
- Many medications may interfere with the test, most commonly alcohol, tricyclic antidepressants, monoamine oxidase inhibitors, methyldopa, phenacetin, acetametaphen, aspirin, phenothiazines, and any phenylalanine-containing product.
- Some foods contain serotonin and may alter test results (see "Client Preparation" below for a partial listing).

Indications

- To evaluate the possibility of carcinoid tumor in clients who present with bronchospasm, diarrhea, and flushing.
- To evaluate clients with known carcinoid tumor by analyzing serial levels of urinary 5-HIAA.

Contraindications

- None.

Procedure

Client preparation

1. The importance of accurately obtaining all urine during the 24-hour collection period is explained to the client.
2. See "Client Preparation" for "Creatinine Clearance Test," (except step 2), p. 181, for the correct method of obtaining the specimen.
3. The client is instructed to refrain from eating serotonin-containing foods (e.g., plums, pineapples, bananas, eggplant, tomatoes, avocados, or walnuts) for several days (usually 3) prior to and during the testing period.
4. The client should be assessed for the ingestion of drugs noted for affecting 5-HIAA levels (see "Deviations from Normal" above). If any of these drugs have been or are being taken, they should be listed on the lab slip and recorded in the client's chart.
5. The client is instructed to preserve the specimen in the refrigerator during the collection period.

Procedure

1. Urine is collected for 24 hours in a large urine container that contains a preservative to keep the specimen at an appropriate pH level.
2. The specimen is refrigerated during the collection period.
3. After the 24-hour collection is completed, the specimen is taken to the chemistry lab.

HUMAN CHORIONIC GONADOTROPIN (HCG)
Normal Values

- Negative.

Deviations from Normal

- Elevated levels are suspicious for tumor progression in clients diagnosed as having gestational or gonadal tumors.
- Decreasing levels indicate effective antitumor treatment.

Indications

- To act as guidelines for evaluation of the success of instituted therapy once gestational or gonadal tumors are detected.
- To aid in detecting gestational tumors and gonadal tumors.

Contraindications

- See "Pregnancy Tests," p. 301.

Procedure

1. See "Pregnancy Tests," p. 301.

Urine Tests
URINE FOR BENCE JONES PROTEIN
Normal Values

- No Bence Jones protein present.

Deviations from Normal

- Bence Jones proteins are commonly found in clients with multiple myelomas.

- They may also be associated with tumor metastases to bone, chronic lymphocytic leukemias, and amyloidosis.

Indications

- To aid in detecting multiple myelomas.

Contraindications

- None.

Procedure
Client preparation

1. The client is told how to obtain an uncontaminated urine specimen and is assisted in doing so as needed. The specimen must not contain stool, menstrual blood, prostatic extractions, or semen.

Procedure

1. An early morning specimen of at least 50 ml of uncontaminated urine is collected in a container.
2. The sample is taken to the lab for analysis.

Nursing implications

1. Ensure that the specimen is taken to the lab as soon as possible. If any delay occurs, refrigerate the specimen because heat-coagulable proteins can decompose, causing a false-positive test.

URINE FOR MELANIN
Normal Values

- No detectable level of melanin in the urine.

Deviations from Normal

- Malignant tumor of the melanocytes (malignant cutaneous melanomas) can produce excessive levels of melanin.

Indications

- To follow the clinical course of clients with melanoma.

Contraindications

- None.

Procedure

1. See "Procedure" for 24-hour urine collection for "Creatinine Clearance Test," p. 181.

Client preparation

1. The client is told how to obtain an uncontaminated specimen.

Procedure

1. The client obtains a spot urine or a 24-hour urine specimen.

Nursing implications

1. Ensure that the specimen is delivered to the lab with minimal delay.

Radiologic Laboratory Tests

X-Ray Tests

LYMPHANGIOGRAPHY (LYMPHANGIOGRAM; LYMPHOGRAPHY)

Normal Values

- Normal lymph nodes and vessels.

Deviations from Normal

- Abnormal nodes or vessels indicate tumor exists.

Indications

- To diagnose causes of edema or signs of tumor (e.g., unexplained fever, weight loss, or enlarged lymph nodes).
- To evaluate the spread of cancer within the body.
- To stage a lymphoma to determine appropriate therapy.
- To evaluate the results of chemotherapy or radiation therapy.

- The contrast medium remains in the lymph nodes for 6 months to 1 year, allowing repeat x-ray examination to follow up disease progression or response to therapy.

Contraindications

- A client allergic to iodine dye who has not been desensitized.
- A client with severe chronic lung disease, cardiac disease, or advanced kidney or liver disease.

Procedure
Client preparation

1. The procedure is explained to the client. The client is told that he or she will need to remain still during the test.
2. The physician obtains a signed informed consent form before the study.
3. The client should be assessed for allergies to iodine, seafood, or any of the dyes used in diagnostic studies (e.g., IVP). If allergies are detected, the physician is notified.
4. The client is told that the dye gives the skin a bluish tinge and may discolor the urine and stool for 2 days.

Procedure

1. The client lies on his or her back.
2. A blue dye is injected between each of the first three toes in each foot to outline the lymphatic vessels. (The dye can also be injected into the web of skin between the fingers.)
3. A local anesthetic is injected before a small incision is made in each foot.
4. A lymphatic vessel is identified, and a cannula is inserted to infuse the iodine contrast agent.
5. The dye is infused into the vessels for approximately 1 to 1½ hours. The infusion is usually accomplished using an infusion pump to inject the dye at a slow, continuous rate.
6. The client must lie very still during the dye injection.
7. Fluoroscopy (moving x-ray films on a television monitor) follows the flow of iodine dye throughout the body.

8. When the contrast medium reaches a certain level of the lumbar vertebrae, the dye is discontinued.
9. Films are taken of the stomach, pelvis, and upper body to demonstrate the filling of the lymphatic vessels.
10. The client must return in 24 hours for additional x-ray films to visualize the lymph nodes.
11. When the injection is given in the hand, the axillary and supraclavicular lymph nodes are evaluated.
12. When the injection is completed, the cannula is removed and the incision is sutured closed.
13. A radiologist performs this procedure in the x-ray department in 3 hours.

Nursing implications

1. After the study the vital signs are taken according to the physician's routine.
2. The client is checked for any signs of shortness of breath, chest pain, fever, or hypotension that microemboli from spillage of the contrast dye into the thoracic duct could cause.

Nurse alert

1. Lipid pneumonia may be a complication of lymphangiography if the contrast medium flows into the thoracic duct and casues microemboli in the lungs. These small emboli usually disappear after several weeks or months. Observe the client for shortness of breath, chest pain, fever, or hypotension.

MAMMOGRAPHY

Normal Values

- Negative; no tumor shadow present.

Deviations from Normal

- Radiographic signs of breast cancer include fine calcific stippling, a localized area of increased radiodensity (nodule) with poorly defined margins (Fig. 12-1), an area of edema surrounding the nodule, or thickening of the skin adjacent to the nodule.

Indications

- To detect nonpalpable breast cancers, especially in clients with large, pendulous breasts.
- To substantiate questionable findings from thermography or breast examination.
- To follow clients at high risk for breast cancer.

Contraindications

- A pregnant client.

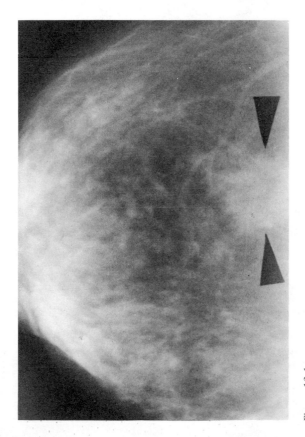

Figure 12-1
Mammogram. Craniocaudal view of breast. Arrows indicate typical breast cancer. Note poorly defined margins.

Procedure
Client preparation

1. The client is told that recent advances in mammography make the risk associated with this study minimal and far outweighed by the advantage of early cancer detection.

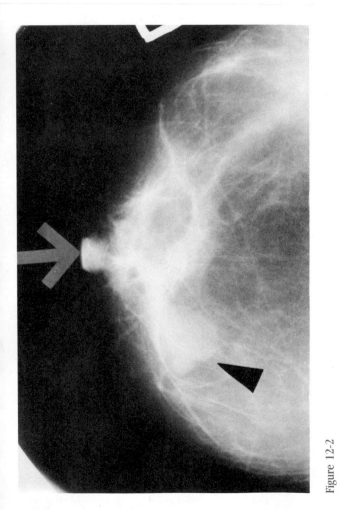

Figure 12-2
Mammogram. Craniocaudal view of breast. Pointer indicates typical benign fibroadenoma with well-circumscribed margin. Arrow indicates nipple. Note large cyst under breast.

2. Some clients are embarrassed by this procedure.
3. Clients are often anxious regarding this examination. Emotional support is provided.

Procedure

1. The client is placed in front of the mammographic x-ray machine.
2. One breast is placed on an x-ray plate, and the x-ray cone is brought down on top of the breast to gently compress it between the broadened cone and the plate.
3. An x-ray film is taken (the craniocaudal view) (Fig. 12-2).
4. Next the x-ray plate is turned perpendicular to the floor and placed laterally on the outer aspect of the breast.
5. The broadened cone is brought in medially, and it again gently compresses the breast (the lateral view).
6. Occasionally oblique views are required.
7. A radiologic technician performs the mammogram in approximately 10 minutes. A radiologist interprets the results and decides whether to use mammography or xeromammography.

Nursing implications

1. Tell the client how and when she can obtain the study results, usually 1 day after the test.

THERMOGRAPHY
Normal Values

■ Avascular pattern with even distribution of temperature patterns. Normal tissues appear as shades of gray.

Deviations from Normal

■ Benign tumors appear as shades of gray.
■ "Hot spots" appear as black areas.
■ Cystic lesions may occasionally appear as cold spots or white areas.
■ Fibrocystic disease and infection may give a false-positive reading.

Indications

- To screen for early breast cancer.
- To detect infection, fibrocystic disease, and benign tumors.

Contraindications

- A premenstrual client with severe vascular engorgement of the breast.
- A client who has recently been exposed to excessive sunlight, causing a sunburn.
- A client who has had recent breast infection.
- A pregnant client.

Procedure

Client preparation

1. This may be a period of high anxiety for the client. She should be encouraged to express any concerns about breast cancer.
2. The client is questioned regarding recent exposure to excessive sunlight, which can cause false-positive results.
3. The client is assessed for the use of any ointment or powder to her breast the day of the test. These will cause false-positive results if not removed prior to the study.
4. A menstrual history is obtained. The client should be postmenstrual for the study. Thermography is not performed if the woman is pregnant, close to her period, or menstruating because the vascularity of the breasts increases at these times.

Procedure

1. The client is instructed to disrobe from the waist up and don an x-ray gown with the opening in the front.
2. She is taken to the thermography room and asked to wait for about 10 minutes.
3. The client is seated with her arms raised above her head.
4. A thermoscope is placed over a small area of breast skin to determine normal breast temperatures.
5. The infrared scanning unit is adjusted to establish a baseline norm.
6. The unit is placed to scan both breasts.

7. Scans are taken from the frontal and lateral views.
8. A technician performs the study in the radiology department in approximately 20 minutes. A radiologist interprets the results.

Nursing implications

1. If the results are positive, explain the other tests that will be necessary to confirm the diagnosis.
2. It may be reasonable to instruct the client in breast self-examination at this time. If, however, the client is anxious, this instruction may be ill-timed.

Computerized Tomography Tests
CT SCAN OF THE BRAIN
See p. 151.

CT SCAN OF THE LIVER
See p. 94.

Nuclear Scanning Tests
BONE SCAN
Normal Values

- No evidence of abnormality.

Deviations from Normal

- Fractures, osteomyelitis, osteoarthritis, areas of bone necrosis, renal osteodystrophy, and Paget's disease produce abnormal scans.
- Tumors appear as abnormal areas often called ''hot spots.''

Indications

- To detect metastatic tumor.
- To detect the body's response to radiation or chemotherapy via repeated scanning.
- To provide valuable information in the evaluation of trauma in clients with unexplained pain, especially in areas where

fractures are not immediately seen on x-ray film (e.g., spine, ribs, face, small bones of the extremities).

■ To evaluate clients with osteomyelitis.
■ To detect secondary changes produced by healing or changes caused by disease (e.g., osteomyelitis) days or weeks before possible to do so on x-ray film.

Contraindications

■ A pregnant or lactating client.

Procedure
Client preparation

1. The client is assured that the dose of radiation he or she will receive is less than the amount of radiation received from regular diagnostic x-rays.
2. The client is told that the injected radionuclide will not affect visitors or hospital staff members. The radioactive substance is usually excreted via the urine in 6 to 24 hours.
3. The client is informed that during the scanning he or she is not exposed to any radiation. The scanning machine detects the radiation emitted *from* the client as opposed to a regular x-ray machine in which radiation is emitted from the machine to the body.
4. The client is instructed to remove jewelry or any metal objects that may obscure x-ray visualization of bones.
5. Sedatives may be given if the client has difficulty remaining still during the procedure.

Procedure

1. The client receives an intravenous injection of an isotope (e.g., sodium pertechnetate Tc 99m) into a vein in the arm.
2. The client is encouraged to drink several glasses of water between the injection of the radioisotope and the actual scanning. The fluids facilitate renal clearance of the circulating tracer not picked up by the bone. The waiting period prior to the scanning is approximately 1 to 3 hours. The client should be told the exact time at which the scanning will occur.

3. The client is instructed to urinate and is positioned subsequently on a scanning table in the x-ray department.
4. A scanning machine is moved back and forth over the client's body, and the machine detects radiation emitted by the skeleton.
5. This information is translated into x-ray film, thus showing a two-dimensional view of the skeleton.
6. Many x-ray pictures are taken, and the client may need to be repositioned several times during the test.
7. Sedatives may be administered if the client has difficulty remaining still during the scanning period.
8. A physician or a nuclear medicine technician performs this study in the radiology department in 30 to 60 minutes.

Nursing implications

1. After the test, check the injection site for redness or swelling. If a hematoma forms, warm soaks can be applied to the area to relieve discomfort.

GALLIUM SCAN
Normal Values

- Gallium uptake in the liver, spleen, bone, and colon. No other concentration noted.

Deviations from Normal

- Gallium scans detect the following types of tumors: sarcomas, lymphomas, and carcinomas of the colon, kidney, uterus, stomach, and testicles.

Indications

- To detect primary or metastatic tumors when cancer is suspected but cannot be located by other diagnostic techniques.
- To demonstrate the source of infection in clients who have fever of unknown origin.

Contraindications

- A client for whom information is needed for therapy earlier than 72 hours.

Procedure
Client preparation

1. The client is reassured that the test is painless and that the dose of radionuclide is safe.
2. Enemas or suppositories are administered as ordered prior to gallium scanning to "wash out" the gallium secreted into the bowel. This process eliminates the possibility that increased uptake in the sigmoid colon would be misread for a pathologic process.
3. The client must be instructed to return for subsequent scanning.

Procedure

1. The client is injected with gallium citrate.
2. Four to six hours later a total body scan may be performed by slowly passing a radionuclide detector over the body. Additional scans are taken 24, 48, and 72 hours later.
3. During the scanning process the client is positioned in the supine, prone, and lateral positions.
4. Because the bowel can take up the gallium, suppositories or enemas are given a few hours prior to each scanning.
5. The client is asked to lie still during the actual scanning.
6. The scan is usually performed by a nuclear medicine technician and interpreted by the nuclear medicine physician. Each scan takes about 30 to 60 minutes and is performed in the nuclear medicine department.

Bibliography

Bouchard-Kurtz, R.E., and Speese-Ownes, N.F.: Nursing care of the cancer patient, ed. 4, St. Louis, 1981, The C.V. Mosby Co.

Brunner, L.S., and Suddarth, D.S.: Textbook of medical-surgical nursing, ed. 5, Philadelphia, 1984, J.B. Lippincott Co.

Couch, W.D.: Combined effusion fluid tumor marker assay, carcinoembryonic antigen (CEA) and human chorionic gonadotropin (HCG), in the detection of malignant tumors, Cancer **48:**2475, 1981.

Cowan, K., and Lippman, M.: Steroid receptors in breast cancer, Arch. Intern. Med. **142:**363, 1982.

DeVita, V.T.: Principles of cancer therapy. In Petersdorf, R.G., editor: Harrison's principles of internal medicine, ed. 10, New York, 1983, McGraw-Hill Book Co.

Egan, R.L.: Multicentric breast carcinomas: clinical-radiographic-pathologic whole organ studies and 10-year survival, Cancer **49:**1123, 1982.

Guidelines for the cancer-related check-up, CA **30:**195-196, 1980.

Henney, J.E., and DeVita, V.T.: Breast cancer. In Petersdorf, R.G., editor: Harrison's principles of internal medicine, ed. 10, New York, 1983, McGraw-Hill Book Co.

Hogan, R., and Xistris, D.M.: Neoplasia. In Phipps, W.J., Long, B.C., and Woods, N.F., editors: Medical-surgical nursing: concepts and clinical practice, ed. 2, St. Louis, 1983, The C.V. Mosby Co.

Kopans, D.B., and others: Palpable breast masses: the importance of preoperative mammography, JAMA **246:**2819, 1981.

Krol, M.A.: The patient with cancer. In Beyers, M., and Dudas, S., editors: The clinical practice of medical-surgical nursing, ed. 2, Boston, 1984, Little, Brown & Co.

Long, B.C., and Molbo, D.M.: Problems of the breast. In Phipps, W.J., Long, B.C., and Woods, N.F., editors: Medical-surgical nursing: concepts and clinical practice, ed. 2, St. Louis, 1983, The C.V. Mosby Co.

Moskowitz, M.: Screening for breast cancer: how effective are our tests? A critical review, CA **33:**26, 1983.

Nolan, H.G., and others: Role of bone scanning in carcinoma of the breast, Ann. Clin. Lab. Sci. **10:**105, 1980.

Reynoso, G.: CEA: basic concepts, clinical applications, Diagn. Med. **4:**41, 1981.

Ultmann, J.E., and Golomb, H.M.: Principles of neoplasia: approach to diagnosis and management. In Petersdorf, R.G., editor: Harrison's principles of internal medicine, ed. 10, New York, 1983, McGraw-Hill Book Co.

Routine Laboratory Tests

13

420

Routine Admission Tests

Clinical Laboratory Tests

Blood Tests

ERYTHROCYTE SEDIMENTATION RATE (SED RATE)

Normal Values (Westergren method)

- Men: up to 15 mm/h.
- Women: up to 20 mm/h.
- Children: up to 10 mm/h.

Deviations from Normal

- Many specific diseases (e.g., toxemia, syphilis, nephritis, pneumonia, and rheumatoid arthritis) can cause an elevated SED rate.
- Decreased values may occur in clients with congestive heart failure, sickle cell anemia, hypofibrinogenemia, and polycythemia vera.

Indications

- To detect disease that is otherwise unsuspected.
- Occasionally to differentiate disease entities or complaints (e.g., with the client with chest pain, the SED rate will be increased with myocardial infarction but normal with angina).

Contraindications

- None.

Procedure

1. Following standard venipuncture technique, venous blood is collected in a lavender-top tube.
2. The blood is immediately taken to the hematology lab because delay may cause retarding of the ESR, thereby causing artificially low results. The study should be performed within 3 hours after the specimen has been obtained.
3. Pressure or a pressure dressing is applied to the puncture site.

Nursing implications

1. Observe the puncture site for bleeding.

SERUM ELECTROLYTE CONCENTRATION TEST

For this study, sodium, potassium, chloride, and carbon dioxide levels are obtained.

Sodium (Na)
Normal values

- 136 to 145 mEq/L.

Deviations from normal

- See boxed material on p. 423.

Potassium (K)
Normal values

- 3.5 to 5.0 mEq/L.

Deviations from normal

- See boxed material on p. 424.

Chloride (Cl)
Normal values

- 90 to 110 mEq/L.

Deviations from normal

- Hypochloremia and hyperchloremia rarely occur alone and usually parallel shifts in sodium levels, the causes of which are listed in the boxed material on p. 423.

Carbon Dioxide (CO_2) Content
Normal values

- 23 to 30 mEq/L.

Deviations from normal

- Increases occur with acidosis.

Causes of Hypernatremia (Increased Serum Sodium Concentration) and Hyponatremia (Decreased Serum Sodium Concentration)

A. Hypernatremia
   1. Increased sodium intake (without access to water)
      a. Excessive dietary intake
      b. Excessive sodium in IV fluid
   2. Decreased sodium loss
      a. Cushing's syndrome
      b. Hyperaldosteronism
   3. Excessive free body water loss (hypernatremic dehydration)
      a. Excessive sweating
      b. Extensive thermal burns
      c. Diabetes insipidus
      d. Osmotic diuresis (as in glucosuria and overzealous mannitol administration)
B. Hyponatremia
   1. Decreased sodium intake
      a. Deficient dietary intake
      b. Deficient sodium in IV fluid
   2. Increased sodium loss
      a. Addison's disease
      b. Diarrhea
      c. Vomiting or nasogastric aspiration
      d. Diuretic administration
      e. Chronic renal insufficiency (inadequate tubular reabsorption of sodium)
   3. Increased free body water (dilutional)
      a. Excessive oral water intake
      b. Excessive IV water intake
      c. Congestive heart failure
      d. Inappropriate secretion of antidiuretic hormone
      e. Osmotic dilution (as in hyperglycemia and hyperproteinemia)
   4. Third-space losses of sodium
      a. Ascites
      b. Peripheral edema
      c. Pleural effusion
      d. Intraluminal bowel loss (ileus or mechanical obstruction)

Causes of Hyperkalemia (Increased Serum Potassium Concentration) and Hypokalemia (Decreased Serum Potassium Concentration)

A. Hyperkalemia
   1. Increased potassium intake
      a. Excessive dietary intake
      b. Excessive IV intake
   2. Decreased potassium loss
      a. Acute or chronic renal failure
      b. Addison's disease
      c. Hypoaldosteronism
      d. Aldosterone-inhibiting diuretics (such as spironolactone and triamterene)
   3. Shift from intracellular space
      a. Acidosis
      b. Infection
      c. Crush injury to tissues
   4. Pseudohyperkalemia
      a. Poor venipuncture technique
      b. Transfusion of hemolyzed blood
B. Hypokalemia
   1. Decreased potassium intake
      a. Deficient dietary intake
      b. Deficient IV intake
   2. Excessive potassium loss
      a. GI disorders (diarrhea, vomiting, and villous adenomas)
      b. Diuretics
      c. Hyperaldosteronism
      d. Cushing's syndrome
      e. Renal tubular acidosis
      f. Licorice ingestion
   3. Shift to intracellular space
      a. Alkalosis
      b. Insulin or glucose administration
      c. Calcium administration

Indications

- To aid in diagnosing conditions listed in the boxed material on p. 423 and ''Deviations from Normal'' above.

Contraindications

- None.

Procedure

1. Following standard venipuncture and using a 20-gauge needle, 7 ml of blood are collected in a red-top tube. The 20-gauge needle prevents hemolysis.
2. If the client has an IV, the venipuncture is performed on the opposite arm to avoid artificial results.
3. Pressure or a pressure dressing is applied to the puncture site.
4. The sample is sent to the chemistry lab for analysis.

Nursing implications

1. Because this study is often performed with a glucose level determination, mark the time of the day the test was performed to avoid confusion in the glucose readings.
2. If the results are abnormal, notify the physician. Occasionally, if the results are unexpectedly abnormal, the physician will repeat the test because the chance of lab error is great in this test, since many specimens are tested at the same time. The machine performing the determinations can malfunction.
3. Observe the puncture site for bleeding.

Special Studies

Culture and Sensitivity (C & S of the Throat, Sputum, Urine, Stool, Blood, Wound, Cervix, and Urethra)

Normal Values

- Negative for all cultures.

Deviations from Normal

- The presence of disease-causing bacteria.

Indications

- To diagnose fever of unknown origin (FVO).
- To determine the causal organism for an obvious infection.
- To determine the source of an epidemic.
- To test for complete resolution of infection, especially in urinary tract infection.

Contraindications

- None.

Procedure
Client preparation

1. The purpose for the culture and the procedure for obtaining the specimen are explained to the client.
2. The instructions are thoroughly explained to the client if he or she is to obtain the specimen.
3. The client must have the necessary cleansing agents and sterile supplies available.
4. If the client cannot obtain the specimen alone, nursing assistance must be provided.
5. The client is draped during the procedure, if necessary, to prevent unnecessary exposure.

General procedure

1. In general, all culture specimens are delivered to the microbiology (bacteriology) lab and cultured as soon as they are obtained. Otherwise overgrowth of the bacteria will occur while the specimen is "sitting around."
2. If the specimen is obtained at night or on weekends and the lab is closed, the specimen should be refrigerated until it can be placed on the culture medium.
3. When an anaerobic infection is suspected, the specimen should be aspirated into a sterile syringe and "topped" until it can be cultured in anaerobic conditions.

Specific procedure
Sputum cultures

1. The client coughs when he or she awakens (see Chapter 4, p. 128.)
2. The cough may be induced by nasotracheal aspiration, nebulizers, or pulmonary physical therapy.
3. The sputum can also be obtained by transtracheal needle aspiration or bronchoscopic aspiration.
4. The specimen is placed in a sterile container and trans ported to the bacteriology lab.

Urine culture

1. The urine culture specimen must be a clean-catch mid- stream collection.
2. The client is asked to wipe the distal urethra with an anti- septic in a front-to-back direction.
3. Voiding is initiated.
4. During midstream, the sterile container is placed into the urine stream to collect between 5 and 50 ml of urine.
5. The container is removed from the stream, and voiding is completed.
6. The urine can also be collected by suprapubic aspiration or directly from an indwelling catheter. The specimen con- tainer is covered, labeled, and transported to the bacteri- ology lab as soon as possible.
7. Frequently culturing the urine of a client who has had an indwelling Foley catheter immediately before the removal of the catheter is beneficial. This procedure is called a "terminal urine for C & S" and is usually more accurate than is culturing the tip of the catheter.

Stool culture

1. Stools for bacteria or parasites are collected in a clean, wide-mouthed plastic or glass container with a tight-fitting lid.
2. The client usually defecates into a clean bed pan and trans- fers either a walnut-sized piece of the feces or the entire specimen (as the lab directs) into the specimen container.

3. Urine and toilet paper should not be mixed with the specimen.
4. Since parasites or bacteria are often found in mucus or blood streaks, some of this material, if present, should be included with the sample.
5. Cultures can also be detected by the "tape test" or by a rectal swab.

Blood cultures

1. At least two culture specimens should be obtained from two different sites to rule out a false-positive culture caused by a contaminant. When both cultures produce the infecting agent, bacteremia exists.
2. If the client is receiving antibiotics, the lab slip should indicate the medication being taken. The blood culture specimen should be taken shortly before the next dose of the antibiotic.
3. Two different peripheral venous sites are carefully prepared with povidone-iodine (Betadine).
4. The tops of the Vacutainer tubes or culture bottles are cleaned with iodine and allowed to dry.
5. The venipuncture is performed aseptically, and enough blood is aspirated (approximately 8 ml) to allow a dilution ratio of blood to culture broth of about 1:10.
6. The culture bottles should be transported to the lab immediately.
7. Culture specimens drawn through an IV catheter are frequently contaminated, and tests using catheters should not be performed unless catheter sepsis is suspected. Then blood culture specimens drawn through the catheter more accurately indicate the causative agent than does a culture specimen from the catheter tip.

Wound culture

1. A sterile cotton swab is aseptically placed into the pus.
2. The swab is put into a sterile, covered test tube.
3. The specimen is transported to the lab as soon as possible.
4. Culturing specimens taken from the skin edge is much less accurate than culturing the suppurative material.

5. If an anaerobic organism is suspected, an anaerobic culture tube is obtained from the microbiologic lab. Routine wound cultures are also performed at the same time.

Cervical cultures

1. The female client should refrain from douching and tub bathing prior to the cervical culture.
2. The client is placed in the lithotomy position.
3. A nonlubricated vaginal speculum is inserted to expose the cervix.
4. Cervical mucus is removed with a cotton ball held in ring forceps.
5. A sterile-tipped swab is inserted into the endocervical canal and moved from side to side.

Urethral culture

1. The urethral specimen should be obtained from the male client prior to his voiding.
2. This is obtained by inserting a sterile swab gently into the anterior urethra.

Nursing implications

1. Obtain the specimens in a sterile manner. Handle all specimens as though they were capable of transmitting disease.
2. Specimens should be transported to the lab immediately (at least within 30 minutes).
3. Obtain the specimens before initiating the prescribed antibiotic therapy. Antibiotics will alter the growth of the organisms in culture media.
4. Carefully label all specimens. Include the precise time at which the specimen was collected. Also indicate any medication the client may be taking that could affect the results.
5. Notify the physician of any positive results so that appropriate antibiotic therapy can be initiated.
6. If wound cultures are to be obtained on a client requiring wound irrigation, obtain the culture *before* the wound is irrigated.

Tuberculin Skin Test (Tuberculin Skin Test with Purified Protein Derivative; PPD)

Normal Values

- Negative; reaction <5 mm.

Deviations from Normal

- If the client is infected with tuberculosis (whether active or dormant), lymphocytes will recognize the PPD antigen and cause a local reaction.

Indications

- To detect tuberculosis infection, although the test cannot indicate whether the infection is active or dormant. A client with a particular complaint and a positive PPD reaction does not necessarily have active tuberculosis. The result may only mean that the client has had tuberculosis in the past, and the infection is now dormant and not causing a problem.
- To assess the immune system when used as part of a series of skin tests (see Table 13-1). If the immune system is non-functioning because of poor nutrition or chronic illness (e.g., neoplasia or infection), the PPD test will be negative despite the fact that the client has had an active or dormant tuberculosis infection.

Contraindications

- A client with known active tuberculosis infections.
- A client who has received bacille Calmette-Guérin (BCG) immunization against PPD because he or she will demonstrate a positive reaction to the PPD vaccination even though he or she may never have had tuberculous infection.

Procedure
Client preparation

1. The client is reassured that he or she will not acquire tuberculosis from this test.
2. The client is assessed for previous tuberculosis.
3. A history of previous PPD results and BCG immunization is obtained from the client.

Table 13-1   Selected skin tests

Disease	Test	Antigen	Time to Read	Positive Reaction
Diphtheria susceptibility	Schick	Diphtheria toxin	3-6 days	>10 mm
Echinococcosis	Casoni	Fluid from hydatid cyst	15-20 min	Immediate erythema and swelling
Lymphogranuloma venereum	Frei	Killed virus	48-72 h	6 × 6 mm raised papule
Sarcoidosis	Kveim-Siltzback	Sarcoid tissue	6 wks	Palpable nodule
Scarlet fever	Schultz-Charlton	Antitoxin	24 h	Blanched area
Scarlet fever susceptibility	Dick	Erythrogenic toxin	24 h	>10 mm
Systemic fungal infection	Histoplasmin, etc.	Killed fungi	48 h	>5 mm
Toxoplasmosis	Toxoplasm	Antigen	24-48 h	>10 mm
Trichinosis	*Trichinella*	Killed larvae	15-20 min	Blanched wheal surrounded by erythema
Tuberculosis	PPD	Tuberculin antigen	48-72 h	>10 mm
Tularemia	Foshay	Killed bacteria	48 h	Erythema and induration

Procedure

1. Prepare the forearm with alcohol and allow it to dry.
2. Intradermally inject the PPD and then circle the area with indelible ink.
3. Record the time at which the PPD was injected.
4. Read the results in 48 to 72 hours and record the results. Some hospitals require readings at 48- and 72-hour intervals.
5. A nurse performs this test.

Nursing implications

1. If the test is positive, be sure the physician is notified and the client is treated appropriately.
2. If the test is positive, check the arm 4 to 5 days after the test to be certain that a severe skin reaction has not occurred.
3. If the client is an outpatient, do not give the PPD test when the reading time (48 to 72 hours later) will fall on a weekend. Frequently no one will be available at such a time to read the results.

Miscellaneous Tests

Clinical Laboratory Tests
Blood Tests
CARBOXYHEMOGLOBIN (CARBON MONOXIDE)
Normal Values

- 3% of the total hemoglobin.
- Up to 15% in tobacco smokers.

Deviations from Normal

- Elevated levels indicating carbon monoxide poisoning.

Indications

- To detect carbon monoxide poisoning.

Contraindications

- None.

Procedure

Client preparation

1. A client history related to any possible source of carbon monoxide inhalation is obtained.
2. The client is assessed for signs and symptoms of mild carbon monoxide toxicity (e.g., headache, weakness, dizziness, malaise, and dyspnea) and moderate to severe carbon monoxide toxicity (e.g., severe headache, bright red mucous membranes, and cherry red blood).

Procedure

1. Following standard venous peripheral venipuncture, as soon as possible 5 to 10 ml of venous blood are collected in a lavender-top tube.
2. Pressure or a pressure dressing is applied to the puncture site.
3. The specimen is sent to the lab for analysis.

Nursing implications

1. Observe the site for bleeding.
2. Treat the client as the physician indicates. Usually the client is treated with high concentrations of oxygen. Encourage respirations to allow the client to clear carbon monoxide from the hemoglobin by breathing.

THERAPEUTIC DRUG MONITORING

Normal Values

- See Table 13-2.

Deviations from Normal

- See Table 13-2.
- The ranges listed in the table may not apply to all clients because many factors influence clinical response (e.g., noncompliance, concurrent drug use, other clinical conditions, age, size, extent and rate of drug absorption, and metabo-

Table 13-2   Therapeutic drug monitoring data

Drug	Use
Acetaminophen	Analgesic, antipyretic
Aminophylline	Bronchodilator
Amitriptyline	Antidepressant
Amikacin	Antibiotic
Carbamazepine	Anticonvulsant
Chloramphenicol	Antiinfective
Desipramine	Antidepressant
Digoxin	Cardiac glycoside
Digitoxin	Cardiac glycoside
Dilantin	Anticonvulsant
Disopyramide	Antiarrhythmic
Ethosuximide	Anticonvulsant
Gentamicin	Antibiotic
Imipramine	Antidepressant
Kanamycin	Antibiotic
Lidocaine	Antiarrhythmic
Lithium	Manic episodes of manic-depression psychosis
Methotrexate	Antitumor
Nortriptyline	Antidepressant
Phenobarbital	Anticonvulsant
Phenytoin	Anticonvulsant
Primidone	Anticonvulsant
Procainamide	Antiarrhythmic
Propranolol	Antiarrhythmic
Quinidine	Antiarrhythmic
Salicylate	Antipyretic, antiinflammatory, analgesic
Theophylline	Bronchodilator
Tobramycin	Antibiotic
Valproic acid	Anticonvulsant

Therapeutic Level	Toxic Level
Depends on use	>250 μg/ml
10-20 μg/ml	>20 μg/ml
120-250 ng/ml	>500 ng/ml
20-25 μg/ml	>35 μg/ml
8-12 μg/ml	>15 μg/ml
10-25 μg/ml	>25 μg/ml
150-250 ng/ml	>500 ng/ml
0.5-2.0 ng/ml	>2.4 ng/ml
5-30 ng/ml	>30 ng/ml
10-20 μg/ml	>30 μg/ml
2-4.5 μg/ml	>6 μg/ml
40-100 μg/ml	>150 μg/ml
4-8 μg/ml	>12 μg/ml
150-250 ng/ml	>500 ng/ml
20-25 μg/ml	>35 μg/ml
1.5-5 μg/ml	>7 μg/ml
0.8-1.4 mEq/L	>1.6 mEq/L
>0.01 μmol	>10 μmol/24 h
50-150 ng/ml	>500 ng/ml
15-30 μg/ml	>40 μg/ml
10-20 μg/ml	>30 μg/ml
5-12 μg/ml	>15 μg/ml
4-10 μg/ml	>16 μg/ml
40-85 ng/ml	>150 ng/ml
1.5-3 μg/ml	>5 μg/ml
20-25 mg/dl	>30 mg/dl
10-20 μg/ml	>20 μg/ml
2-8 μg/ml	>12 μg/ml
50-100 μg/ml	>200 μg/ml

lism). Furthermore, different labs use different units for reporting test results and normal ranges. Last, sufficient time must pass between the administration of the drug and the collection of the blood sample to allow for therapeutic levels to occur.

Indications

- To determine the effective drug dosage.
- To prevent drug toxicity.

Contraindications

- None.

Procedure
Client preparation

1. The nurse assures that blood is drawn at the appropriate peak or trough (see ''Procedure'' step 3) level. If a peak level is needed, the nurse should record the exact time at which the drug was administered and then either draw the blood at the appropriate time or notify the lab technologist to obtain the specimen. If a residual level is needed, the next dose of the drug is usually held until the blood specimen is drawn approximately 15 minutes before the scheduled dose. After the blood is drawn, the dose is administered. Unless the exact time is given for obtaining the specimen and administering the drug, drug levels cannot be properly interpreted and may be grossly misleading.

2. Prior to drawing the blood specimen, the nurse determines that the appropriate concentrations have been reached by consulting the pharmacist about the half-life of the drug. Drug blood levels should have reached a steady state or equilibrium that generally takes five drug half-lifes (the time required to decrease the drug blood concentration by 50%).

Procedure

1. Following standard venipuncture technique, blood is collected in the type of tube specified by the lab.

2. Pressure or a pressure dressing is applied to the puncture site.
3. Blood samples can be taken at the drug's *peak* level (the highest concentration) or at the *trough* level (the lowest concentration). Peak levels are useful when testing for toxicity, and trough levels are helpful for demonstrating a satisfactory therapeutic level. Peak levels are usually obtained about 1 to 2 hours after oral intake, about 1 hour after IM administration, and about 30 minutes after IV administration. *Residual* or trough levels are usually obtained shortly before (0 to 15 minutes) the next scheduled dose.

Nursing implications

1. All blood samples should be clearly marked with the following information: client's name, diagnosis, name of drug, time of last drug ingestion, time of sample, and list of any other drugs the client is currently taking.
2. Assess the venipuncture site for bleeding.
3. Observe the client for signs of toxicity related to the appropriate drug. Record all observations and notify the physician as needed.

TOXICOLOGY SCREENING

Normal Values

■ See Tables 13-3 and 13-4.

Deviations from Normal

■ See Tables 13-3 and 13-4.

Indications

■ To determine the cause of acute drug toxicity.
■ To help monitor drug dependency.
■ To detect the presence of narcotics in the body for medicolegal purposes.

Contraindications

■ None.

Table 13-3 Blood toxicology screening

Drug	Type	Therapeutic Level	Toxic Level
Acetaminophen	Analgesic, antipyretic	Depends on use	>250 µg/ml
Alcohol		None	80-200 mg/dl (mild to moderate intoxication)
			250-400 mg/dl (marked intoxication)
			>400 mg/dl (severe intoxication)
Amobarbital	Sedative, hypnotic	0.5-3.0 µg/ml	>10 µg/ml
Butabarbital	Sedative, hypnotic	0.5-3.0 µg/ml	>10 µg/ml
Carbon monoxide	Gas	None	>30% COHb (beginning of coma)
Dilantin	Anticonvulsant	10-20 µg/ml	>30 µg/ml
Glutethimide	Sedative	0.5-3.0 µg/ml	>10 µg/ml
Lead		None	>40 µg/dl
Lithium	Manic episodes of manic-depression psychosis	0.8-1.4 mEq/L	>1.6 mEq/L
Meprobamate	Antianxiety agent	0.5-3.0 µg/ml	>10 µg/ml
Methyprylon	Hypnotic	0.5-3.0 µg/ml	>10 µg/ml
Phenobarbital	Anticonvulsant	15-30 µg/ml	>40 µg/ml
Salicylate	Antipyretic, antiinflammatory, analgesic	20-25 mg/dl	>30 mg/dl

Table 13-4   Urine toxicology screening for amphetamines

Drug	Therapeutic Level	Toxic Level
Amphetamine	2-3 µg/ml	>3 µg/ml
Dextroamphetamine	1-1.5 µg/ml	>15 µg/ml
Methamphetamine	3-5 µg/ml	>40 µg/ml
Phenmetrazine	5-30 µg/ml	>50 µg/ml

Procedure

Client preparation

1. As much information as possible is obtained about the type, amount, and time of consumed drugs.
2. The client is carefully assessed for respiratory distress, which is commonly a side effect of drug overdose.
3. Gastric lavage is performed as needed.
4. If the specimen is obtained for medicolegal testing, the client or family member must sign a consent form.
5. The client should be approached in a nonjudgmental way.

Procedure

1. Following standard venipuncture technique, venous blood is collected in the type of tube specified by the lab.
2. Pressure or a pressure dressing is applied to the puncture site.
3. The blood is usually drawn immediately after the client is admitted to the emergency department.
4. Random urine specimens may be collected.
5. Gastric contents may be aspirated or lavaged for analysis.
6. The hair and the nails are used for detecting or documenting long-term exposure to arsenic or mercury.

Nursing implications

1. The client may be referred for appropriate drug or psychiatric counseling.

Radiologic Laboratory Tests

X-Ray Tests

SIALOGRAPHY

Normal Values

- No evidence of pathology in salivary ducts and related structures.

Deviations from Normal

- Evidence of strictures, tumors, or inflammatory disease.

Indications

- To examine the salivary ducts and related glandular structures in clients complaining of pain, tenderness, or swelling in these areas.

Contraindications

- None.

Procedure

Client preparation

1. The client is told to remove jewelry, hairpins, and dentures that could obscure x-ray visualization.
2. The client is instructed to rinse his or her mouth with an antiseptic solution to reduce the possibility of introducing bacteria into the ductal structures.

Procedure

1. Preinjection x-ray films are taken to ensure that stones are not present that could prevent the contrast material from entering the ducts.
2. After the client is placed in a supine position on an x-ray table, the contrast medium is injected directly into the desired orifice via a cannula or a special catheter.
3. X-ray films are taken with the client in various positions.
4. The client is given a sour substance (e.g., lemon juice) to stimulate salivary excretion.

5. Another set of x-ray films is taken to evaluate ductal drainage.
6. A radiologist performs the study in less than 30 minutes in the radiology department.

Special Studies
Nuclear Magnetic Resonance (NMR)
Possible Indications

- To visualize areas at the base of the skull and the interior of the spine.
- To detect cerebral infarctions, arteriovenous (AV) malformations, hemorrhage, and subdural hematoma.
- To detect atherosclerotic plaques in large arteries.
- To depict lesions in degenerative diseases (e.g., multiple sclerosis).
- To determine the extent of chronic myocardial infarction.
- To identify coronary arteries and bypass grafts.
- To diagnose diseases of the kidney, pancreas, and prostate gland.
- To detect tumors.
- To evaluate trauma clients because the vertebral column, spinal cord, and adjacent soft tissue can be visualized in multiple projections without moving the client.
- To differentiate between normal and degenerated discs.
- To detect aortic aneurysm, aortic dissection, aortic occlusion and stenosis, and aortic AV malformation.
- To assess the response of cancer and lymphoma to radiotherapeutics and chemotherapy by performing serial studies.

Procedure

1. During NMR the client is placed inside a giant, doughnut-shaped electromagnet to align the magnetic nuclei of hydrogen atoms in the water of the body cells. Short bursts of alternating energy are then introduced to knock the nuclei out of alignment. As the nuclei flip back into alignment, tiny radio-frequency signals are emitted, which are then detected by the NMR machine and computer-processed into cross-sectional images of the area under study.

Positron-Emission Tomography (PET)

Possible Indications

- To determine regional metabolism of the heart and brain.
- To study tissue permeability.
- To measure the size of infarcts left in the heart by a coronary attack.
- To investigate the physiology of psychosis.
- To assess the effects of drugs on tissues that are diseased or malfunctioning.
- To attempt to measure the effect of cancer treatment by noting changes in malignant tissues and by biochemical reactions in the normal tissues around it.

Procedure

1. For positron-emission tomography (PET), a chemical compound with the desired biologic activity is labeled with a radioactive isotope that decays by emitting a positron (or positive electron). The positron combines with an electron, and the two are mutually annihilated with emission of two gamma rays. The rays penetrate the surrounding tissue and are recorded outside the body by a circular array of detectors. Their source can be established with a high degree of accuracy.

Bibliography

Alford, R.H.: Histoplasmosis. In Conn, H.F.: Current therapy, 1982, Philadelphia, 1982, W.B. Saunders Co.

Brunner, L.S., and Suddarth, D.S.: Textbook of medical-surgical nursing, ed. 5, Philadelphia, 1984, J.B. Lippincott Co.

Cassmeyer, V.L.: Mechanisms for maintaining dynamic equilibrium. In Phipps, W.J., Long, B.C., and Woods, N.F., editors: Medical-surgical nursing: concepts and clinical practice, St. Louis, 1983, The C.V. Mosby Co.

Crooks, L.E.: Magnetic resonance imaging: effects of magnetic field strength, Radiology **151**(1):127-133, April 1984.

Davis, P.L.: Contemporary nuclear magnetic resonance imaging, Cont. Diag. Rad. **7**(11):1-5, 1984.

Fincher, J.: New machines may soon replace the doctor's black bag, Smithsonian **14**(10):64-71, Jan. 1984.

Goodwin, P.N.: Recent developments in instrumentation for emission computed tomography, Semin. Nucl. Med. **10**(4):322-334, Oct. 1980.

Govoni, L.E., and Hayes, J.E.: Drugs and nursing implications, ed. 4, Norwalk, Conn., 1982, Appleton-Century-Crofts.

Gunby, P.: The new wave in medicine: nuclear magnetic resonance, JAMA **247**:151, 1982.

Harms, S.E., and others: Principles of nuclear magnetic resonance imaging, RadioGraphics **4**(special ed.):26-43, Jan. 1984.

Juhl, P.: Paul and Juhl's essentials of modern roentgen interpretation, ed. 4, Hagerstown, Md., 1981, Harper & Row Publishers, Inc.

Partain, C.L., and others: Nuclear magnetic resonance imaging, RadioGraphics **4** (special ed.):5-25, Jan. 1984.

Petersdorf, R.G., and others, editors: Harrison's principles of internal medicine, ed. 10, New York, 1983, McGraw-Hill Book Co.

Phipps, W.J., and Daly, B.J.: Problems of the lower airway. In Phipps, W.J., Long, B.C., and Woods, N.F., editors: Medical-surgical nursing: concepts and clinical practice, St. Louis, 1983, The C.V. Mosby Co.

Rudy, E.B.: Advanced neurological and neurosurgical nursing, St. Louis, 1984, The C.V. Mosby Co.

Stroot, V.R., Lee, C.A., and Barrett, C.A.: Fluid and electrolytes—a practical approach, ed. 3, Philadelphia, 1984, F.A. Davis Co.

Ter-Pogossian, M.M., and others: Positron emission tomography, Sci. Am. **243**(4):171-181, Oct. 1980.

Van Assendelft, O.W.: NCCLS document ASH-3: standard procedures for collection of diagnostic blood specimens by venipuncture, Villanova, Pa., 1980, NCCLS.

Abbreviations
and Symbols

<	Less than
≤	Less than or equal to
>	Greater than
≥	Greater than or equal to
C	Celsius
cc	Cubic centimeter
cg	Centigram
cm	Centimeter
cm H_2O	Centimeter of water
cu	Cubic
dl	Deciliter (100 ml)
g	Gram
h	Hour
IU	International unit
ImU	International milliunit
IμU	International microunit
K	Kilo
kg	Kilogram
L	Liter
m	Meter
m^2	Square meter
m^3	Cubic meter
mEq	Milliequivalent
mEq/L	Milliequivalent per liter
mg	Milligram
min	Minute
ml	Milliliter
mm	Millimeter
mm^3	Cubic millimeter
mM	Millimole
mm H_2O	Millimeter of water
mol	Mole
mmol	Millimole

mOsm	Milliosmole
mμ	Millimicron
mU	Milliunit
mV	Millivolt
ng	Nanogram
nmol	Nanomole
Pa	Pascal
pg	Picogram (or micromicrogram)
pl	Picoliter
pm	Picomole
S	Second (SI)
sec	Second
SI units	International System of Units
torr	Millimeter of mercury
μm	Micrometer
μm^3	Cubic micrometer
μg	Microgram
μIU	Microinternational unit
μmol	Micromole
μU	Microunit
U	Unit
yr	Year

Blood, Plasma, or Serum Values

	Reference Range	
Test	Conventional Values	SI Units*
Acetoacetate plus acetone	0.3-2.0 mg/dl	
Acetone	Negative	Negative
Acid phosphatase	Adults: 0.10-0.63 U/ml (Bessey-Lowry) 0.5-2.0 U/ml (Bodansky) 1.0-4.0 U/ml (King-Armstrong) Children: 6.4-15.2 U/L	28-175 nmol/s/L
Activated partial thromboplastin time (APTT)	30-40 sec	
Adrenocortico-tropic hormone (ACTH)	15-100 pg/ml	
Albumin	3.2-4.5 g/dl	35-55 g/L
Alcohol	Negative	Negative
Aldolase	Adults: 3.0-8.2 Sibley-Lehninger units/dl Children: approximately 2 × adult values	22-59 mU/L at 37°C

*The use of the System of International Units (SI) was recommended at the 30th World Health Assembly in 1977 to implement an international language of measurement. Because this system is being adopted by many laboratories, many of the common values are expressed in both conventional and SI units. SI units are calculated by multiplying the conventional unit by a number factor. The SI measurement system uses *moles* as the basic unit for the amount of a substance, *kilograms* for its mass, and *meter* for its length.

	Reference Range	
Test	Conventional Values	SI Units
	Newborns: approximately 4 × adult values	
Aldosterone	Peripheral blood: Supine: 7.4 ± 4.2 ng/dl Upright: 1-21 ng/dl Adrenal vein: 200-800 ng/dl	
Alkaline phosphatase	Adults: 30-85 ImU/ml Children and adolescents: <2 years: 85-235 ImU/ml 2-8 years: 65-210 ImU/ml 9-15 years: 60-300 ImU/ml (active bone growth) 16-21 years: 30-200 ImU/ml	
Alpha-aminonitrogen	3-6 mg/dl	2.1-3.9 mmol/L
Alpha-1-antitrypsin	>250 mg/dl	
Alpha fetoprotein (AFP)	<25 ng/ml	
Ammonia	Adults: 15-110 µg/dl Children: 40-80 µg/dl Newborns: 90-150 µg/dl	47-65 µmol/L
Amylase	56-190 IU/L 80-150 Somogyi units/ml	111-296 U/L
Alanine aminotransferase (ALT)	5-35 IU/L	
Angiotensin-converting enzyme (ACE)	23-57 U/ml	

| | Reference Range | |
Test	Conventional Values	SI Units
Antinuclear anti-bodies (ANA)	Negative	
Antistreptolysin O (ASO)	Adults: ≤160 Todd units/ml	
	Children:	
	Newborns: similar to mother's value	
	6 months-2 years: ≤50 Todd units/ml	
	2-4 years: ≤160 Todd units/ml	
	5-12 years: ≤200 Todd units/ml	
Antithyroid microsomal antibody	Titer <1:100	
Antithyroglobulin antibody	Titer <1:100	
Ascorbic acid (vitamin C)	0.6-1.6 mg/dl	23-57 μmol/L
Aspartate aminotransferase (AST, SGOT)	12-36 U/ml 5-40 IU/L	0.10-0.30 μmol/s/L
Australian antigen (hepatitis-associated antigen, HAA)	Negative	Negative
Barbiturates	Negative	Negative
Base excess	Men: −3.3 to +1.2 Women: −2.4 to +2.3	
Bicarbonate (HCO_3^-)	22-26 mEq/L	
Bilirubin		
Direct (conjugated)	0.1-0.3 mg/dl	1.7-5.1 μmol/L
Indirect (unconjugated)	0.2-0.8 mg/dl	3.4-12.0 μmol/L

Test	Reference Range	
	Conventional Values	SI Units
Total	Adults and children: 0.1-1.0 mg/dl	5.1-17.0 μmol/L
	Newborns: 1-12 mg/dl	
Bleeding time (Ivy method)	1-9 min	
Blood count (see complete blood count)		
Blood gases (arterial)		
pH	7.35-7.45	
Pco_2	35-45 torr	4.7-6.0 kPa
HCO_3^-	22-26 mEq/L	21-28 nmol/L
Po_2	80-100 torr	11-13 kPa
O_2 saturation	95%-100%	
Blood urea nitrogen (BUN)	5-20 mg/dl	3.6-7.1 mmol/L
Bromide	Up to 5 mg/dl	0-63 mmol/L
Bromosulfophthalein (BSP)	<5% retention after 45 min	
C-reactive protein (CRP)	<6 μg/ml	
Calcitonin	<50 pg/ml	<50 pmol/L
Calcium (Ca)	9.0-10.5 mg/dl (total)	
	3.9-4.6 mg/dl (ionized)	
Carbon dioxide (CO_2) content	23-30 mEq/L	21-30 mmol/L
Carboxyhemoglobin (COHb)	3% of total hemoglobin	
Carcinoembryonic antigen (CEA)	<2 ng/ml	
Carotene	50-200 μg/dl	0.74-3.72 mol/L
Chloride (Cl)	90-110 mEq/L	98-106 mmol/L
Cholesterol	150-250 mg/dl	3.90-6.50 mmol/L
Clot retraction	50%-100% clot retraction in 1-2 hours, complete retraction within 24 hours	

| Test | Reference Range | |
	Conventional Values	SI Units
Complement	C_3: 70-176 mg/dl	0.55-1.20 g/L
	C_4: 16-45 mg/dl	0.20-0.50 g/L
Complete blood count (CBC)		
Red blood cell (RBC) count	Men: 4.7-6.1 million/ mm^3	
	Women: 4.2-5.4 million/mm^3	
	Infants and children: 3.8-5.5 million/mm^3	
	Newborns: 4.8-7.1 million/mm^3	
Hemoglobin (Hgb)	Men: 14-18 g/dl	8.7-11.2 mmol/L
	Women: 12-16 g/dl (pregnancy: >11 g/dl)	7.4-9.9 mmol/L
	Children: 11-16 g/dl	
	Infants: 10-15 g/dl	
	Newborns: 14-24 g/dl	
Hematocrit (Hct)	Men: 42%-52%	
	Women: 37%-47% (pregnancy: >33%)	
	Children: 31%-43%	
	Infants: 30%-40%	
	Newborns: 44%-64%	
Mean corpuscular volume (MCV)	Adults and children: 80-95 μm^3	
	Newborns: 96-108 μm^3	
Mean corpuscular hemoglobin (MCH)	Adults and children: 27-31 pg	
	Newborns: 32-34 pg	
Mean corpuscular hemoglobin concentration (MCHC)	Adults and children: 32-36 g/dl	
	Newborns: 32-33 g/dl	
White blood cell count (WBC)	Adults and children >2 years: 5000-10,000/cm^3	

Test	Reference Range	
	Conventional Values	SI Units
	Children ≤2 years: 6200-17,000/mm^3	
	Newborns: 9000-30,000/mm^3	
Differential count		
Neutrophils	55%-70%	
Lymphocytes	20%-40%	
Monocytes	2%-8%	
Eosinophils	1%-4%	
Basophils	0.5%-1%	
Platelet count	150,000-400,000/mm^3	
Coombs' test		
Direct	Negative	Negative
Indirect	Negative	Negative
Copper (Cu)	70-140 µg/dl	11.0-24.3 µmol/L
Cortisol	6-28 µg/dl (AM)	
	2-12 µg/dl (PM)	
CPK isoenzyme (MB)	<5% total	
Creatinine	0.7-1.5 mg/dl	<133 µmol/L
Creatinine clearance	Males: 95-104 ml/min	
	Females: 95-125 ml/min	
Creatinine phosphokinase (CPK)	5-75 mU/ml	
Cryoglobulin	Negative	
Differential (WBC) count		
Neutrophils	55%-70%	
Lymphocytes	20%-40%	
Monocytes	2%-8%	
Eosinophils	1%-4%	
Basophils	0.5%-1%	
Digoxin	Therapeutic level: 0.5-2.0 ng/ml	40-79 µmol/L
	Toxic level: >2.4 ng/ml	>119 µmol/L

	Reference Range	
Test	Conventional Values	SI Units
Erythrocyte count (see complete blood count)		
Erythrocyte sedimentation rate (ESR)	Men: up to 15 mm/h	
	Women: up to 20 mm/h	
	Children: up to 10 mm/h	
Ethanol	80-200 mg/dl (mild to moderate intoxication)	17-43 mmol/L
	250-400 mg/dl (marked intoxication)	54-87 mmol/L
	>400 mg/dl (severe intoxication)	>87 mmol/L
Euglobulin lysis test	90 min-6 h	
Fats	Up to 200 mg/dl	
Ferritin	15-200 ng/ml	15-200 μg/L
Fibrin degradation products (FDP)	<10 μg/ml	
Fibrinogen (factor I)	200-400 mg/dl	0.5-1.4 μmol/L
Fibrinolysis/euglobulin lysis test	90 min-6 h	
Fluorescent treponemal antibody (FTA)	Negative	Negative
Fluoride	<0.05 mg/dl	<0.027 mmol/L
Folic acid (Folate)	5-20 μg/ml	14-34 mmol/L
Follicle-stimulating hormone (FSH)	Men: 0.1-15.0 ImU/ml	
	Women: 6-30 ImU/ml	
	Children: 0.1-12.0 ImU/ml	
	Castrate and postmenopausal: 30-200 ImU/ml	
Free thyroxine index (FTI)	0.9-2.3 ng/dl	

Test	Reference Range	
	Conventional Values	SI Units
Galactose-1-phosphate uridyl transferase	18.5-28.5 U/g hemoglobin	
Gammaglobulin	0.5-1.6 g/dl	
Gamma-glutamyl transpeptidase (GGTP)	Men: 8-38 U/L Women: <45 years: 5-27 U/L	5-40 U/L 37°C
Gastrin	40-150 pg/ml	40-150 ng/L
Glucagon	50-200 pg/ml	14-56 pmol/L
Glucose, fasting (FBS)	Adults: 70-115 mg/dl Children: 60-100 mg/dl Newborns: 30-80 mg/dl	
Glucose, 2-hour postprandial (2-hour PPG)	<140 mg/dl	
Glucose-6-phosphate dehydrogenase (G-6-PD)	8.6-18.6 IU/g of hemoglobin	
Glucose tolerance test (GTT)	Fasting: 70-115 mg/dl 30 min: <200 mg/dl 1 hour: <200 mg/dl 2 hours: <140 mg/dl 3 hours: 70-115 mg/dl 4 hours: 70-115 mg/dl	
Glycosylated hemoglobin	Adults: 2.2%-4.8% Children: 1.8%-4.0% Good diabetic control: 2.5%-6% Fair diabetic control: 6.1%-8% Poor diabetic control: >8%	
Growth hormone	<10 ng/ml	<10 µg/L
Haptoglobin	100-150 mg/dl	1.3 ± 0.2 g/L
Hematocrit (Hct)	Men: 42%-52% Women: 37%-47% (pregnancy: >33%)	

Test	Reference Range	
	Conventional Values	SI Units
Hematocrit (Hct) —cont'd	Children: 31%-43% Infants: 30%-40% Newborns: 44%-64%	
Hemoglobin (HgB)	Men: 14-18 g/dl Women: 12-16 g/dl (pregnancy: >11 g/dl) Children: 11-16 g/dl Infants: 10-15 g/dl Newborns: 14-24 g/dl	8.7-11.2 mmol/L 7.4-9.9 mmol/L
Hemoglobin electrophoresis	Hgb A_1: 95%-98% Hgb A_2: 2%-3% Hgb: F: 0.8%-2% Hgb S: 0 Hgb C: 0	
Hepatitis B surface antigen (HB_sAG)	Nonreactive	
Heterophil antibody	Negative	
HLA-B27	None	None
Human chorionic gonadotropin (IICG)	Negative	Negative
Human placental lactogen (HPL)		
5-Hydroxyindole-acetic acid (5-HIAA)	2.8-8.0 mg/24 hours	
Immunoglobulin quantification	IgG: 565-1765 mg/dl IgA: 85-385 mg/dl IgM: 55-375 mg/dl	
Insulin	4-20 μU/ml	0.17-1.00 μg/L
Iron (Fe)	60-190 μg/dl	19 ± 6 μmol/L
Iron-binding capacity, total (TIBC)	250-420 μg/dl	55 ± 6 μmol/L
Iron (transferrin) saturation	30%-40%	

	Reference Range	
Test	Conventional Values	SI Units
Ketone bodies	Negative	Negative
Lactic acid	0.6-1.8 mEq/L	
Lactic dehydrogenase (LDH)	90-200 ImU/ml	0.4-1.7 μmol/s/L
LDH isoenzymes	LDH-1: 17%-27%	
	LDH-2: 28%-38%	
	LDH-3: 19%-27%	
	LDH-4: 5%-16%	
	LDH-5: 6%-16%	
Lead	20 μg/dl or less	<1.0 μmol/L
Leucine aminopeptidase (LAP)	Men: 80-200 U/ml	
	Women: 75-185 U/ml	
Leukocyte count (see complete blood count)		
Lipase	Up to 1.5 units/ml	0-417 U/L
Lipids		
Total	400-1000 mg/dl	4-8 g/L
Cholesterol	150-250 mg/dl	3.9-6.5 mmol/L
Triglycerides	40-150 mg/dl	1.09-20.7 mmol/L
Phospholipids	150-380 mg/dl	48-81 mmol/L
Lithium (see Table 13-2)		
Long-acting thyroid stimulating hormone (LATS)	Negative	Negative
Magnesium (Mg)	1.6-3.0 mEq/L	0.8-1.3 mm/L
Methanol	Negative	
Mononucleosis spot test	Titer: >1:56	
Nitrogen, nonprotein	15-35 mg/dl	0.15-0.35 g/L
Nuclear antibody (ANA)	Negative	
5'-Nucleotidase	Up to 1.6 units	27-233 nmol/s/L
Osmolality	275-300 mOsm/kg	
Oxygen saturation (arterial)	95%-100%	
Parathormone (PTH)	<2000 pg/ml	

Test	Reference Range	
	Conventional Values	SI Units
Partial thrombo-plastin time, activated (APTT)	30-40 sec	
P_{CO_2}	35-45 torr	
pH	7.35-7.45	
Phenylalanine	Up to 2 mg/dl	
Phenylketonuria (PKU)	Negative	
Phenytoin (Dilantin)	Therapeutic level: 10-20 µg/ml	
Phosphatase (acid)	0.10-0.63 U/ml (Bessey-Lowry) 0.5-2.0 U/ml (Bodansky) 1.0-4.0 U/ml (King-Armstrong)	28-175 nmol/s/L
Phosphatase (alkaline)	Adults: 30-85 ImU/ml Children and adolescents: <2 years: 85-235 ImU/ml 2-8 years: 65-210 ImU/ml 9-15 years: 60-300 ImU/ml (active bone growth) 16-21 years: 30-200 ImU/ml	
Phospholipids (see Lipids)		
Phosphorus (P, PO_4)	Adults: 2.5-4.5 mg/dl Children: 3.5-5.8 mg/dl	0.78-1.52 mmol/L 1.29-2.26 mmol/L
Platelet count	150,000-400,000/mm^3	
P_{O_2}	80-100 torr	
Potassium (K)	3.5-5.0 mEq/L	3.5-5.0 mmol/L
Progesterone	Men, prepubertal girls, and postmenopausal women: <2 ng/ml	6 nmol/L
	Women, luteal: peak >5 ng/ml	>16 nmol/L

Test	Reference Range	
	Conventional Values	SI Units
Prolactin	2-15 ng/ml	2-15 µg/L
Protein (total)	6-8 g/dl	55-80 g/L
Albumin	3.2-4.5 g/dl	35-55 g/L
Globulin	2.3-3.4 g/dl	20-35 g/L
Prothrombin time (PT)	11.0-12.5 sec	
Pyruvate	0.3-0.9 mg/dl	34-103 µmol/L
Red blood cell count (see complete blood count)		
Red blood cell indexes (see complete blood count)		
Renin		
Reticulocyte count	Adults and children: 0.5%-2% of total erythrocytes	
	Infants: 0.5%-3.1% of total erythrocytes	
	Newborns: 2.5%-6.5% of total erythrocytes	
Rheumatoid factor	Negative	Negative
Rubella antibody test		
Salicylates	Negative	
	Therapeutic: 20-25 mg/dl (to age 10: 25-30 mg/dl)	1.4-1.8 mmol/L
	Toxic: >30 mg/dl (after age 60: >20 mg/dl)	>2.2 mmol/L
Schilling test (vitamin B_{12} absorption)	8%-40% excretion/24 h	
Serologic test for syphilis (STS)	Negative (nonreactive)	
Serum glutamic oxaloacetic transaminase (SGOT, AST)	12-36 U/ml 5-40 IU/L	0.10-0.30 µmol/s/L

Test	Reference Range	
	Conventional Values	SI Units
Serum glutamic-pyruvic trans-aminase (SGPT, ALT)	5-35 IU/L	0.05-0.43 μmol/s/L
Sickle cell	Negative	
Sodium (Na$^+$)	136-145 mEq/L	136-145 mmol/L
Sugar (see glucose)		
Syphilis (see serologic test for, fluorescent treponemal antibody, venereal disease research laboratory)		
Testosterone	Men: 300-1200 ng/dl	10-42 nmol/L
	Women: 30-95 ng/dl	1.1-3.3 nmol/L
	Prepubertal boys and girls: 5-20 ng/dl	0.165-0.70 nmol/L
Thymol flocculation	Up to 5 units	
Thyroglobulin antibody (see antithyroglobulin antibody)		
Thyroid-stimulating hormone (TSH)	1-4 μU/ml	5 m U/L
	Neonates: <25 μIU/ml by 3 days	
Thyroxine (T$_4$)	Murphy-Pattee: neonates: 10.1-20.1 μg/dl	50-154 nmol/L
	1-6 years: 5.6-12.6 μg/dl	
	6-10 years: 4.9-11.7 μg/dl	
	>10 years: 4-11 μg/dl	
	Radioimmunoassay: 5-10 μg/dl	

| Test | Reference Range | |
	Conventional Values	SI Units
Thyroxine-binding globulin (TBG)	12-28 µg/ml	
Toxoplasmosis antibody titer	See Chapter 8	
Transaminase (see serum glutamic-oxaloacetic transaminase, serum glutamic pyruvic trans-aminase)		
Triglycerides	40-150 mg/dl	
Triiodothyronine (T$_3$)	110-230 ng/dl	1.2-1.5 nmol/L
Triiodothyronine (T$_3$) resin up-take	25%-35%	
Tubular phosphate reabsorption (TPR)	80%-90%	
Urea nitrogen (see blood urea ni-trogen)		
Uric acid	Males: 2.1-8.5 mg/dl	0.15-0.48 mmol/L
	Females: 2.0-6.6 mg/dl	0.09-0.36 mmol/L
	Children: 2.5-5.5 mg/dl	
Venereal Disease Research Labo-ratory (VDRL)	Negative	Negative
Vitamin A	20-100 g/dl	0.7-3.5 µmol/L
Vitamin B$_{12}$	200-600 pg/ml	148-443 pmol/L
Vitamin C	0.6-1.6 mg/dl	23-57 µmol/L
Whole blood clot retraction (see Clot retraction)		
Zinc	50-150 µg/dl	

Urine Values

	Reference Range	
Test	Conventional Values	SI Units*
Acetone plus aceto-acetate (ketone bodies)	Negative	Negative

Addis count (12-hour)	Adults:
	  WBCs and epithelial cells: 1.8 million/12 h
	  RBCs: 500,000/12 h
	  Hyaline casts: up to 5000/12 h
	Children:
	  WBCs: <1 million/12 h
	  RBCs: <250,000/12 h
	  Casts: <5000/12 h
	  Protein: <20 mg/12 h	

Albumin	Random: ≤8 mg/dl 24-hour: 10-100 mg/24 h	Negative
Aldosterone	2-16 μg/24 h	5.5-72 nmol/24 h
Alpha-aminonitrogen	0.4-1.0 g/24 h	28-71 nmol/24 h
Amino acid	50-200 mg/24 h	

*The use of the System of International Units (SI) was recommended at the 30th World Health Assembly in 1977 to implement an international language of measurement. Because this system is being adopted by many laboratories, many of the common values are expressed in both conventional and SI units. SI units are calculated by multiplying the conventional unit by a number factor. The SI measurement system uses *moles* as the basic unit for the amount of a substance, *kilograms* for its mass, and *meter* for its length.

	Reference Range	
Test	Conventional Values	SI Units
Ammonia (24-hour)	30-50 mEq/24 h 500-1200 mg/24 h	30-50 nmol/ 24 h
Amylase	≤5000 Somogyi units/ 24 h 3-35 IU/h	6.5-48.1 U/h
Arsenic (24-hour)	<50 μg/L	<0.65 mol/L
Ascorbic acid (vitamin C)	Random: 1-7 ng/dl 24-hour: >50 mg/24 h	0.06-0.40 mmol/L >0.29 mmol/24 h
Bacteria	None	None
Bence Jones protein	Negative	Negative
Bilirubin	Negative	Negative
Blood or hemoglobin	Negative	Negative
Borate (24-hour)	<2 mg/L	<32 μmol/L
Calcium	Random: 1 + turbidity 24-hour: 1-300 mg (diet dependent)	1 + turbidity
Catecholamines (24-hour)	Epinephrine: 5-40 μg/ 24 h Norepinephrine: 10-80 μg/24 h Metanephrine: 24-96 μg/24 h Normetanephrine: 75- 375 μg/24 h	
Chloride (24-hour)	140-250 mEq/24 h	140-250 mmol/24 h
Color	Amber-yellow	
Concentration test (Fishberg test)	Specific gravity: >1.025 Osmolality: 850 mOsm/L	>1.025 >850 mOsm/L
Copper (Cu) (24-hour)	Up to 25 μg/24 h	0-0.4 μmol/ 24 h
Coproporphyrin (24-hour)	100-300 μg/24 h	150-460 nmol/ 24 h

| | Reference Range | |
Test	Conventional Values	SI Units
Creatine	Adults: <100 mg/24 h or <6% creatinine	
	Pregnant women: ≤12%	
	Infants <1 year: equal to creatinine	
	Older children: ≤30% of creatinine	
Creatinine (24-hour)	12-25 mg/kg body wt/ 24 h	
Creatinine clearance (24-hour)	Men: 90-140 ml/min Women: 85-125 ml/ min	
Crystals	Negative	
Cystine or cysteine	Negative	Negative
Delta-aminolevulinic acid (ΔALA)	1-7 mg/24 h	
Epinephrine (24-hour)	5-40 μg/24 h	
Epithelial cells and casts	Occasional	Occasional
Estriol (24-hour)	>12 mg/24 h	
Fat	Negative	
Fluoride (24-hour)	<1 mg/24 h	0.053 mmol/ 24 h
Follicle-stimulating hormone (FSH) (24-hour)	Men: 2-12 IU/24 h Women:	
	During menses: 8-60 IU/24 h	
	During ovulation: 30-60 IU/24 h	
	During menopause: >50 IU/24 h	
Glucose	Negative	Negative
Granular casts	Occasional	Occasional
Hemoglobin and myoglobin	Negative	Negative
Homogentisic acid	Negative	Negative
Human chorionic gonadotropin (HCG)	Negative	Negative

| | Reference Range | |
Test	Conventional Values	SI Units
Human placental lactogen (HPL)		
Hyaline casts	Occasional	Occasional
17-Hydroxycortico-steroids (17-OCHS) (24-hour)	Men: 5.5-15.0 mg/24 h Women: 5.0-13.5 mg/24 h Children: lower than adult values	
5-Hydroxyindole-acetic acid (5-HIAA, serotonin) (24-hour)	Men: 2-9 mg/24 h Women: lower than men	10-47 μmol/24 h
Ketones (see acetone plus acetoacetate)		
17-Ketosteroids (17-KS) (24-hour)	Men: 8-15 mg/24 h Women: 6-12 mg/24 h Children: 12-15 yr: 5-12 mg/24 h <12 yr: <5 mg/24 h	
Lactose (24-hour)	14-40 mg/24 h	41-116 μm
Lead	<0.08 g/ml or <120 g/24 h	0.39 μmol/L
Leucine aminopepti-dase (LAP)	2-18 U/24 h	
Magnesium (24-hour)	6.8-8.5 mEq/24 h	3.0-4.3 mmol/24 h
Melanin	Negative	Negative
Odor	Aromatic	Aromatic
Osmolality	500-800 mOsm/L	
pH	4.6-8.0	4.6-8.0
Phenolsulfon-phthalein (PSP)	15 min: at least 25% 30 min: at least 40% 120 min: at least 60%	
Phenylketonuria (PKU)	Negative	Negative
Phenylpyruvic acid	Negative	Negative
Phosphorus (24-hour)	0.9-1.3 g/24 h	29-42 mmol/24 h

Test	Reference Range	
	Conventional Values	SI Units
Porphobilinogen	Random: negative 24-hour: up to 2 mg/ 24 h	Negative
Porphyrin (24-hour)	50-300 mg/24 h	
Potassium (K^+) (24-hour)	25-100 mEq/24 h	25-100 nmol/ 24 h
Pregnancy test	Positive in normal pregnancy or with tumors producing HCG	Positive in normal pregnancy or with tu- mors pro- ducing HCG
Preganediol	After ovulation: >1 mg/24 h	
Protein (albumin)	Random: ≤8 mg/dl 10-100 mg/24 h	<0.05 g/24 h
Sodium (Na^+) (24-hour)	100-260 mEq/24 h	100-260 nmol/ 24 h
Specific gravity	1.010-1.025	
Steroids (see 17-Hy- droxycorticoste- roids and 17- Ketosteroids)		
Sugar (see Glucose)		
Titratable acidity (24-hour)	20-50 mEq/24 h	20-50 mmol/ 24 h
Turbidity	Clear	Clear
Urea nitrogen (24-hour)	6-17 g/24 h	0.21-0.60 mol/ 24 h
Uric acid (24-hour)	250-750 mg/24 h	1.48-4.43 mmol/24 h
Urobilinogen	0.1-1.0 Ehrlich units/ dl	
Uroporphyrin	Negative	Negative
Vanillylmandelic acid (VMA) (24-hour)	1-9 mg/24 h	<40 μmol/day
Zinc (24-hour)	0.20-0.75 mg/24 h	

Common Drugs Affecting
Clinical Laboratory Tests

Table 1 Drugs affecting thyroid function tests*

Drug	Free Thyroxine Index	^{131}I Uptake	T_3 Uptake	T_4 (Murphy-Pattee)
Ampicillin		−		
Aspirin	−†	−	+	−
Barium		−		
Bromides		−		
Cascara		−		
Chlordiazepoxide		−	−	
Corticosteroids	−	−	+	
Coumarin			+	
Dicumarol			+	
Digitalis		−		
Digitoxin		−		
Heparin			+	−
Levodopa				+
Oral contraceptives	+		−	−
Penicillin		−	+	−
Pentobarbital		−		
Phenylbutazone	−	−	+	
Phenytoin sodium	−		+	+
(Pregnancy)			−	−

From Tilkian, S.M., Conover, M.B., and Tilkian, A.G.: Clinical implications of laboratory tests, ed. 3, St. Louis, 1983, The C.V. Mosby Co.
*Sources for the material in these tables are as follows: Davies, D.M., editor: Textbook of adverse drug reactions, New York, 1977, Oxford University Press, Inc.; Wallach, J.: Interpretation of diagnostic tests, ed. 3, Boston, 1978, Little, Brown & Co.; Young, D.S., Pestaner, L.C., and Gibberman, V.: Effects of drugs on clinical laboratory tests, Clin. Chem. **21**(5):240D-399D, 1975.
† +, increased value; −, decreased value; blank, no effect.

Continued.

Table 1   Drugs affecting thyroid function tests—cont'd

Drug	Free Thyroxine Index	^{131}I Uptake	T_3 Uptake	T_4 (Murphy-Pattee)
Propylthiouracil	−	−	−	
Quinidine	−			
Secobarbital	−			
Sulfonamides	−		+	
Thiazides			−	
Thyroid	−		+	

Drugs Affecting Prothrombin Time

Drugs such as salicylates, phenylbutazone, oxyphenbutazone, indomethacin, and some sulfonamides can displace the anticoagulants from the plasma protein to which they are bound. This will make more anticoagulants available, thus increasing the prothrombin time.

Other drugs, such as barbiturates, griseofulvin, and glutethimide, induce the formation of enzymes by the liver that metabolize coumarin and phenindione derivatives, thus decreasing the prothrombin time. If any of these drugs is withdrawn from a patient who has been stabilized on an anticoagulant plus the drug, a critical fall in prothrombin level may result.

Additionally, vitamin K may be suppressed by broad-spectrum antibiotics and some oral sulfonamides that change the intestinal flora and inhibit the microorganisms responsible for vitamin K production, thus increasing the prothrombin time. By the same token, the patient who is taking vitamin K or daily mineral oil (which enhances vitamin K absorption) may have prothrombin time decreased.

The commonly used drugs affecting prothrombin time are listed in Table 2.

Table 2   Most common drugs affecting prothrombin time

Increased Time	Comment
Acenocoumarol	
Acetaminophen	
Allopurinol	Patients on coumarin
Aminosalicylic acid	Suppresses prothrombin formation
Anabolic steroids	
Aspirin	In large doses
Cathartics	
Chloral hydrate	Displaces anticoagulants from albumin
Chloramphenicol	May lower prothrombin
Chlorthalidone	Patients on coumarin
Clofibrate	
Diazoxide	Displaces anticoagulants from albumin
Dicumarol	
Disulfiram	Patients on coumarin
Diuretics	May prolong action of anticoagulants
Erythromycin	
Ethacrynic acid	Patients on coumarin
Glucagon	Patients on coumarin
Guanethidine	
Heparin	
Indomethacin	Displaces anticoagulants from binding proteins
Mefenamic acid	Displaces coumarin from albumin
Mercaptopurine	
Methyldopa	
Methylphenidate	Inhibits metabolism of coumarin
Monoamide oxidase (MAO) inhibitors	
Nalidixic acid	Displaces coumarin from albumin
Neomycin	
Oxyphenbutazone	Displaces anticoagulants from albumin

Continued.

Table 2   Most common drugs affecting prothrombin time—
cont'd

Increased Time	Comment
Phenylbutazone	
Phenyramidol	
Propylthiouracil	
Quinidine	
Quinine	
Streptomycin	May decrease vitamin K synthesis
Sulfinpyrazone	
Sulfonamides	
Thyroid	
Tolbutamide	

Decreased Time	Comment
Anabolic steroids	
Antacids	May shorten anticoagulant action
Antihistamines	Anticoagulant metabolism accelerated
Ascorbic acid	Anticoagulant action may shorten
Aspirin	In small doses
Barbiturates	Patients on coumarin
Chloral hydrate	Patients on coumarin
Colchicine	Patients on coumarin
Corticosteroids	Anticoagulant metabolism accelerated
Cortisone	Patients on coumarin
Diuretics	Patients on anticoagulant
Ethchlorvynol	Patients on coumarin
Glutethimide	Patients on coumarin
Griseofulvin	
Heptabarbital	Anticoagulants metabolized by liver
Oral contraceptives	
Phenobarbital	
Secobarbital	Patients on coumarin
Tetracycline	May partially counteract action of heparin
Vitamin K	

Table 3   Drugs affecting urinalysis

Test	Increased Value	Decreased Value
Creatine	Caffeine Methyltestosterone PSP	Anabolic steroids Androgens Thiazides
Creatinine	Ascorbic acid* Corticosteroids Levodopa* Methyldopa* Nitrofurans* PSP*	Anabolic steroids Androgens Thiazides
Diagnex blue excretion	Aluminum salts Barium salts Calcium salts Iron salts Kaolin Magnesium salts Methylene blue* Nicotinic acid Quinacrine* Quinidine* Quinine* Riboflavin* Sodium salts* Vitamin B*	Caffeine benzoate
Glucose	Aminosalicylic acid Aspirin Corticosteroids Ephedrine Furosemide Phenytoin sodium	With glucose-oxidase method Ascorbic acid* Aspirin* Levodopa* Mercurial diuretics* Tetracycline*
Hematuria or hemoglobinuria	Acetanilid Acetophenetidin Acetylsalicylic acid Amphotericin B Bacitracin Coumarin Indomethacin Phenylbutazone	

*Method-affected.   *Continued.*

Table 3 Drugs affecting urinalysis—cont'd

Test	Increased Value	Decreased Value
17-Hydroxy-corticosteroids	Acetazolamide Chloral hydrate Chlordiazepoxide Chlorpromazine Colchicine Erythromycin Etryptamine Meprobamate Oleandomycin Paraldehyde Quinidine Quinine Spironolactone	Estrogens Oral contraceptives Phenothiazines Reserpine
17-Ketosteroids	Chloramphenicol Chlorpromazine Cloxacillin Dexamethasone Erythromycin Ethinamate Meprobamate Nalidixic acid Oleandomycin Penicillin Phenaglycodol Phenazopyridine Phenothiazines Quinidine Secobarbital Spironolactone	Chlordiazepoxide Estrogens Meprobamate Metyrapone Probenecid Promazine Reserpine
pH	Aldosterone Parathyroid extract Prolactin Sodium bicarbonate	
Porphyrins (fluorometric method)	Acriflavine Antipyretics Barbiturates Ethoxazene Phenazopyridine Phenylhydrazine	

Table 3 **Drugs affecting urinalysis—cont'd**

Test	Increased Value	Decreased Value
	Sulfamethoxazole Sulfonamides Tetracycline	
Pregnancy test (DAP test)	False positive Chlorpromazine (frog, rabbit; immunologic) Phenothiazines (frog, rabbit; immunologic) Promethazine (Gravindex)	False negative Promethazine
Protein	Drugs causing nephrotoxicity, such as: Aminosalicylic acid Ampicillin Aspirin Bacitracin Cephaloridine Corticosteroids Insecticides Mercurial diuretics Neomycin Penicillin (large doses) Phenylbutazone Radiographic agents (post-aortography) Streptomycin Sulfonamides Turbidimetric procedures* (false positive) Aminosalicylic acid Cephaloridine Chlorpromazine Penicillin (large doses) Promazine Sulfisoxazole Thymol	

Continued.

Table 3   Drugs affecting urinalysis—cont'd

Test	Increased Value	Decreased Value
Specific gravity	Dextran* (Diurnal variation) Radiographic agents Sucrose*	
Vanillylman- delic acid (VMA)	Aminosalicylic acid* Aspirin* Bromsulphalein (BSP) Glyceryl guaiacolate* Mephenesin* Nalidixic acid* Oxytetracycline* Penicillin* Phenazopyridine* PSP* Sulfa drugs*	Clofibrate* Guanethidine an- alogs Imipramine Methyldopa Monoamine oxi- dase (MAO) inhibitor

Table 4   Drugs affecting blood tests

Test	Increased Value	Decreased Value
Amylase	Cholinergics Codeine Drugs inducing acute pancreatitis Ethanol Meperidine Methacholine Morphine Oral contraceptives	
Bilirubin	Ajmaline Antimalarials Aspirin Cholinergics Coumarin Ethoxazene Morphine Oral contraceptives Penicillin	Barbiturates Corticosteroids Phenobarbital Sulfonamides Thioridazine

Table 4   Drugs affecting blood tests—cont'd

Test	Increased Value	Decreased Value
	Phenylbutazone	
	Primaquine	
	Procainamide	
	Quinidine	
	Quinine	
	Radiographic agents	
	Rifampin	
	Streptomycin	
	Sulfa drugs	
	Tetracycline	
Calcium	Thiazides	Corticosteroids
	Anabolic steroids	Diuretics (mercurial)
	Antacids (Ca containing)	Gastrin
	Calcium gluconate (newborns)	Insulin
	Estrogens	Laxatives (excess)
	Hydralazine	Mestranol
	Oral contraceptives	Oral contraceptives
	Secretin	Phenytoin sodium (chronic use)
	Thiazides	Sulfates
Chloride	Chlorothiazide (prolonged therapy)	Aldosterone
		Bicarbonates
	Corticosteroids	Corticosteroids
	Guanethidine	Corticotropin
	Marijuana	Cortisone
	Phenylbutazone	Diuretics
		Laxatives (chronic abuse)
		Prednisolone
Cholesterol	Anabolic steroids	Allopurinol
	Cinchophen	Azathioprine
	Cortisone	Clofibrate
	Epinephrine	Clomiphene
	Heparin (after cessation)	Corticotropin
	Oral contraceptives	Erythromycin
		Garlic

Continued.

Table 4   Drugs affecting blood tests—cont'd

Test	Increased Value	Decreased Value
Cholesterol—cont'd	Phenytoin sodium (Pregnancy) Promazine Sulfadiazine Sulfonamides Thiazides Thiouracil	Isoniazid Kanamycin MAO inhibitors Neomycin Tetracycline Thiouracil
CO_2 content	Aldosterone Bicarbonates Ethacrynic acid Hydrocortisone Laxatives (chronic abuse) Metolazone Prednisone Thiazides Tromethamine Viomycin	Acetazolamide Dimercaprol Dimethadione Methicillin Nitrofurantoin Phenformin Tetracycline Triamterene
Coombs' test	Positive Chlorpromazine Chlorpropamide Dipyrone Ethosuximide Hydralazine Isoniazid Levodopa Mefenamic acid Melphalan Oxyphenisatin Phenylbutazone Phenytoin sodium Procainamide Quinidine Quinine Streptomycin Sulfonamides Tetracycline	

Table 4   Drugs affecting blood tests—cont'd

Test	Increased Value	Decreased Value
Creatinine	Clofibrate Clonidine Colistimethate Colistin Doxycycline Drugs causing nephrotoxicity, such as: Amphotericin B Capreomycin Carbutamide Cephaloridine Chlorthalidone	
Erythrocyte sedimentation rate (ESR)	Dextrans Methyldopa Methysergide Penicillamine Theophylline Trifluperidol Vitamin A	Quinine Salicylates Steroids
Glucose	Aminosalicylic acid Aspirin Caffeine Chlorpromazine Chlorthalidone Coffee Corticosteroids Cortisone Dopamine Ephedrine Epinephrine Estrogens Ethacrynic acid Furosemide Hydralazine Levodopa Phenylbutazone Phenytoin	Dicumarol Erythromycin Ethacrynic acid Guanethidine Insulin Sulfaphenazole Sulfonamides Sulfonylureas

Continued.

Table 4   Drugs affecting blood tests—cont'd

Test	Increased Value	Decreased Value
Glucose—cont'd	Prednisolone Reserpine Secretin Thiazides Thyroid	
Lactic dehydrogenase (LDH)	Anesthetic agents Codeine Dicumarol Morphine (Muscular exercise)	
Leucine aminopeptidase	Estrogens Morphine Oral contraceptives (Pregnancy) Thorium dioxide	
Lipase	Cholinergics Codeine Heparin (10 min postinjection) Meperidine Methacholine Morphine Narcotics	Protamine Saline (at molar concentrations)
Phosphate	Anabolic steroids Methicillin Phosphates Phospho-Soda	Alkaline antacids Anticonvulsants Calcitonin Epinephrine Insulin (Menstruation) Oral contraceptives Phenobarbital
Potassium	Amphotericin B Epinephrine Heparin Histamine (IV) Marijuana Methicillin	Aldosterone Amphotericin B Aspirin Bicarbonates Corticosteroids Cortisone

Table 4   Drugs affecting blood tests—cont'd

Test	Increased Value	Decreased Value
	Spironolactone	Diuretics
	Tetracycline	Ethacrynic acid
		Furosemide
		Gentamicin
		Insulin
		Licorice
		Polythiazide
		Sodium bicarbonate
		Thiazides
Protein	Anabolic steroids	Estrogens
	Androgens	Oral contraceptives
	Corticosteroids	
	Corticotropin	
	Digitalis	
	Epinephrine	
	Insulin	
	Thyroid	
SGOT/SGPT	Ascorbic acid	
	Cholinergics	
	Codeine	
	Guanethidine	
	Hydralazine	
	Isoniazid	
	Meperidine	
	Morphine	
	Tolbutamide	
Sodium	Anabolic steroids	Ammonium chloride
	Bicarbonate	Cathartics (excessive)
	Clonidine	Chlorpropamide
	Corticosteroids	Ethacrynic acid
	Cortisone	Furosemide
	Estrogens	Mannitol
	Guanethidine	Metolazone
	Marijuana	Spironolactone
	Methoxyflurane	Thiazides
	Oral contraceptives	Triamterene
	Phenylbutazone	
	Prolactin (IM)	
	Tetracycline	

Continued.

Table 4   Drugs affecting blood tests—cont'd

Test	Increased Value	Decreased Value
Triglycerides	Birth control pills Cholestyramine Estrogens	Ascorbic acid Asparaginase Clofibrate Metformin Phenformin
Urea nitrogen (BUN)	Drugs causing nephrotoxicity, and also the following: Anabolic steroids Androgens Arginine Bacitracin Calcium salts Clonidine Dextran Guanethidine Licorice Marijuana Mephenesin Methoxyflurane Methsuximide Metolazone Minocycline	Glucose (Muscular exercise) Paramethasone (Pregnancy)
Uric acid	Acetazolamide Aspirin Ethacrynic acid Furosemide Hydralazine Propylthiouracil Thiazides	Allopurinol Chlorpromazine Cinchophen Clofibrate Corticosteroids Corticotropin Cortisone Coumarin Dicumarol Phenylbutazone Probenecid Radiographic agents

Index

Critical Limits (Panic Values) for Laboratory Tests and Drug Levels

The following laboratory values indicate potentially life-threatening situations. When such values are encountered and confirmed, the nurse and the physician responsible for the patient's care should be notified immediately. Sometimes these values are called "panic values." It should be clearly understood, however, that the patient's overall condition and clinical status ultimately determine the significance of these extreme laboratory variations.

In addition to the values listed here, results of all laboratory studies ordered "stat," as well as all positive blood, acid-fast, and cerebrospinal fluid cultures, should be reported immediately to the responsible nurse and physician.